THE A TO Z OF

BREAST CANCER

Carol Turkington
Karen Krag, M.D.

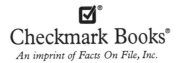

Checkmark Books®
An imprint of Facts On File, Inc.

The A to Z of Breast Cancer

Checkmark Books
An imprint of Facts On File, Inc.
132 West 31st Street
New York NY 10001

For Library of Congress Cataloging-in-Publication data, please contact the publisher.
ISBN 0-8160-6690-6

Checkmark Books are available at special discounts when purchased in bulk quantities for businesses, associations, institutions or sales promotions. Please call our Special Sales Department in New York at
(212) 967-8800 or (800) 322-8755.

You can find Facts On File on the World Wide Web at http://www.factsonfile.com

Text design by Cathy Rincon

Printed in the United States of America

VB FOF 10 9 8 7 6 5 4 3 2 1

This book is printed on acid-free paper.

To all those who have lost the fight against breast cancer
and to the memory of

Linda Buser Leber
Grace Turkington Merchant
Eleanor Turkington Roulston
Florence Turkington Haas
Nancy Turkington Cluelow
Robert Dayton Turkington
Mabel Crowley Turkington

CONTENTS

FOREWORD

Breast cancer is the most common cancer among American women after skin cancer, affecting more than 200,000 women each year and making up almost a third of all cancer diagnoses in women. Fortunately, breast cancer mortality continues to fall as better treatments are utilized and as cancers are diagnosed earlier due to more widespread use of mammography. Yet breast cancer continues to affect women of all ethnic groups, all ages, and all walks of life. Knowledge—of risk factors, screening tools, and treatments—is essential to continue the fight against this cancer.

Over the past 20 years our understanding of this disease has grown immensely. Radical mastectomy was once the treatment of choice because we thought that aggressive local treatment would cure the majority of women, but we now understand that cells often break off and spread to other organs early in the growth of this cancer. This has led to broader and earlier use of systemic adjuvant therapy (chemotherapy and hormone therapy that reaches all parts of the body). As a result, more women are cured when their disease is confined to the breast or breast plus lymph nodes at diagnosis.

Also, our tools to treat this disease have increased in number. We initially had few chemotherapy drugs, but we now have many; we once used mainly tamoxifen for hormonal therapy, but we now have options, including the aromatase inhibitors. Although women in the past who chose chemotherapy often became deathly ill from the treatments, today many women experience only minimal nausea. New medications support red cells and white cells, thus avoiding anemia and infec-tions. There are even medications to strengthen the bones of women who suffer from treatment-induced bone thinning or fragile bones due to the tumor.

Although all women are at risk for breast cancer, we can now predict those who are at highest risk. Doctors can test for genes found in some families that significantly increase risk, and the search for other such genes continues. We also understand the hormonal risks—early onset of periods, late preg-nancies, use of hormone replacement therapy—as well as other risks such as postmenopausal obesity and excessive alcohol use.

We also know how to decrease the risk of devel-oping breast cancer, by maintaining normal body weight, taking folic acid if alcohol is frequently used, and possibly getting plenty of exercise. We know that women at very high risk for breast cancer may halve that risk by using tamoxifen, and other med-ications to reduce the risk of breast cancer are being investigated. We also know the importance of yearly mammograms so that cancer can be caught earlier, treated more easily, and hopefully cured.

We all hope for a magic bullet that will either eradicate cancer or cure all women when they are diagnosed with the disease, but that is unlikely. Yet, each small step we make improves survival. These steps have included better screening, better under-standing of those at risk, more aggressive local treat-ment, more widespread use of adjuvant treatment, and better drugs for these treatments.

Most women diagnosed with breast cancer will not die of their disease. However, they will face the agony of hearing the diagnosis, the pain of surgery and radiation therapy, and the side effects of hormonal therapy or chemotherapy.

Afterward, they must live with the knowledge that the cancer can return. Someday we will be able to prevent most breast cancers, diagnose earlier those we cannot prevent, treat with less morbidity, and assure patients that their cancer has been eradicated. Understanding of this disease is key. Knowledge provides tremendous power, both to those who treat and those who suffer from this disease.

—Karen Krag, M.D.

ACKNOWLEDGMENTS

As always, the creation of a detailed encyclopedia involves the help and guidance of a wide range of experts. Without their assistance this book could not have been written.

First of all, thanks to all the staff at Fox Chase Cancer Center in Philadelphia and to Dr. Mary Daly at the Fox Chase Family Risk Assessment Program. Also thanks to the staffs of the National Institute of Mental Health, the National Institute of Nursing Research, the American Medical Association, National Institutes of Health, American Association of People with Disabilities, American College of Obstetricians and Gynecologists, American Heart Association, American Psychiatric Association, American Psychological Association, American Society of Hematology, Cancer Information Service, Centers for Disease Control and Prevention, the Food and Drug Administration, the National Cancer Institute, American Board of Plastic and Reconstructive Surgeons. Thanks also to the Look Good . . . Feel Better program, National Bone Marrow Transplant Link, National Marrow Donor Program, American Brachytherapy Society, ENCORE plus, National Alliance of Breast Cancer Associations, National Breast Cancer Coalition, National Lymphedema Network, Susan G. Komen Breast Cancer Foundation, Y-Me, Cancer Care, Cancer Hope Network, Cancer Information and Counseling Line, Cancer Information Service, Cancer Net, Cancer Research Institute, Cancer Survivors Network, CanSurmount, I Can Cope, and International Union Against Cancer. Thanks also to James Chambers and Vanessa Nittoli at Facts On File, to Bert Holtje and Gene Brissie at James Peter Associates, and to Michael and Kara.

INTRODUCTION

Breast cancer is the most common type of cancer among women in the United States after skin cancer. According to the National Cancer Institute, a woman in the United States has a one-in-eight chance of developing breast cancer during her lifetime.

But statistics can be misleading. A one-in-eight chance seems very high—but if you reverse that statistic, it indicates that an average woman has a seven-out-of-eight chance of *never* developing breast cancer. In addition, the one-in-eight statistic does not mean that a woman has a one-in-eight chance of developing breast cancer at each stage of her life. These numbers are weighted, which means that the risk of having breast cancer changes as a woman gets older.

A woman's actual chance of being diagnosed with breast cancer from age 30 to age 40 is only one out of 252. From age 40 to age 50, her risk is one out of 68, and from age 50 to age 60 it is one out of 35. From age 60 to age 70, a woman's risk is one out of 27.

Every woman has *some* chance of developing breast cancer during her lifetime, but that particular risk depends a great deal on a variety of issues, including genetics and lifestyle. The biggest risk factor, of course, is simply age—as women get older, their chances of being diagnosed increase. But although breast cancer is more common in older women, it also occurs in younger women and even in a small number of men.

Just as it is important to understand a woman's true breast cancer risk, it is also important to remember that once breast cancer has been diagnosed, there is no single treatment that is right for all women.

New treatments are available today that were not even imagined a few years ago, and medical researchers continue to find better ways to prevent and treat breast cancer. If women have any doubts about their care, they should feel comfortable in asking more than one doctor about their diagnosis and treatment plan. In fact, a woman's doctor can help her arrange an appointment with another specialist. Many health insurance companies pay for other opinions, and some even require it.

All of this information about breast cancer treatments and statistics—plus much, much more—is available in *The A to Z of Breast Cancer,* which includes the most up-to-date information designed as a guide and reference to a wide range of subjects important to the understanding of breast cancer. The book also includes a wide variety of contact information for organization and governmental agencies affiliated with breast cancer issues, including current Web site addresses and phone numbers. The book is not designed as a substitute for prompt assessment and treatment by oncologic experts in the prevention, diagnosis, and treatment of breast cancer.

In this encyclopedia, we have tried to present the latest information in the field, based on the newest research. Although information in this book comes from the most up-to-date medical journals and research sources, readers should keep in mind that changes occur very quickly in the field of oncology. A bibliography has been included for those who seek additional sources of information.

—Carol Turkington

ENTRIES A–Z

accessory breast tissue An unusual appearance of extra breast tissue located in the underarm area. Because this area is not usually included in standard mammograms, women who have this condition often require an extra MAMMOGRAM view.

acini The parts of the breast gland where fluid or milk is produced.

acitretin A drug used in cancer prevention that belongs to the family of drugs called RETINOIDS.

acupressure A noninvasive treatment for CHEMOTHERAPY-related nausea. While it is based on the same principles as ACUPUNCTURE, in acupressure a therapist presses on acupuncture points with the fingers instead of using needles. (Some therapists use electrical impulses, heat, laser beams, sound waves, friction, suction, or magnets instead of their fingers at the acupressure points, but the goal is still the same.)

Although acupressure is not used to treat breast cancer, studies have shown that it may be effective in relieving symptoms such as nausea that follows chemotherapy treatment or surgery. The technique can be used alone or as part of another system of manual healing such as shiatsu massage.

See also ACUSTIMULATION.

acupuncture A technique in which very thin needles of varying lengths are inserted through the skin to treat a variety of conditions. Although there is no evidence that acupuncture is effective as a treatment for breast cancer, clinical studies have found it to be effective in treating NAUSEA caused by chemotherapy drugs and surgical anesthesia. This finding was supported by a National Institutes of Health expert panel consisting of scientists, researchers, and health-care providers. There is also some evidence that acupuncture may lessen the need for conventional pain-relieving drugs. Some studies are currently studying whether acupuncture is effective in easing nausea, hot flashes, and pain in patients with breast cancer.

Acupuncture has been practiced for the past 2,000 years and is an important component of traditional Chinese medicine. Practitioners of traditional Chinese medicine believe that health depends on a vital energy called *qi* (pronounced "chee"), which they say flows through pathways in the body called meridians. Practitioners think that pain and disease occur when an obstruction along a meridian blocks the natural flow of energy. Also important to Chinese physicians is the idea of the opposing forces of yin and yang, which, when balanced, are said to work together with *qi* to promote physical and mental wellness. The insertion of needles into precise points on the skin is believed to unblock energy flow, balance yin and yang, and restore health. Originally, 365 acupuncture points were identified, corresponding to the number of days in a year, but gradually the number of acupoints grew to more than 2,000.

Some practitioners in the West reject the traditional philosophies of Chinese medicine and claim that acupuncture works by stimulating the production of natural painkiller substances in the body called endorphins. Because Western scientists have found it difficult to study meridians (because they do not correspond exactly to nerve or blood circulation pathways), some conclude that meridians do not exist at all. Nevertheless, several studies have found that acupuncture used along with mainstream medicine can have real benefits.

Traditional acupuncture needles were made of bone, stone, or metal (including silver and gold), but modern disposable acupuncture needles are made of very thin stainless steel. In 1996 the U.S. Food and Drug Administration approved the use of acupuncture needles by licensed practitioners; by law, needles must be labeled for one-time use only.

The procedure should cause little or no discomfort because the needles are as thin as a strand of hair. They usually are left in place for less than half an hour. Some acupuncturists twirl the needles or apply low-voltage electricity to them as a way to enhance the results. When conducted by a trained professional, acupuncture is generally considered safe. Relatively few complications have been reported, but there is a risk that a patient may be harmed if the acupuncturist is not well trained.

There are more than 10,000 acupuncturists in the United States, and about 32 states have established training standards for licensing the practice of acupuncture. Medicare does not cover acupuncture, but it is covered by some private health insurance plans and health maintenance organizations (HMOs). Consumers should consult an experienced, qualified practitioner who is state licensed or board certified. The American Academy of Medical Acupuncture (http://www.medicalacupuncture.org) can refer patients to physicians (M.D.s or D.O.s) who practice acupuncture.

See also ACUSTIMULATION; ACUPRESSURE.

acustimulation Mild electrical stimulation of ACUPUNCTURE points to control symptoms such as nausea and vomiting.

See also ACUPRESSURE.

adenocarcinoma Cancer that begins in cells that line certain internal organs and that have glandular properties (*adeno* means "gland"). Almost all breast cancers are adenocarcinomas. Depending on what the cells look like under the microscope and where in the breast they originate, they may be described as DUCTAL CARCINOMA, LOBULAR CARCINOMA, MEDULLARY CARCINOMA, or TUBULAR CARCINOMA. More than 75 percent of all adenocarcinomas are ductal carcinomas; 15 percent are lobular carcinomas.

adenoma A noncancerous tumor that occasionally appears in the inner surface of the breast. Although the diagnosis is often made by exam and radiologic studies, these tumors are often removed to be absolutely certain there is no malignancy.

adenovirus A virus group used in gene therapy that is altered so it can carry a specific tumor-fighting gene.

adjuvant treatment Treatment for breast cancer that is used in addition to surgery to decrease the chance that cancer will return. It usually refers to the use of CHEMOTHERAPY, HORMONAL THERAPY, or RADIATION therapy after surgery.

Adriamycin (doxorubicin) An anthracycline CHEMOTHERAPY drug that belongs to the family of drugs called ANTINEOPLASTIC ANTIBIOTICS. This drug works by disrupting the growth of cancer cells and destroying them. It is given intravenously and can cause scarring and tissue damage if it leaks from the vein during administration. Because Adriamycin can injure the heart, a heart function test is performed before and during treatment. This drug also can cause radiation recall (a reddening of skin that has been exposed to prior radiation treatment).

This drug can cause severe NAUSEA and vomiting, which can often be completely controlled by a variety of medications. Other side effects include decreased white blood cell count and increased risk of infection, decreased platelet count with increased risk of bleeding, loss of appetite, and hair loss. It can temporarily turn the urine red, which may stain clothes. This normal reddening of the urine lasts just a day or so after treatment.

advance directives A document that is completed and signed when a person is legally competent, explaining what the person would or would not want if unable to make decisions about medical care. Common advance directives include the following:

• Health care proxy (or health care power of attorney), which gives another person the authority to make decisions for the patient when the patient is unable to do so

- Living will, which directs a doctor to use, not start, or stop treatment that is keeping a dying patient alive when the patient cannot make his or her wishes known
- Nonhospital DO NOT RESUSCITATE ORDER, which directs emergency staff not to resuscitate a person who is not in a hospital or other health-care facility

Advance directives are an important part of any patient's financial affairs, since such a document allows someone else to make treatment decisions on a patient's behalf when the person is no longer capable of making those decisions.

Patients should prepare and sign advance directives that comply with state law and give copies to family, friends, and doctors. The document should reflect the patient's wishes and appoint someone to make decisions who is willing to carry out those wishes.

African-American women and breast cancer
African-American women experience higher death rates from breast cancer than any other racial or ethnic group, even though Caucasians have higher incidence rates. Such disparities may be due to multiple factors, such as late stage of disease at diagnosis, barriers to health-care access, history of other diseases, biological and genetic differences in tumors, health practices, and presence of risk factors.

In addition, breast cancer is the most common cancer in African-American women (100.2 cases per 100,000) and the second leading cause of cancer death among African-American women, exceeded only by lung cancer.

African-American women have a higher breast cancer death rate (31.4 per 100,000) than women of any other racial or ethnic population. It is about 28 percent higher than that for white women.

Nevertheless, African-American women's survival rate for breast cancer has increased in recent decades. The five-year survival rate for breast cancer among African-American women is 71 percent compared to 87 percent among Caucasian women.

Annual MAMMOGRAPHY screening and treatment of the disease at its earliest stages offer the best opportunity for decreasing the mortality rate and improving the survival rate of African-American women.

See also RACE AND BREAST CANCER.

age The most important factor in determining the risk for breast cancer is a woman's age; the older a woman is, the greater her chance of developing breast cancer. About 80 percent of breast cancers occur in women age 50 or older; the risk is especially high in women older than age 60. Breast cancer is uncommon before age 35.

A woman's chance of having breast cancer by age 30 is one in 2,525; by age 40 it is one in 217; by age 50, one in 50; by age 60, one in 24; by age 70, one in 14; by age 80 one in 10.

A projection based on present rates finds that each year, of 100,000 women

- In their 30s, 43 women will be diagnosed with breast cancer and eight will die of the disease
- In their 40s, 163 women will be diagnosed with breast cancer and 29 will die of the disease
- In their 50s, 263 women will be diagnosed with breast cancer and 59 will die of the disease
- In their 60s, 374 women will be diagnosed with breast cancer and 91 will die of the disease

age bias Older women who have breast cancer tend to be denied lifesaving treatment and access to promising new experimental treatments, according to an Ohio State University Medical Center study. Researchers say women older than age 50 are six to 62 times less likely to receive chemotherapy treatment, even after controlling for identified age-related compounding and modifying factors. This suggests possible age bias in offering older women adjuvant therapy, although researchers note that prior studies suggest that clinical considerations such as risk of spreading, treatment efficacy, and other illnesses a woman may have, as opposed to age, influence adjuvant treatment decisions in older women.

Previous studies have shown that older women are less likely to receive standard care than younger women. It could be that the benefits of adjuvant chemotherapy decline with age; the risk of drug toxicity outweighs the benefits of treatment; the risk of dying of other coexisting medical conditions may be greater than the risk of dying of cancer—or the decision not to treat is based solely on chronological age, a decision that would indicate age bias.

The authors investigated 480 women with non-metastatic breast cancer. Compared to women younger than age 50, women between 50 and 65 who had ESTROGEN-RECEPTOR-POSITIVE TUMORS were six times less likely to receive adjuvant chemotherapy. Meanwhile, women above age 65 with ER-positive tumors were 62 times less likely to receive chemotherapy. Women older than 65 with estrogen-receptor-negative tumors were almost seven times less likely to receive chemotherapy than younger women.

alcohol   The risk for development of breast cancer appears to rise with increased alcohol consumption. While having just one or two one-ounce drinks a day is not associated with an increased risk for breast cancer, women who have three or more drinks per day have twice the usual risk of development of breast cancer. This level of risk is similar in proportion to that associated with other well-established risk factors. For example, breast cancer risk is reported to be about 25 percent higher in women whose age at menarche was 12 years or younger versus 15 years or older. Also, the risk of breast cancer among women whose mother or sister had breast cancer is increased about 50 percent or more compared to that of women who do not have a family history of the disease.

To guard against development of alcohol-related cancers, some experts suggest women at normal risk for breast cancer should have no more than two one-ounce drinks a day. Taking a folate supplement such as in a multivitamin may help lower the risk for breast cancer if a woman does drink alcohol.

Women on hormone replacement therapy who have just 1.5 drinks a day may nearly double their risk of breast cancer, according to results published in 2002 from the Nurses' Health Study, based on 44,187 participating women. From 1980 to 1994 breast cancer developed in 1,722 women. Researchers found that hormone replacement and alcohol separately increased a woman's risk for breast cancer by about 30 percent. Women who took hormone replacement for at least five years and had more than one drink per day doubled their lifetime risk for breast cancer. Researchers say that a good compromise for women on hormone replacement therapy who want to get the health benefits of moderate alcohol consumption would be to have no more than one drink per day.

Although not all research supports an alcohol link to breast cancer, most does; in a recent summary of 63 published studies, 65 percent of these studies reported that consuming alcohol was associated with an increased risk of breast cancer. These studies involved different populations of women in several countries.

Women who drink alcohol may be different in many ways from those who do not drink alcohol. In order to determine whether the consumption of alcohol is associated with breast cancer, researchers must take into account other factors that have been previously shown to influence breast cancer risk. For example, getting older, having a family history of breast cancer, and having an earlier age at menarche (the age when a girl has her first menstrual period) are established risk factors for breast cancer. When assessing the influence of alcohol consumption on breast cancer risk, it is important that researchers account for these as well as other potential risk factors. These factors may be more common among women who drink alcoholic beverages and may actually be contributing to the reported association between alcohol and breast cancer.

Many of the studies of alcohol consumption and breast cancer risk have taken established breast cancer risk factors into account, and some have also included other types of habits and behavioral differences, such as diet and SMOKING. The results of most of these studies suggest that the consumption of alcohol may have an independent and direct effect on a woman's risk of development of breast cancer.

However, other researchers are not convinced that alcohol is acting independently, and they are continuing to analyze the relationship between alcohol and other lifestyle and personal characteristics.

Age and Alcohol

Some studies have reported that alcohol use before the age of 30 is more closely tied to breast cancer risk than recent or current drinking habits. Others have reported that current or recent drinking habits have a greater influence on breast cancer rates than drinking at an early age. Lifetime consumption of alcohol, regardless of the age at which the habit starts, has also been suggested as an important factor when determining breast cancer risk. Although researchers have not been able to establish the age at which consumption of alcohol has the greatest effect, drinking at any age may contribute to the risk.

There are no studies that compare the effects of drinking every day to the effects of drinking only occasionally. Experts do not know whether drinking one drink every day, such as drinking wine with a meal, has the same relationship to breast cancer risk as binge drinking (such as having seven drinks on a Saturday night).

Current evidence also suggests that it is probably the alcohol in wine, beer, and liquor and not some other component of these beverages that is associated with the risk of breast cancer. Some researchers reported that the consumption of beer and hard liquor, such as vodka and gin, had a greater association with breast cancer risk than the consumption of wine. Others have reported no difference in the type of alcoholic beverage consumed. Studies in European countries, such as Italy, where wine is consumed regularly at dinner have also reported that the drinking of alcohol is associated with increased breast cancer risk.

There are several possible ways that alcohol consumption could influence the risk of breast cancer. Many researchers are analyzing the influence of alcohol on the levels of hormones in the body—particularly of ESTROGEN. Estrogen is important for normal development of the reproductive system, and many experts believe that lifetime estrogen exposure influences the development of breast cancer. In some studies, drinking alcohol was shown to increase the level of estrogen in a woman's body, either because of an increase in production of estrogen or because of a decrease in the breakdown of estrogen.

Researchers are also studying other ways that alcohol may influence biological systems that affect breast cancer risk. For example, alcohol has a strong effect on the liver, an organ that helps rid the body of potentially harmful substances. If the liver is not able to function properly, it may not be able to get rid of potentially cancer-causing agents.

Benefits of Alcohol

Researchers have reported that women who drink light to moderate amounts of alcohol have a lower risk of development and death of heart disease. Since more women die of cardiovascular diseases than breast cancer, the recommendations about alcohol and breast cancer may seem to contradict the reports on cardiovascular disease.

The 1996 Guidelines on Diet, Nutrition and Cancer Prevention of the American Cancer Society suggest that most adults can drink safely, but they should limit their intake. Given the complex relationship between alcohol consumption and different diseases, any recommendations should be based on an individual's health risks and benefits.

Ultimately, experts say that the decision whether or not to drink alcoholic beverages needs to be made by a woman herself with the help of her physician. Women who have other well-established risk factors for breast cancer, such as a family history of the disease, may want to consider seriously limiting their alcohol consumption. Certainly, they should take a multivitamin.

alkaline phosphatase test   A test that measures the amount of an enzyme called alkaline phosphatase (ALP) in the blood, which may be elevated if breast cancer has spread to the bone or liver.

ALP is found in all tissues, especially in the liver, bile ducts, placenta, and bone. Since damaged or diseased tissue releases enzymes into the blood, ALP level measurements can be abnormal in many conditions, including metastatic breast cancer. But serum ALP level is also high in some normal circumstances, and may be elevated or in response to a variety of drugs.

alkylating agents   A family of CHEMOTHERAPY drugs used to treat breast cancer. They inhibit cancer cell growth by directly interfering with a cell's DNA. Alkylating agents cause the most damage to cells in the active phase of the cell cycle, but they are active in all phases of the cycle. In high doses, they can also kill cells in the "resting" phase.

Cyclophosphamide (CYTOXAN) is the most common alkylating agent used in breast cancer treatment.

Side Effects

Alkylating drugs may cause NAUSEA, mouth sores, low blood counts, and hair loss. They also may cause early menopause, and very rarely, leukemia.

allicin A phytochemical found in onions and garlic that experts suspect may help protect against cancer. Allicin is most widely recognized for its action as an antiviral, antifungal, and antibacterial agent with the ability to block the toxins produced by bacteria and viruses. It is also an ANTIOXIDANT and helps to eliminate toxins from the body.

See also BIOFLAVONOIDS; DIET.

allogeneic bone marrow transplant See BONE MARROW TRANSPLANT.

alopecia See HAIR LOSS.

American Brachytherapy Society (ABS) A nonprofit professional organization founded in 1978 that seeks to provide insight and research into the use of BRACHYTHERAPY in malignant and benign conditions. Members include physicists, physicians, and other health-care providers interested in brachytherapy. The mission of the ABS is to provide information directly to the consumer, promote the highest standards of practice of brachytherapy, and help health-care professionals by encouraging improved and continuing education for RADIATION ONCOLOGISTS and other health-care professionals involved in the treatment of cancer. In addition, the ABS promotes clinical and laboratory research into the practice of brachytherapy. For contact information, see Appendix I.

American Cancer Society (ACS) A nationwide community-based organization dedicated to eliminating cancer as a major health problem, providing research, education, advocacy, and service. It is one of the oldest and largest voluntary health agencies in the United States, involving more than 2 million

Americans. Headquartered in Atlanta, Georgia, the ACS has state divisions throughout the country and more than 3,400 local offices.

To ease the impact of cancer on patients and their families, the American Cancer Society provides printed materials, service and rehabilitation programs, as well as education and support programs. Cancer Society staff members accept calls and distribute publications in Spanish. The ACS also sponsors a number of related support groups, including CANCER SURVIVORS NETWORK, I CAN COPE, LOOK GOOD . . . FEEL BETTER, and REACH TO RECOVERY. A local ACS group may be listed in the white pages of the telephone directory.

To date, the society has invested more than $2.5 billion in cancer research and has provided grant support to 32 Nobel Prize winners early in their career. The society's overall annual expenditure in research grew steadily from $1 million in 1946 to more than $125 million in 2002. The research program focuses primarily on peer-reviewed projects initiated by beginning investigators working in leading medical and scientific institutions across the country. The research program consists of three components: extramural grants, intramural epidemiology and surveillance research, and the intramural behavioral research center. The society's prevention programs focus primarily on tobacco control, the relationship between diet and physical activity and cancer, promoting comprehensive school health education, and reduction of the risk of skin cancer.

In order to ensure that all cancers are found at the earliest possible stage, when there is the greatest chance for successful treatment, the society provides patients and professionals with early detection guidelines and offers detection education and advocacy programs.

The ACS also sponsors national conferences and workshops, audiovisual and print publications, a Web site, and the National Call Center, as well as clinical awards, professorships, and scholarships. For contact information, see Appendix I.

American Cancer Society Web site This Web site (http://www.cancer.org) is sponsored by the AMERICAN CANCER SOCIETY to provide lifesaving information to the public. The site includes an interactive cancer resource center containing in-depth information on breast cancer and every other major cancer type. Through the resource center, visitors can order American Cancer Society publications, gain access to recent news articles, and find additional on- and off-line resources. Other sections on the Web site include a directory of medical resources, links to other sites organized by cancer type or topic, resources for media representatives, and information on the society's research grants program, advocacy efforts, and special events.

American Institute for Cancer Research (AICR)
A nonprofit group founded in 1982 that provides educational programs and printed materials on cancer prevention, particularly through DIET and nutrition. It also supports research at sites throughout the country. The institute offers a toll-free nutrition hotline, a pen pal support network, and a wide array of brochures for consumers and health professionals.

The AICR also supports the CancerResource, an information and resource program for cancer patients. A limited selection of Spanish-language publications is available. For contact information, see Appendix I.

American Society of Clinical Oncology (ASCO)
A nonprofit organization dedicated to supporting all types of cancer research, but especially patient-oriented clinical research. ASCO's mission is to facilitate the delivery of high-quality health care, foster the exchange of information, further the training of researchers, and encourage communication among the various cancer specialties.

ASCO has more than 16,000 professional members worldwide, including clinical ONCOLOGISTS in medical oncology, therapeutic radiology, surgical oncology, pediatric oncology, gynecologic oncology, urologic oncology, and hematology; students; oncology nurses; and other health-care practitioners. International members make up 20 percent of the total membership and represent 75 countries worldwide. For contact information, see Appendix I.

American Society of Plastic and Reconstructive Surgeons
See AMERICAN SOCIETY OF PLASTIC SURGEONS.

American Society of Plastic Surgeons
The largest plastic surgery specialty organization in the world, the society was founded in 1931 to promote high-quality care for plastic surgery patients, to provide educational programs, and to support the activities of its members. Formerly the American Society of Plastic and Reconstructive Surgeons, the name was changed in 1999. The society is composed of PLASTIC SURGEONS certified by the American Board of Plastic Surgery, who perform cosmetic and reconstructive surgery, such as BREAST RECONSTRUCTION.

In addition to its professional activities, the society maintains a speakers' bureau and a patient referral service to help patients choose a plastic surgeon. The society acts as an advocate for patient safety—for example, by encouraging its members to operate in surgical facilities that have passed rigorous external review of equipment and staffing. For contact information, see Appendix I.

aminoglutethimide (Cytadren, Elipten)
A type of CHEMOTHERAPY drug that belongs to a class of hormone and hormone-inhibiting drugs called adrenal steroid inhibitors. These drugs stop the adrenal glands from making steroid hormones, including ESTROGEN. Aminoglutethimide is given orally and must be taken with hydrocortisone.

A33 monoclonal antibody
A type of MONOCLONAL ANTIBODY used in breast cancer detection or therapy. Monoclonal antibodies are laboratory-produced substances that can locate and bind to cancer cells.

anastrozole
See ARIMIDEX.

androgens
Male sex hormones that may be used as medications for patients with breast cancer to treat recurrence of the disease. Androgens seem to change the cancer cell's hormonal environment, blunting the stimulus to grow so that the cancer cell does not divide. Exactly how they work is not known.

Androgen medications include the following:

- Calusterone (Methosarb)
- Dromostanolone propionate (Drolban, Masteril, Macleron, Permastril)

- Fluoxymesteron (Halotestin, Ora-Testryl)
- Nandrolone decanoate (Deca-Durabolin)
- Testosterone propionate (Neohombreol-M, Orator)

Side Effects

Androgens may cause patients to retain salt and water. Women who receive androgens notice a deepening of their voice after a period of use. Patients who take androgens for more than three months may experience decreased sexual interest, increased body hair, and acne.

anemia   A condition in which the blood does not have enough red blood cells, in hemoglobin (the part of blood that carries oxygen to the body's tissues) or in total volume. Anemia is common in patients with cancer and may contribute to debilitating FATIGUE. About three in four cancer patients experience fatigue caused by anemia or by cancer treatment.

Anemia can be caused by decreased formation of red blood cells. If the cancer is in the bone marrow, it can crowd out the cells that would ordinarily become red blood cells. Anemia also can be caused by loss of red blood cells; for example, if a cancer is bleeding. Blood cells also can be destroyed as a side effect of chemotherapy or radiation.

Several other forms of anemia may occur in patients with cancer. *Hemolytic anemia* occurs when red blood cells are destroyed prematurely (rarely as a result of some types chemotherapy). *Iron-deficiency anemia* occurs when there is too low a level of iron in the blood, which leads to a lack of hemoglobin. In those with cancer, iron deficiency may be a result of bleeding (such as from a tumor in the colon). *Pernicious anemia* occurs when there is a lack of vitamin B_{12} in the diet. People who have some types of intestinal cancer may have trouble absorbing B_{12}. In addition, many cancer patients often have a poor appetite and may not eat enough foods with vitamin B_{12}.

aneuploid   Cells that contain an unusual amount of deoxyribonucleic acid (DNA).

angiogenesis   The formation of blood vessels. The walls of blood vessels are formed by cells that divide only about once every three years. However, when the body requires it, angiogenesis can stimulate them to divide.

Angiogenesis is regulated by both activator and inhibitor molecules. Normally, the inhibitors predominate, blocking growth. Should a need for new blood vessels arise (such as to repair a wound), angiogenesis activators increase in number and inhibitors decrease. This prompts the formation of new blood vessels.

In tumor angiogenesis, blood vessels penetrate cancerous growths, supplying nutrients and oxygen and removing waste products. This process helps cancer to spread. Tumor angiogenesis starts when cancerous tumor cells release activator molecules that send signals to surrounding normal host tissue, which then activate certain genes that in turn make proteins to encourage growth of new blood vessels.

Because cancer cannot grow or spread without the formation of new blood vessels, scientists are trying to find ways to stop angiogenesis. They are studying natural and synthetic angiogenesis inhibitors (also called antiangiogenesis agents) in the hope that these chemicals will prevent the growth of cancer by blocking the formation of new blood vessels. In animal studies, angiogenesis inhibitors have successfully stopped the formation of new blood vessels, causing the cancer to shrink and die.

When researchers realized that cancer cells can release molecules to activate the process of angiogenesis, the challenge became to find and study these angiogenesis-stimulating molecules in animal and human tumors. From such studies more than a dozen different proteins, as well as several smaller molecules, have been identified as angiogenic, meaning that they are released by tumors as signals for angiogenesis. Among these molecules, two proteins appear to be the most important for sustaining tumor growth: vascular endothelial growth factor (VEGF) and basic fibroblast growth factor (bFGF). VEGF and bFGF are produced by many kinds of cancer cells and by certain types of normal cells, too.

Although many tumors produce angiogenic molecules such as VEGF and bFGF, their presence is not enough to begin blood vessel growth. For angiogenesis to begin, these activator molecules must overcome a variety of angiogenesis inhibitors that normally restrain blood vessel growth. Almost a dozen naturally occurring proteins can inhibit angiogenesis, including proteins called angiostatin, endostatin, and thrombospondin. A finely tuned balance between the concentration of angiogenesis inhibitors and that of activators such as VEGF and bFGF determines whether a tumor can induce the growth of new blood vessels. To trigger angiogenesis, the production of activators must increase as the production of inhibitors decreases.

The discovery that angiogenesis inhibitors such as ENDOSTATIN can restrain the growth of primary tumors raises the possibility that such inhibitors may also be able to slow tumor spread.

It has been known for many years that cancer cells originating in a primary tumor can spread to another organ and form tiny, microscopic tumor masses that may remain dormant for years. A likely explanation for this tumor dormancy is that no angiogenesis occurred, so the small tumor lacked the new blood vessels needed for continued growth. One possible reason for this tumor dormancy may be the fact that some primary tumors secrete the inhibitor angiostatin into the bloodstream; which then circulates throughout the body and inhibits blood vessel growth at other sites. This process could prevent microscopic cancer cells from growing into visible tumors.

Researchers are now studying whether interfering with angiogenesis can slow or prevent the growth and spread of cancer cells in humans. To answer this question scientists are currently testing almost two dozen ANGIOGENESIS INHIBITORS in patients with cancers of the breast. If the results of clinical trials show that angiogenesis inhibitors are both safe and effective in treating cancer in humans, these agents may be approved by the U.S. Food and Drug Administration and made available for widespread use. The process of producing and testing angiogenesis inhibitors is likely to take several years.

angiogenesis inhibitor Substance (also called antiangiogenesis agent) that may prevent the growth of blood vessels from surrounding tissue to a solid tumor (ANGIOGENESIS).

anorexia and breast cancer Young women who have suffered from anorexia have a lower risk of developing breast cancer, according to one recent study. This suggests that calorie intake early in life may play a significant role in development of the disease.

In the study by scientists in Sweden and Harvard medical school, young women hospitalized for anorexia were found to be about half as likely to develop breast cancer as women overall. The finding does not prove that calorie deprivation is the reason, however. The next study needs to discover what the real mechanisms may be to explain the connection.

Researchers examined breast cancer incidence in 7,303 Swedish women who were under 40 when they underwent hospital treatment for anorexia between 1965 and 1998. Most developed anorexia before age 20. Only seven women developed breast cancer by the study's end in 2000. Nearly 15 cases would have been expected in the general population—a difference of 53 percent. That translates to about one anorexic woman developing breast cancer out of 1,000, compared with two out of 1,000 in the general population.

Weight gain has long been known to be a risk factor for breast cancer. It could be that calorie restriction during early adolescence might stunt breast-cell reproduction and reduce the chance for mutations to occur that could lead to cancer. Also, calorie restriction during crucial phases of development might reduce levels of estrogen and other hormones linked to tumor development. Girls with anorexia often stop menstruating, which reduces their estrogen levels.

Once the link is better understood, scientists might be able to design an intervention, including medication, that is more practical than just generalized starvation.

antibiotics and breast cancer The use of antibiotics may be linked to an increase in breast cancer risk, but it is not yet clear if taking the drugs actually causes the disease, according to a study released in February 2004. In the study, women who took antibiotics for more than 500 days or who took more than 25 different antibiotics over about 17 years had twice the risk of breast cancer as women who never took antibiotics. The risk was smaller (about one and a half times) for women who took between one and 25 antibiotics. All classes of antibiotics were linked to the increase in risk. The study's findings were remarkable in their strength and consistency; the association between breast cancer risk and antibiotic use was similar no matter what antibiotic was used. The risk was also closely related to dose—women who consumed the most antibiotics had the highest risk.

However, researchers insisted that they could not say that antibiotics *cause* breast cancer. Instead, it could be that the increased risk may be linked to the diseases women are using antibiotics to treat. In fact, compelling evidence links breast cancer to the inflammation that can result from chronic infection. Such infections are routinely treated with antibiotics. Or it may be that women who use many antibiotics have a weak immune response or a hormonal imbalance that may be an underlying cause of breast cancer. Still other theories suggest that since antibiotics affect intestinal bacteria, this might interfere with the metabolism of certain foods known to protect the body against cancer.

In addition, the control group—the women who did not take any antibiotics—may represent a uniquely healthy group either in general well-being or lifestyle characteristics, which could account for some of the difference between the two groups. In addition, women who took lots of antibiotics saw their doctors more often and may have been screened more carefully.

Doctors hastened to reassure women who are taking antibiotics for serious infections that they should not stop taking these medications. Instead, doctors suggest that there is an urgent need for everyone to take fewer antibiotics when they are not needed. Indeed, experts note that the over-reliance on antibiotics to treat conditions for which they are not effective, such as colds and other viral infections, has contributed to a universal problem of drug-resistant germs. Alarmingly, the U.S. Centers for Disease Control and Prevention reports that virtually all significant bacterial infections are becoming resistant to their antibiotic treatment of choice.

antibodies Proteins produced by certain white blood cells in response to foreign substances called antigens. Each antibody can only bind to—and therefore destroy—a specific antigen. Antibodies can work in several ways, depending on the nature of the antigen they target. Some antibodies disable antigens directly; others make the antigen more vulnerable to destruction by white blood cells.

See also ANTIBODY THERAPY.

antibody therapy Treatment with an antibody, a substance that can directly kill specific tumor cells or stimulate the immune system to kill tumor cells.

See also ANTIBODIES, MONOCLONAL ANTIBODY THERAPY.

anticancer antibiotics See ANTINEOPLASTIC ANTIBIOTICS.

anti–carcinoembryonic antigen antibody An antibody against CARCINOEMBRYONIC ANTIGEN (CEA), a protein present on certain types of cancer cells.

antiemetics See ANTINAUSEA MEDICATION.

antiestrogen A substance that blocks the activity of ESTROGENS, the family of hormones that promote the development and maintenance of female sex characteristics. Several antiestrogen drugs have been developed to treat estrogen-receptor-positive breast cancers (cancers that grows in response to estrogen). SELECTIVE ESTROGEN-RECEPTOR MODULATORS such as TAMOXIFEN (Nolvadex), toremifene, and EVISTA (raloxifene) inhibit the effects of estrogen on breast cancer cells.

Tamoxifen is taken in pill form for five years after breast cancer surgery to prevent the recurrence of cancer. The most common side effect of this medication is HOT FLASHES. Other side effects include mild NAUSEA, leg cramps and vaginal dryness. Very rare side effects can include uterine cancer, blood clots, and strokes.

Evista is also a SERM, but it is used to treat osteopenia and osteoporosis. It also may reduce the risk for breast cancer. Side effects are very similar to tamoxifen.

Fulvestrant (FASLODEX) destroys estrogen receptors in breast cancer cells; it is used to treat metastatic breast cancer in postmenopausal women whose condition has not responded to tamoxifen. Fulvestrant is administered once a month by intramuscular injection. Side effects include nausea, hot flashes, and pain at the infection site.

Goserelin (Zoladex) is a synthetic form of luteinizing hormone–releasing hormone that is prescribed to treat metastatic breast cancer in premenopausal women. This medication signals the body to stop producing estrogen, depriving the tumor of the estrogen it needs to grow. Several weeks or months of treatment is needed before periods stop and tumor growth slows. Side effects include hot flashes, sexual dysfunction, increased pain, and rash.

AROMATASE INHIBITORS (such as anastozole [ARIMIDEX], letrozole [FEMARA], and exemestane [AROMASIN]) inhibit the action of the enzyme aromatase, which is involved in estrogen production in postmenopausal women. These drugs may be prescribed for postmenopausal women who have advanced breast cancer. Like tamoxifen, these drugs are well tolerated, although some women may have muscle or joint aches, as well as hot flashes. Rare side effects include cough and gastrointestinal upsets.

antimetabolite   A type of breast cancer CHEMOTHERAPY drug that interferes with the normal metabolic processes within cells, preventing cell division. Because antimetabolites are similar to nutrients, they fool the cancer cell, which ingests them. The chemotherapy drugs 5-fluorouracil and methotrexate are antimetabolites that prevent growth of a cell at a short, specific time in its reproduction cycle by interfering with important enzyme reactions within the cell.

Side Effects

Side effects of antimetabolites include NAUSEA, DIARRHEA, mouth sores, and low blood counts. Hair loss is less common with these drugs than with other chemotherapies.

antinausea medication   A type of drug that can prevent or reduce NAUSEA and vomiting, common side effects of CHEMOTHERAPY and RADIATION THERAPY. Popular antinausea drugs include dexametha-

sone (DECADRON), prochlorperazine (COMPAZINE), Toracan, chlorpromazine (Thorazine), metoclopramide, lorazepam (ATIVAN), dronabinol (Marinol), granisetron (KYTRIL), dolasetron mesylate (Anzemet), and ondansetron (ZOFRAN). Often a combination of these drugs is prescribed; if the first combination does not work, others may be effective. Antinausea medications are often given along with chemotherapy drugs, and sometimes for several days after, to prevent nausea before it begins. It is usually much easier to prevent nausea and vomiting than to try to treat them once they occur.

antineoplastic antibiotics   A group of CHEMOTHERAPY drugs used to treat a variety of cancers, including breast cancer. They work by interfering with DNA, the genetic material in cells, thereby blocking cell growth. Also called anticancer antibiotics or antitumor antibiotics, these drugs include bleomycin, doxorubicin (ADRIAMYCIN), and epirubicin (ELLENCE).

Side effects of these medications include NAUSEA, low blood counts, HAIR LOSS, and, rarely, cardiac problems.

antioxidants   Compounds that fight cell damage caused by highly reactive oxygen radicals (FREE RADICALS), a rogue type of highly reactive oxygen molecule that can attack cells throughout the body. Although free radicals serve important functions, such as helping the immune system fight off disease, at excessive levels they can cause problems.

Free radicals are formed both during normal metabolism and in response to infection and some chemicals. They cause damage to fatty acids in cell membranes, and the products of this damage can then damage proteins and DNA. They can promote malignant changes and may play an important role in the development of breast cancer.

A number of different mechanisms are involved in protection against, or repair after, free radical damage, including a number of nutrients—especially vitamin E, beta-carotene, vitamin C, and selenium. Collectively known as antioxidant nutrients, they limit the cell and tissue damage caused by toxins and pollutants. However, antioxidants are not known to prevent or treat breast cancer.

Because high doses of antioxidant supplements can cause side effects, consuming antioxidants as part of a healthy diet is safer. Antioxidants are found in

- Fruits and vegetables (especially blueberries and yellow fruits and vegetables)
- Brown rice
- Whole grains
- Meats
- Eggs
- Dairy products

Side Effects

Supplements containing high doses of antioxidants can cause severe side effects, including internal bleeding, and may be harmful in patients taking blood thinners. No one should take these or any supplements without consulting a doctor. They also may interfere with the effects of RADIATION THERAPY.

antiperspirants and breast cancer   See DEODORANTS AND BREAST CANCER.

antitumor antibiotics   See ANTINEOPLASTIC ANTIBIOTICS.

appetite loss   Lack of interest in eating is frequently a problem experienced by patients with breast cancer as a direct result of cancer and as a side effect of treatment. People also may lose their appetite while struggling with cancer because of mouth sores (STOMATITIS), taste changes, or because pain from the cancer itself can trigger appetite loss.

Appetite loss is a serious problem among cancer patients because it can lead to poor nutrition, which can interfere with tissue healing and recovery. Loss of appetite and weight loss can lead to CACHEXIA, a type of malnutrition.

Treatment

Drugs such as megestrol (Megace) or dronabinol (MARINOL) (derived from marijuana) may be used to improve appetite. Patients also should eat

- Small, frequent meals
- Nutritious snacks
- High-calorie, high-protein food
- Attractive, appetizing meals

In addition, patients should eat during the times when they feel most comfortable. Often, appetite is best in the morning, so eating a good breakfast may help. Patients also may stimulate appetite with light exercise, take medications with high-calorie drinks, and eat at a friend's home or a good restaurant. Patients should also try using lemon-flavored drinks, rinsing their mouth before eating, and eating cold, white food (ice cream, milk shakes, boiled chicken). Many patients find that eating meat becomes unpleasant at this time; other high-protein foods may be more palatable.

Aredia (pamidronate disodium)   A CHEMOTHERAPY drug approved in 1996 to treat the spread of breast cancer to the bone. It belongs to a class of blood calcium–lowering drugs called BISPHOSPHONATES. Aredia stops bone breakdown so that calcium is not released from the bones into the blood.

Aredia was originally developed to treat high levels of calcium in the blood (hypercalcemia), a condition that is associated with malignancy, bone lesions of multiple myeloma, and Paget's disease of bone.

Side Effects

Common side effects include pain at the injection site and fever that last a few days after infusion. Less common side effects include NAUSEA, CONSTIPATION, and APPETITE LOSS. Rarely, patients may experience vomiting or stomach discomfort.

areola   The circular field of dark-colored skin surrounding the nipple.

Arimidex (anastrozole)   A chemotherapy drug given accelerated approval in September 2002 for the adjuvant treatment of postmenopausal women who have ESTROGEN-sensitive early breast cancer. Arimidex works by inhibiting production of estrogen in postmenopausal women, which has been linked to the development of breast cancer. Most cases of breast cancer occur in postmenopausal women. Arimidex belongs to a class of drugs known as hormone antagonists, which prevent the body's adrenal glands from producing estrogen.

The U.S. Food and Drug Administration approved Arimidex just six months after the application was submitted. It was quickly approved because early test results in one of the largest cancer trials ever conducted showed the drug was as good as, or better than, TAMOXIFEN for postmenopausal women—and that it had fewer side effects. Up until 2002, tamoxifen had been the standard treatment for older women who had estrogen-sensitive tumors.

In studies of 9,366 postmenopausal women who had operable breast cancer, anastrozole was compared to tamoxifen for five years or until recurrence of the cancer. The study showed that for women with early breast cancer, anastrozole was better than tamoxifen in preventing a tumor in the other breast. Anastrozole reduced the occurrence of contralateral breast cancers in women with hormone-sensitive tumors by nearly 60 percent more than tamoxifen.

Research suggests that neither tamoxifen nor estrogen should be given together with Arimidex.

On the basis of preliminary findings reported in the British medical journal *The Lancet,* doctors believe the drug could help to prevent the disease in high-risk women. A trial to determine how effective the drug would be in preventing cancer is currently being undertaken in Britain.

Side Effects

Anastrozole has fewer side effects than tamoxifen, which is associated with an increased risk of endometrial cancer, HOT FLASHES, and blood clots. But it does not work in young women, and it may increase the risk of bone fractures. Most common side effects include weakness and decreased energy level.

Aromasin (exemestane) CHEMOTHERAPY drug approved in 1999 for the treatment of advanced breast cancer in postmenopausal women whose disease had progressed after TAMOXIFEN therapy. Aromasin is the only oral AROMATASE INHIBITOR being studied for treatment of breast cancer both before and after surgery.

Aromasin is currently used to treat advanced breast cancer in postmenopausal women whose tumors have stopped responding to anti-estrogen therapy such as tamoxifen. It is the first in a new class or oral hormonal inactivator therapies.

Aromatase inactivators permanently bind with the aromatase enzyme, preventing it from producing estrogen, which some breast cancer tumors need for growth. This effect contrasts with that of aromatase inhibitors, which only temporarily interfere with the aromatase enzyme.

Early results from a Phase II study comparing Aromasin with tamoxifen in advanced breast cancer indicate Aromasin outperformed tamoxifen, slowing tumor growth and spread by several months. Additionally, women treated with Aromasin experienced fewer side effects (FATIGUE, pain, HOT FLASHES, sweating, and NAUSEA) than did those treated with tamoxifen. The NATIONAL CANCER INSTITUTE began a trial in 2001 to explore whether exemestane might eventually replace tamoxifen as a standard postsurgical treatment to prevent cancer recurrence. The drug may also have potential to prevent breast cancers of women who are at high risk for the disease.

Although tamoxifen is widely used after surgical and radiation treatment to prevent recurrence of breast tumors that grow in response to the HORMONE ESTROGEN, it seems to be effective for only five years. Studies have shown that continued use of tamoxifen beyond five years may actually increase the risk of recurrence.

Tamoxifen works by blocking estrogen, preventing it from stimulating the growth of breast tumors. That effect can prevent tumor growth, but it also sensitizes any remaining tumor cells to estrogen. After five years the cells are so sensitized that tamoxifen, which has some estrogenic activity, may actually spur new tumor growth. But halting tamoxifen therapy carries risks, too. Women whose breast cancer has spread to their lymph nodes and who have completed tamoxifen therapy still face a 30 percent chance of recurrence.

Aromasin does not block estrogen but actually stops most of the body's production of the hormone by targeting an enzyme called aromatase, which is necessary for estrogen production. Before menopause, most of the body's estrogen is produced in the ovaries. But fatty tissues, adrenal glands, and other tissues throughout the body also produce estrogen, so even postmenopausal women produce some estrogen.

In a separate study, Aromasin was able to shrink primary breast cancers before surgical removal; that effect would be important for women considering breast-conserving surgical options rather than mastectomy. In a sample of 13 postmenopausal women with estrogen-receptor-positive breast cancer, over three months Aromasin reduced tumor volume by 83 percent.

aromatase inhibitors   A new type of hormonal medication used to treat ESTROGEN-sensitive breast cancer in postmenopausal women that dramatically suppresses estrogen production by blocking the effects of the enzyme aromatase. The new aromatase inhibitor drugs may be superior to TAMOXIFEN, the current post-chemotherapy preventive treatment, which binds to specific tumor cell sites to keep estrogen from attaching and directing the cells to multiply.

Currently, there are several approved aromatase inhibitors for breast cancer: anastrozole (ARIMIDEX), exemestane (AROMASIN), and letrozole (FEMARA). These drugs are used by postmenopausal women to prevent the recurrence of breast cancer or to treat metastatic disease.

Normally, early-stage breast cancer is treated by surgery to remove the tumor (plus radiation, if part of the breast is conserved). If tumor cells have spread to underarm lymph nodes, cell-killing cancer drugs often are given, particularly in the United States. Then, if the cancer is undetectable and it is the type fueled by estrogen, women take daily tamoxifen pills for five years—to prevent any microscopic cancer cells lurking in the body from later triggering cancer in another spot. Such metastasized cancer is virtually incurable. But cancer cells grow resistant to tamoxifen in many patients, sometimes within 12 months, and prolonged use can cause uterine cancer and dangerous blood clots. Those problems sparked interest in aromatase inhibitors.

Aromatase inhibitors have been known since the 1970s, but high toxicity limited use. Today's third-generation aromatase inhibitors—including Aromasin, Femara, and Arimidex—work better and are less toxic but still increase bone loss, a serious problem for elderly women.

More than two-thirds of breast cancers are considered "estrogen sensitive" because they need estrogen to grow. Hormone therapy that can stop this growth is the basis of regimens designed to prevent cancer recurrences and improve survival. Although tamoxifen prevents estrogen from acting on tumors, aromatase inhibitors actually block an enzyme the body uses to make estrogen, thereby slashing the body's production of estrogen altogether. New studies suggest that aromatase's different mechanism of action to decrease estrogen levels may mean that these drugs can shrink tumors better and longer with fewer side effects.

In fact, a 2003 study published in *The New England Journal of Medicine* showed that women could cut their risk of recurrence by nearly half by taking the aromatase inhibitor Femara after they completed about five years on tamoxifen.

Femara was so effective that an international committee decided to disclose the results early in order to offer the drug to all women in the trial. The international study compared Femara against a placebo for nearly 5,200 women who had completed five years of tamoxifen therapy. Four years after the start of the study, cancer came back in 13 percent of the women on placebo but only in 7 percent of those on Femara.

Another recent study showed that postmenopausal women who switch to another aromatase inhibitor (Arimidex) after two or three years of tamoxifen therapy had fewer recurrences of cancer than those who continued to take tamoxifen for the full recommended five years.

In the Arimidex trial, women who switched to the aromatase inhibitor fared better than if they stayed on standard tamoxifen. The study followed 448 postmenopausal women who had been taking tamoxifen for at least two years after breast cancer surgery. The women were randomly assigned to continue taking tamoxifen or switch to Arimidex for five years. Three years later, cancer was 64 percent less likely to have recurred in the group of women who had switched to Arimidex, the study showed.

Yet another trial showed that women who took Arimidex instead of tamoxifen were slightly less likely to see their cancer recur after four years compared with those who took tamoxifen. And in another study of nearly 300 women, those who took Arimidex before surgery were significantly more likely to become candidates for breast-conserving surgery than those who took standard tamoxifen.

Aromasin

This drug for advanced breast cancer is better than tamoxifen at preventing localized tumors from returning after surgery, according to a large international study published in March 2004 that promises new hope and treatment strategies for many patients. Recurrence of such early cancer was reduced by one-third in women who started on tamoxifen and who then switched after two and one-half years to Aromasin, compared to those who took tamoxifen the whole time.

The women switching to Aromasin also had less serious side effects, were 56 percent less likely to get cancer in the other breast and were half as likely to develop unrelated cancer in other body areas. Moreover, a recent study on Aromasin's cousin letrozole showed important advantages over tamoxifen. Researchers predict doctors will give Aromasin to many women at high risk for recurrence, such as those whose breast cancer spreads to multiple lymph nodes.

The study, which included 4,742 postmenopausal women in 37 countries, focused on women with breast cancer in which the hormone estrogen fuels tumor growth—the type causing about 70 percent of breast cancer. The results do not apply to premenopausal women or those with tough-to-treat breast cancer not driven by estrogen. Among the women switching to exemestane, 54 died of breast cancer, compared with 67 in the tamoxifen-only group. Overall, 91.5 percent of women in the exemestane group were cancer-free three years after switching drugs, compared with 86.8 percent for women who stayed on tamoxifen.

Several smaller trials also had showed that Aromasin also may be effective for the treatment of hormone-responsive metastatic breast cancer. It may be useful after the other aromatase inhibitors stop working; in one study of 105 women who had previously been on aromatase inhibitors, about one-fourth appeared to benefit from the newer drug.

Faslodex

Faslodex is not an aromatase inhibitor but is another type of hormonal therapy that is given as a monthly injection instead of a daily pill. Like Aromasin, the trials so far show only that Falsodex is effective for the treatment of metastatic breast cancer, not for newly diagnosed women undergoing surgery. One study reported earlier this month showed that Faslodex is about as effective as Arimidex in the treatment of postmenopausal women with advanced breast cancer whose disease continues to spread after treatment with tamoxifen. Faslodex works by destroying the estrogen receptor on the surface of breast cancer cells.

Ongoing studies are looking at both Aromasin and Faslodex in the treatment of early breast cancer.

Aromatase Inhibitors vs. Tamoxifen

Experts still believe tamoxifen still has a major place in the prevention and treatment of breast cancer. For example, aromatase inhibitors (AIs) only work for postmenopausal women. And tamoxifen is the only treatment approved to prevent breast cancer.

In addition, doctors have decades of experience with tamoxifen, whereas the aromatase inhibitors are still relatively new. Experts still do not know, therefore, whether the AIs should be used instead of tamoxifen, or whether two or five years of tamoxifen should be followed by the AIs. Ongoing Studies are addressing these issues.

Side Effects

Tamoxifen is associated with a higher risk of uterine cancer than the newer aromatase inhibitors. But some studies have shown that women taking aromatase inhibitors are more prone to bone fractures than those taking tamoxifen. In general, however, side effects from aromatase inhibitors—both Femara and Arimidex—are mild.

The AIs may worsen bone density and raise cholesterol, but they are not associated with the increased risk of blood clots, strokes, or uterine cancer. They seem to cause fewer hot flashes than tamoxifen and less vaginal bleeding, but they may cause more muscle and bone aches.

ascites The presence of excess fluid in the abdomen, usually caused by liver disease, also can be a symptom of breast cancer. If cancer cells have spread to the lining of the abdomen, they can cause irritation that leads to fluid buildup. It is also possible for cancer cells to block the lymphatic system—

which is responsible for draining off excess fluid into the urine—resulting in fluid buildup.

Symptoms

Ascites may cause the abdomen to become painfully swollen. It can make patients feel tired and breathless or cause NAUSEA, indigestion, and APPETITE LOSS.

Treatment

The best treatment of ascites caused by cancer is to treat the cancer. If the treatment is effective, the ascites will resolve. If the cancer cannot be treated, diuretics may help, or the fluid can be drained by a needle placed into the abdomen. Unfortunately, relief is usually temporary unless the cancer can be treated.

Ashkenazi Jews and breast cancer Although all women are at risk for breast cancer, some groups have higher risks than others. Breast and ovarian cancer are somewhat more common among women of Ashkenazi Jewish descent, whose ancestors emigrated from Central or Eastern Europe. In the United States, nine out of every 10 Jewish Americans are of Ashkenazi descent. Their elevated risk may be due to mutations in two breast cancer genes, *BRCA1* and *BRCA2*, which appear more often among Ashkenazi Jews than in the general population.

Researchers have long known that some inherited diseases occur more commonly in certain ethnic groups than they do in the general population because of the "founder effect": In groups that have been isolated for religious, cultural, or geographical reasons and that have originated from a small group of common ancestors, disease-associated mutations are passed down with greater frequency. This is because any mutations present in the founders become common in their offspring.

Researchers believe the *BRCA1* and *BRCA2* mutations that today occur with a relatively high degree of frequency in Ashkenazi Jews originated in common ancestors approximately 600 years ago. The word *Ashkenazi* is derived from the Hebrew word for "Germany." The term is now used to refer to Jews who have ancestors from Eastern or Central Europe, such as Germany, Poland, Lithuania, Ukraine, and Russia. Although today Ashkenazi

Jews all over the world are intermarrying with non-Jewish people, for centuries political and religious factors ensured their genetic isolation from the population at large.

Every woman has the *BRCA1* and *BRCA2* genes, but some women have inherited a mutated form of one or both genes and thus are at higher risk for breast and ovarian cancer. Among the Ashkenazi population, three *BRCA* mutations predominate.

About 2.3 percent of Ashkenazi Jews carry one of three *BRCA1* or *BRCA2* mutations, whereas approximately one in 500 members of the general population carries a *BRCA1* or *BRCA2* mutation. Moreover,

- Of Ashkenazi Jews who have been diagnosed with breast cancer before the age of 40, 20 percent have a *BRCA1* mutation.
- Of Ashkenazi Jews with a family history of two or more breast cancers, 29 percent carry one of these mutations.
- Of Ashkenazi Jews with a family history that includes two or more cases of breast cancer and at least one case of ovarian cancer, 73 percent carry one of these mutations.

See also BREAST CANCER SUSCEPTIBILITY GENES; RACE AND BREAST CANCER.

Asian-American women and breast cancer Breast cancer is the most common type of cancer among Asian-American women. Among Asian and Pacific Islander women, breast cancer incidence (72.6 per 100,000) and mortality (11.4 per 100,000) rates are lower than for Caucasian and African-American women. Still, breast cancer is the leading cancer among Chinese, Filipina, Hawaiian, Japanese, and Korean women, although incidence and mortality rates vary from group to group. However, for particular subgroups such as immigrants, native Hawaiians, the economically disadvantaged, and the elderly, breast cancer incidence and mortality risk may be higher.

When Asian women immigrate to the United States, their risk of breast cancer rises sixfold compared to that of the women in their native country; those Asian-American women who immigrated to the United States at least a decade ago have a risk of breast cancer that is 80 percent higher than that of new immigrants. For those born in the United States, the breast cancer risk is similar to that of U.S. Caucasian women. Exposure to Western lifestyles (especially DIET and nutrition) has been the most popular explanation for the dramatic differences in incidence rates for Asian women living in the United States and in Asia.

Asian-American women have the lowest breast cancer mortality rate of all ethnic groups in America. Among ethnic populations in the United States, Asian-American women are the least likely to have ever had a MAMMOGRAM, probably because of barriers due to cultural beliefs and practices, mistrust of Western medicine, and socioeconomic factors.

The breakdown among Asian-American women for the incidence of breast cancer per 100,000 women is as follows:

- Korean women: 29
- Vietnamese women: 38
- Chinese women: 55
- Filipina women: 73
- Japanese women: 82
- Native Hawaiian women: 106

(In comparison, Caucasian women had a reported breast cancer incidence of 92 per 100,000 women.)

Despite this, they have the lowest breast cancer mortality rate of all ethnic groups in America. Asian-American women have a combined mortality rate of 13 deaths for every 100,000 women, compared to a rate of 27 per 100,000 Caucasian women and 15 per 100,000 Latina women. Among Asian Americans, the mortality ranged from 7 per 100,000 for Korean and Southeast-Asian women to 12 for Filipino and 13 for Japanese women. For Chinese women the deaths were 11 per 100,000. The lower number of Asian-American women who die of breast cancer reflects the lower incidence of the disease.

The NATIONAL ASIAN WOMEN'S HEALTH ORGANIZA-TION created the Asian American Women's Breast and Cervical Cancer Program as a means to address the problem of breast cancer in their community. This program aims to improve screening outreach and cancer education and eliminate the threat of these diseases in Asian-American communities nationwide.

See also RACE AND BREAST CANCER.

aspiration   Removing fluid or cells from tissue by inserting a needle and drawing the fluid or cells into the syringe.

Association of Community Cancer Centers (ACCC)   The nation's leading oncology policy organization for the cancer care team, dedicated to helping cancer professionals adapt to the complex challenges of program management, reimbursement, legislation, and regulations. In the 1970s the ACCC presented the first U.S. meeting devoted to hospital oncology units and HOSPICE care; throughout the 1990s, association support resulted in passage of ACCC's off-label drug legislation in 39 states. The association focuses on helping to ensure that cancer programs are adequately funded. ACCC priorities also include cancer patient advocacy and the development of guidelines for standard patient care.

ACCC members include medical and radiation ONCOLOGISTS, surgeons, cancer program administrators, hospital executives, practice managers, oncology nurses and social workers, and cancer program data managers. ACCC Institution/Group Practice members include more than 650 medical centers, hospitals, oncology practices, and cancer programs across the United States. For contact information, see Appendix 1.

ataxia telangiectasia (AT)   An inherited autosomal recessive condition characterized by shaky movements, spidery red veins, sensitivity to radiation, and a predisposition to breast cancer and lymphoma. The abnormal AT gene, which is located on chromosome 11, is carried by one in 100 Americans. Among women with no family history of AT but who carry the AT gene, studies have suggested a twofold increased risk for breast cancer.

Genetic testing for AT carrier status is not yet available, although it may become available soon. The gene for AT is considered to be a "non-*BRCA*" ONCOGENE.

See also BREAST CANCER SUSCEPTIBILITY GENES; COWDEN DISEASE.

atypical cells Cells that are abnormal. Cancer is the result of division of atypical cells.

atypical hyperplasia A condition, considered to be a risk factor for breast cancer, in which abnormal-looking extra cells appear in the lining of the inside of the milk ducts (atypical ductal hyperplasia) and lobules of the breast (ATYPICAL LOBULAR HYPERPLASIA).

The term *hyperplasia* indicates that there are extra normal cells lining the breast ducts and lobules. However, if the excess cells look abnormal, the condition is described as "atypical hyperplasia." Atypical hyperplasia increases the risk of developing breast cancer by two to four times, but if a woman has family members with breast cancer and atypical hyperplasia, her risk is eight to 11 times greater.

Historically, atypical hyperplasia has been diagnosed during a biopsy. Today it also can be identified by using a technique called DUCTAL LAVAGE, in which fluid from the nipple is examined in the laboratory.

atypical lobular hyperplasia Excessive multiplication of abnormally shaped cells in the normal tissue of a breast lobule.

automated tissue excision and collection system A new device that allows a woman to have a breast BIOPSY in the doctor's office using only local anesthesia. Unlike other methods, the automated tissue excision and collection (ATEC) system removes the entire suspicious area in the breast, not just a bit of the mass. The device, which was approved by the U.S. Food and Drug Administration in March 2002, is believed to be more accurate than needle biopsy because it removes more tissue.

The device is compatible with ULTRASOUND, stereotactic, and MAGNETIC RESONANCE IMAGING (MRI) technologies.

The vacuum-assisted device pulls the tissue into the needle, which then cuts off the tissue and collects it in a filter. A local anesthetic provides an almost pain-free biopsy.

axillary lymph node dissection A type of diagnostic procedure typically performed during surgery for breast cancer in which the LYMPH NODES located in the armpit are removed, usually during a modified radical MASTECTOMY or a breast conservation procedure such as a LUMPECTOMY. The lymph node tissue is sent to the pathologist to determine whether the breast cancer has spread outside the breast.

The number of nodes dissected varies. The standard breast cancer operation calls for removal of these nodes to determine further treatment and prognosis, depending on whether the nodes are "positive" (contain malignant cells) or "negative" (no cancer cells).

Unfortunately, removing the lymph nodes under the arm also slows the flow of lymph fluid. In some women, after removal of lymph nodes fluid builds up in the arm and hand and causes swelling (LYMPHEDEMA). To prevent this, women need to protect the arm and hand on the treated side from injury or pressure, even years after surgery. This is why women should not have blood pressure measured or injections given on the side where lymph nodes have been removed. Doctors can explain how women should handle any cuts, scratches, insect bites, or other injuries to the arm or hand.

See also SENTINEL NODE BIOPSY, BLUE NODES, AXILLARY NODES.

axillary lymph nodes The LYMPH NODES that form a chain from the underarm (axilla) to the collarbone. Level 1 nodes are found in the underarm and receive most of the lymph fluid from the breast. Level 2 nodes are located farther up and receive the fluid from level 1 and some fluid from the breast and chest wall. Level 3 nodes are located below the collarbone and receive fluid from levels 1 and 2, and sometimes from the upper part of the breast.

When breast cancer develops, level 1 nodes are usually affected first. To determine whether or not lymph nodes are involved in the breast cancer, axillary nodes are often removed from levels 1 and 2 during surgery so they can be examined under a microscope for cancer cells. If cancer cells are found, there is a higher chance the cancer may have spread to other parts of the body. Finding out whether or not the cancer has spread to the axillary nodes helps determine the stage of the breast cancer and the type of treatment needed.

Sometimes, instead of a total removal of axillary nodes, the doctor performs a SENTINEL LYMPH NODE BIOPSY, which is becoming a standard procedure used to determine whether axillary lymph nodes contain cancer. In this procedure, a radioactive substance and/or a blue dye is injected into the cancer site to locate the first axillary node (called the sentinel node) that receives drainage from the breast. A Geiger counter is used to measure the activity of the radioactive substance in the first draining lymph node (or, if the dye is used, the sentinel node appears blue). The surgeon removes the first axillary node for examination to see whether cancer cells are present. If cancer is present, more lymph nodes are removed. If cancer is not present, no more lymph nodes are taken. This procedure can reduce the number of lymph nodes that are removed, thus reducing the risk of infection and of LYMPHEDEMA (swelling) of the arm.

Whether the axillary lymph nodes contain cancer is one of three factors used to determine breast cancer stage (tumor size and spread to other areas of the body are the other two). Lymph node involvement is rated in the following way:

• *NX:* Nodes cannot be evaluated.
• *N0:* Axillary nodes do not have cancer.
• *N1:* Axillary nodes have cancer but are not attached to one another nor to the chest wall.
• *N2:* Axillary nodes have cancer and have attached to one another or to the chest wall; also clinically evident internal mammary nodes without clinically evident axillary nodes.
• *N3:* Infraclavicular, supraclavicular, or a combination of axillary and intermammary nodes have cancer.

benign breast lump A harmless growth in the breast that is not cancer and does not spread to other parts of the body. Fluid-filled CYSTS are typical benign breast lesions often found in breast tissue.

beta-carotene A common plant chemical within a group of more than 600 called CAROTENOIDS. Beta-carotene is converted by the body into vitamin A, which has many vital functions, including the growth and repair of body tissues, formation of bones and teeth, resistance of the body to infection, and development of healthy eye tissues. While vitamin A supplements can be toxic, excess beta-carotene is safely stored away and converted to vitamin A only when the body needs it. Epidemiologic studies have linked high intake of foods rich in beta-carotene and high blood levels of the micronutrient to a lower risk of cancer (particularly LUNG CANCER).

Beta-carotene acts as an ANTIOXIDANT and immune-system booster and is found in bright orange fruits and vegetables such as carrots, pumpkins, peaches, and sweet potatoes. Some experts suspect it may be possible to shield the body's immune system from the risk of cancer by supplementing the diet with beta-carotene. Most, but not all, beta-carotene in supplements is synthetic, consisting of only one molecule (natural beta-carotene found in food is made of two molecules). Researchers originally saw no meaningful difference between natural and synthetic beta-carotene, but this view was questioned when the link between beta-carotene-containing foods and LUNG CANCER prevention wasn't duplicated in studies using synthetic pills.

The most common beta-carotene dosage is 25,000 international units (IU) (15 mg) per day,

but some people take as much as 100,000 IU (60 mg) per day. Excessive level of beta-carotene (more than 100,000 IU, or 60 mg per day) sometimes tints the skin yellow-orange. Individuals who take beta-carotene for long period should also supplement with vitamin E, as beta-carotene may reduce vitamin E level.

biochanin A An isoflavone found in SOY PRODUCTS and other legumes, currently being studied as a possible cancer preventative. It is a phytoestrogen, a plant product with weak estrogenic activity.

bioflavonoids Chemical compounds related to vitamin C that have demonstrated an ability to slow cancer growth. These naturally occurring plant compounds act primarily as plant pigments and ANTIOXIDANTS, substances that fight cell damage caused by FREE RADICALS (rogue oxygen molecules that can attack cells throughout the body).

Lemons, grapes, plums, grapefruit, cherries, blackberries, and rosehips are some of the richest dietary sources of bioflavonoids. Other sources include citrus fruits, green peppers, broccoli, tomatoes, green tea, and some herb teas (especially stinging nettle tea). Bioflavonoids belong to a large group of more than 2,000 PHYTOCHEMICALS called phenols that are known to be very powerful antioxidants. Many studies have identified their unique role in protecting vitamin C from oxidation in the body, thereby allowing the body to reap more benefits from the vitamin.

Different bioflavonoids tend to have different health effects on the body, but in general, a diet high in bioflavonoids is associated with a lower incidence of many diseases, including cancer. Anyone who takes bioflavonoid supplements should inform a doctor before undergoing surgery, because they may interfere with the results of some blood and urine tests.

biological response modifier (BRM) Treatments that modify the body's natural response to infection and disease. There are many types of these modifiers, some produced by the body and others created in the lab. Many ongoing studies are investigating the use of these substances in BIOLOGICAL THERAPY to treat a wide variety of cancers.

The primary biological response modifiers include antibodies, COLONY-STIMULATING FACTORS, CYTOKINES (including INTERFERONS and INTERLEUKINS), MONOCLONAL ANTIBODIES, and vaccines. Researchers continue to discover new BRMs, learn more about how they function, and develop ways to use them in cancer therapy. All of these substances alter the interaction between cancer cells and the body's immune defenses, restoring the body's ability to fight cancer.

Biological therapies may be used to stop or control processes that allow cancer cells to grow, make cancer cells more recognizable to the immune system, boost the killing power of immune system cells, or alter malignant growth patterns to make them more like healthy cells. They can block or reverse the process that turns a normal cell into a cancerous cell and enhance the body's ability to repair normal cells damaged by other forms of cancer treatment, such as chemotherapy or radiation. BRMs also are being investigated to decrease chances of cancer cells spreading to other parts of the body. Some BRMs are a standard part of treatment for certain types of cancer, such as interferons for melanoma. Others are being studied as new types of treatments, either alone or in combination with each other.

The colony-stimulating factors are often used to prevent anemia and low white blood cell counts during chemotherapy.

biological therapy A relatively new type of cancer treatment, sometimes called immunotherapy, biotherapy, or BIOLOGICAL RESPONSE MODIFIER (BRM) therapy, that is designed to enhance the body's natural defenses against cancer. Biological therapies may be used to stop or suppress processes that allow cancer growth or to make cancer cells

more recognizable and therefore more susceptible to destruction by the immune system. Biological therapies also boost the killing power of immune system cells and alter cancer cells' growth patterns to make them more like healthy cells. They can be used to block or reverse the process that changes a normal cell into a cancerous cell, and to enhance the body's ability to repair normal cells damaged by other forms of cancer treatment, such as chemotherapy or radiation. Biological therapy also can help prevent cancer cells from spreading to other parts of the body.

Biological Response Modifiers
These immune-system-related substances are produced in the lab for use in cancer treatment and alter the interaction between the body's immune defenses and cancer cells to boost the body's ability to fight the disease. BRMs include INTERFERONS, INTERLEUKINS, COLONY-STIMULATING FACTORS, CYTOKINES, MONOCLONAL ANTIBODIES, and vaccines.

Interferons An interferon is a kind of naturally occurring cytokine. There are three major types: interferon alfa, interferon beta, and interferon gamma. Interferon alfa is the type most widely used in cancer treatment.

Interferons can improve the way a cancer patient's immune system fights cancer cells and may slow the growth of cancer cells or promote their transformation into more normal cells. Researchers believe that some interferons may also stimulate other components of the immune system, such as NATURAL KILLER (NK) CELLS, T cells, and macrophages, boosting the immune system's anticancer function.

Interleukins These cytokines occur naturally in the body and also can be produced synthetically. There are many different kinds of interleukins, but interleukin-2 (IL-2 or aldesleukin) has been the most widely studied in cancer treatment. IL-2 stimulates the growth and action of cancer-killing immune cells such as lymphocytes. The Food and Drug Administration (FDA) has approved IL-2 for the treatment of kidney cancer and melanoma. Interleukins are also being studied as potential treatments for BREAST CANCER.

Colony-stimulating factors (CSFs) Because chemotherapy drugs can damage the body's ability to make white blood cells, red blood cells, and platelets, patients who are receiving these drugs have an increased risk of infections, anemia, and bleeding more readily. Colony-stimulating factors may help these patients by encouraging stem cells in bone marrow to divide and develop into white blood cells, platelets, and red blood cells.

Also, by using CSFs to stimulate blood cell production, doctors can increase the dosages of anticancer drugs without increasing the risk of infection or the need for transfusion with blood products. As a result, researchers have found CSFs particularly useful when combined with high-dose chemotherapy.

CSFs include the following:

- GRANULOCYTE COLONY-STIMULATING FACTOR (G-CSF) (filgrastim) and granulocyte-macrophage colony-stimulating factor (GM-CSF) (sargramostim) can increase the number of white blood cells, thereby reducing the risk of infection in patients who are receiving chemotherapy. G-CSF and GM-CSF can also stimulate the production of stem cells in preparation for stem cell or bone marrow transplantation.
- ERYTHROPOIETIN can increase the number of red blood cells and reduce the need for red blood cell transfusions in patients who receive chemotherapy.
- Oprelvekin can reduce the need for platelet transfusions in patients who are receiving chemotherapy.

Researchers are studying CSFs in clinical trials to treat some types of leukemia, metastatic colorectal cancer, melanoma, lung cancer, and other types of cancer.

MONOCLONAL ANTIBODIES (MOABS) These are antibodies made in the laboratory that are produced by a single type of cell and attack a single type of antigen. Researchers currently are studying how to create MOABs specific to the antigens found on the surface of cancer cells in order to enhance a patient's immune response to the cancer. MOABs can be programmed to interfere with the growth of cancer cells. In addition, MOABs may be linked to CHEMOTHERAPY drugs, radioactive substances, other biological response modifiers, or other toxins so that when the antibodies latch onto cancer cells, they deliver these poisons directly to the tumor, helping to destroy it. MOABs may help destroy cancer cells in bone marrow that has been removed from a patient in preparation for bone marrow transplantation. MOABs carrying radioisotopes may also prove useful in diagnosing certain cancers, such as colorectal, ovarian, and prostate cancers.

Rituximab (Rituxan) and trastuzumab (Herceptin) are examples of monoclonal antibodies that have been approved for treatment by the FDA. Rituxan, the first MOAB approved for treatment, is used in patients with B-cell non-Hodgkin's lymphoma. Herceptin is used to treat metastatic breast cancer in 25 percent of patients whose tumor cells produce large amounts of a protein called human epidermal growth factor receptor-2 (HER-2). By blocking HER-2, Herceptin slows or stops the growth of these cells. Herceptin may be used alone or with chemotherapy.

Cancer Vaccines

Researchers are developing VACCINES to be used in cancer treatments that may encourage the patient's immune system to recognize and reject cancer cells, preventing cancer from recurring. In contrast to vaccines against infectious diseases, cancer vaccines are designed to be injected after the disease is diagnosed, rather than before it develops.

Cancer vaccines given when a tumor is small may be able to cure the cancer. Early cancer vaccine studies focused on patients with melanoma, but today vaccines are also being studied in the treatment of many other types of cancer, including lymphomas and cancers of the breast, among others. Researchers are also investigating ways that cancer vaccines can be used in combination with other BRMs.

Side Effects

Biological therapies can cause a number of side effects. Interferons and interleukins, may cause flu-like symptoms, including fever, chills, NAUSEA, vomiting, and APPETITE LOSS. FATIGUE is another common side effect, and blood pressure may be affected. The side effects of IL-2 can often be severe, depending on the dosage given. Patients need to be closely monitored during treatment.

Side effects of CSFs may include bone pain, fatigue, fever, and appetite loss. The side effects of MOABs vary, and serious allergic reactions may occur. Cancer vaccines can cause muscle aches and fever.

biomarker A substance that may indicate the presence of cancer when it is present in high levels in blood, other body fluids, or tissues. Examples of biomarkers related to breast cancer include CA 2729, CA 15-3, and CARCINOEMBRYONIC ANTIGEN (CEA), a marker for colon cancer. There is no benefit to assessing these markers after ADJUVANT THERAPY. They are most useful to help determine growth or response of cancer during therapy for metastatic disease.

biopsy The surgical removal of a small piece of tissue or a small tumor for microscopic examination to determine if cancer cells are present. If a woman or her doctor finds a suspicious breast lump, or if imaging studies show a suspicious area, the woman must have a biopsy—the most important procedure in diagnosing cancer.

There are two types of biopsies: needle biopsy and open biopsy. The particular method chosen depends on the nature and location of the abnormality and on the patient's general health and preference. Each type of biopsy has advantages and disadvantages.

Needle Biopsy

There are several different types of needle biopsies. Because it is fast and simple, a needle biopsy is often used first. In a needle biopsy, the area involved is numbed and cleaned, and a sterile hollow needle is inserted through the skin to take a tissue or cell sample.

In a FINE NEEDLE ASPIRATION, the doctor uses a thin, hollow needle to remove a few cells from the breast lump. It can be done in an outpatient setting and takes only a few minutes. Fine needle aspiration can also be used to remove fluid from a CYST.

In a *core needle biopsy*, a thicker hollow needle is used to remove a larger amount of tissue. The skin is nicked with a scalpel so the needle can enter. This type of biopsy is done in an outpatient setting. A core needle biopsy provides more tissue than fine needle aspiration, and estrogen receptors can be obtained with this method. (See CORE BIOPSY.)

In a *vacuum-assisted biopsy,* a thicker hollow needle is used to remove cores of tissue by inserting a single vacuum-assisted probe. A vacuum-assisted breast biopsy is done with a local anesthetic in an outpatient setting. This type of biopsy may also be done with the guidance of stereotactic mammography or ultrasound imaging. The MAMMOTOME breast biopsy system is a type of vacuum-assisted biopsy that was approved in 1996; the handheld version of the Mammotome received clearance from the Food and Drug Administration in September 1999. In this method, a large needle is inserted into the suspicious area by using ultrasound or stereotactic guidance. The Mammotome is then used gently to vacuum tissue from the suspicious area. Additional tissue samples can be obtained by rotating the needle. This procedure can be performed with the patient lying on her stomach on a table. If the handheld device is used, the patient may lie on her back or in a seated position. There have been no reports of serious complications that resulted from the Mammotome breast biopsy system.

In most cases, if it is possible, a needle biopsy is preferred to an open biopsy as the first step in a cancer diagnosis because it provides a quicker diagnosis and causes less discomfort. It also gives the woman an opportunity to discuss treatment options with her doctor before any surgery is performed. However, in some instances, an open surgical biopsy must be done instead. The surgeon can perform a core needle biopsy or fine needle aspiration if the lump can be felt; but often these procedures are done by a radiologist using ultrasound or mammogram to guide the needle, as the biopsy is of a visible, but not palpable, change.

The mammogram-directed technique is called STEREOTACTIC NEEDLE BIOPSY. In this procedure, computerized mammogram breast images help the radiologist map the exact location of the breast lump and guide the tip of the needle to the right spot. Ultrasound images can be used in the same way to guide the needle.

The choice between a mammogram-directed stereotactic needle biopsy and ultrasound-guided biopsy depends on the type of breast change and the experience and preference of the doctor.

The time required of a biopsy varies according to the specific type of biopsy procedure. Open biopsies that require general surgery can take much longer than others.

Open (Surgical) Biopsy

In a surgical biopsy, a sample of tissue can be cut directly from the tumor that has been exposed with a surgical incision. The surgeon usually removes the entire tumor together with a margin of normal-looking breast tissue surrounding the malignant area. If the tumor cannot be felt, needle localization is done before the biopsy. After numbing the area with a local anesthetic, the surgeon places a small, hollow needle in the abnormal spot in the breast. A thin wire is inserted through the center of the needle, the needle is removed, and the wire is used to guide the surgeon to the right spot.

A surgical biopsy may be either incisional or excisional. In an incisional surgical biopsy, only a portion of the lump is removed. It is most often performed on women who have advanced stage cancer whose tumor is too large to be removed by excisional biopsy. Excisional biopsies remove the entire lump plus some surrounding normal tissue. This is the most common type of open biopsy. Although the primary purpose is to diagnose cancer, a biopsy can also be a surgical treatment to remove cancer.

Lab Analysis

Once inside the lab, the biopsy sample is stained and examined under a microscope. Microscopic examination can determine whether the tissue sample is part of a benign process or if it is malignant. Laboratory examination can also identify the type of cancer and may be used to evaluate the probability that cancer has spread to other parts of the body.

Risks

Most limited biopsy procedures are very safe and carry only a small risk of bleeding or infection at the biopsy site. For larger open biopsies, there are additional risks.

When to Call the Doctor

Patients should consult a doctor after a biopsy in the event of a fever or pain, swelling, redness, pus, or bleeding at the biopsy site or at the site of the surgical wound.

biotherapy   See BIOLOGICAL THERAPY.

birth control pills and breast cancer   About 80 percent of U.S. women born since 1945 have used oral contraceptives, but researchers are still unclear about whether they are linked to BREAST CANCER.

Studies of birth control pills and cancer have been ongoing since the early 1970s and have reached conflicting conclusions. A 1996 review of 54 small studies conducted over the previous 25 years found a slightly increased risk of breast cancer in women who were current or recent users of oral contraceptives.

Other studies have not found an increased risk of breast cancer among oral contraceptive users. According to findings from the National Institute of Child Health and Human Development (NICHD) Women's Contraceptive and Reproductive Experiences Study, women between 35 and 64 who had taken oral contraceptives at some point in their life were no more likely than other women to develop breast cancer. The study appeared in the June 27, 2002, issue of the *New England Journal of Medicine*. The women studied were members of the first generation of American women to use birth control pills. Researchers interviewed more than 9,200 white and black women between the ages of 35 and 64 living in Atlanta, Detroit, Philadelphia, Los Angeles, and Seattle. About half of the participants had recently been diagnosed with breast cancer; the other half had not. The women were asked a series of questions in person about their use of oral contraceptives and other hormones as well as reproductive, health, and family issues.

The Pill and BRCA1

However, a separate study published in the *Journal of the National Cancer Institute* found that while women with certain gene mutations have more than a 60 percent lifetime risk of development of breast cancer, they are at even greater risk if they used oral contraceptives at an early age and before 1975. Early birth control pill use increases the lifetime breast cancer risk up to about 85 percent for women with the *BRCA1* mutation when compared to women without the mutation. Further, among women who had the *BRCA1* gene mutation, taking the pill years ago increased the probability for development of breast cancer by 33 to 42 percent when compared to mutation carriers who did not take it. Oral contraceptive use was not found to increase the risk among *BRCA2* mutation carriers, however.

The study does not mean that birth control pills now on the market are dangerous for women who have the BREAST CANCER SUSCEPTIBILITY GENE, but it adds a note of caution about how these women should use the Pill. In this data, the only women who had an increased risk of breast cancer were those who started taking the Pill before 1975, those who were under age 25 when they started taking the Pill, and those who took oral contraceptives for longer than five years.

Currently available birth control pills have only a fraction of the hormones that were found in birth control pills routinely used before 1975.

The study suggests that women with the BRCA mutations should approach oral contraceptive use with caution. Decisions about oral contraceptive use among mutation carriers are complex because the Pill protects to some degree against ovarian cancer, a deadly cancer that is much more difficult to detect.

Other studies have shown that for healthy women who do not smoke, the health benefits of oral contraceptives far exceed the risks. Women who had used an oral contraceptive did not have a greater risk of development of breast cancer than women who had never used oral contraceptives.

A Mayo Clinic study found an elevated risk of breast cancer among high-risk women who had taken older versions of the Pill. Researchers believed that the high amounts of ESTROGEN and progestin in these drugs were the factor that seemed to be increasing risk. Mayo researchers studied thousands of women from 426 families with a history of breast cancer. Their study, published in the *Journal of the American Medical Association*, is thought to be the first to evaluate the link between Pill use and an inherited risk for breast cancer. Among women who took birth control pills before 1975 and had daughters and sisters who had breast cancer, the researchers found a threefold increase in the disease. There was an 11-fold breast cancer increase among Pill users

with an "excessive" family history (that is, five or more close relatives who had breast or ovarian cancer).

Birth control pills are among the leading forms of contraception, second only to sterilization, used by about 100 million women around the world. The Mayo researchers agree that more research is needed to evaluate any link between use of current birth control pills and breast cancer in families at risk for the disease. There was no increase in risk in women who took birth control pills after 1975, when the hormone dose was lowered.

birth size   There appears to be an association between large size at birth (as measured by length and head size) and risk of premenopausal breast cancer, according to one Swedish study.

More than 5,000 women born in Sweden during 1915 to 1929 were included in the study; 63 had breast cancer before age 50. In addition, a shorter pregnancy was independently associated with an increased risk of breast cancer before the age of 50, indicating that the rate of fetal growth may underlie the association between birth size and risk of early breast cancer. There was no evidence of an association between birth size and breast cancer in postmenopausal women.

However, large birth size appears to be responsible for only a small proportion of the total number of cases of breast cancer in any population, as the incidence at premenopausal ages is low.

bisphosphonates   A family of drugs (also called disphosphonates) used to treat BREAST CANCER when it spreads to the bone. These drugs, given intravenously once a month, decrease the chances of bone metastases causing harm: they decrease fractures and the need for radiation. They also may decrease pain.

AREDIA (Pamidronate) and Zometa (zolen-dronate) are the two types of bisphosphonates typically used for this purpose, and they are generally well tolerated. They may cause brief flulike symptoms and, rarely, kidney damage.

If Zometa is used, the doctor must monitor the patient's blood chemistry and kidney function monthly.

These drugs are also used to treat high calcium levels, which occur rarely in advanced cancer.

black cohosh A dietary supplement herbal extract containing PHYTOESTROGENS that is one of the most widely used alternative therapies for women who are experiencing menopause symptoms. At this point, there is little data evaluating the effectiveness of phytoestrogens in the treatment of HOT FLASHES, or their safety in women and breast cancer.

blood count A test to measure the number of red blood cells, white blood cells, and platelets in a blood sample.

blue node The first LYMPH NODE that is stained blue after injection of blue dye into a breast cancer tumor and its surrounding tissue, as part of a SENTINEL NODE BIOPSY.

bone cancer, metastatic Tumors in the bone usually have spread from another organ—often the breast. Once spread to the bone, they grow and compress healthy bone tissue and absorb it or replace it with abnormal tissue. The bones are the most common site of secondary cancer from the breast. The bones most commonly affected are the spine, skull, pelvis, hipbones, or upper bones of the arms and legs.

Bone contains two types of living cells, osteoclasts and osteoblasts, which help to form new bone. Osteoclasts destroy and remove small amounts of old bone; osteoblasts help build up new bone. In secondary bone cancer, the breast cancer cells that have spread to the bone produce chemicals that disturb this process, so that the osteoclasts become overactive. This overactivity causes more bone destruction than bone replacement, leading to the symptoms of secondary bone cancer.

Symptoms

Pain is the most common symptom of bone cancer, but symptoms may vary, depending on the location and size of the cancer. Tumors that occur in or near joints may cause swelling or tenderness in the affected area. Bone cancer can interfere with normal movements and can weaken the bones, occasionally leading to fracture. If a bone weakens, radiation or surgery can prevent it from fracturing. A weak bone can be secured with a metal screw or plate; a compromised joint can be replaced. If a bone has already fractured, the surgeon can try to repair the break. In rare cases a whole section of bone can be replaced. If an area of the vertebrae should fracture or collapse, pressing on the spinal cord, this may need to be treated as an emergency. If symptoms appear very rapidly, surgery may be the first choice of treatment. If the symptoms appear over a period of time, radiation may be recommended at first. Either treatment also includes the administration of steroids (drugs that help to reduce inflammation). Sometimes a combination of all three treatments may be used.

Hypercalcemia is another symptom of secondary bone cancer. Bone is a living tissue made up of calcium and various proteins that make it strong. Secondary bone cancer can alter the bone structure so that calcium is released into the bloodstream. If the calcium level gets too high, it can cause NAUSEA, vomiting, CONSTIPATION, or drowsiness. In more severe cases, there may be excessive thirst, weakness, or confusion. To ease these symptoms, the patient can drink plenty of water or be admitted to a hospital, where fluids will be given to flush the calcium out of the body.

Diagnosis

In addition to a personal and family medical history and a complete medical exam, the doctor may suggest a blood test to determine the level of an enzyme called ALKALINE PHOSPHATASE. A high level of alkaline phosphatase can be found in the blood when the cells that form bone tissue are very active—when children are growing, when a broken bone is mending, or when a tumor triggers the production of abnormal bone tissue.

X-rays can show the location, size, and shape of a bone tumor. If X-rays suggest that a tumor may be cancer, the doctor may recommend special imaging tests such as a bone scan, computed tomography scan, MAGNETIC RESONANCE IMAGING, or angiogram.

Either a needle BIOPSY or an incisional biopsy can detect bone cancer. During a needle biopsy, the surgeon uses a needlelike instrument to make a small hole in the bone and remove a sample of tissue from the tumor. In an incisional biopsy, the surgeon cuts into the tumor and removes a sample of tissue.

Treatment

Secondary bone cancer can be treated effectively, although it cannot be cured. The aim is to relieve symptoms and improve the quality of life by controlling the growth of the cancer.

Treatment options depend on the type, size, location, and stage of the cancer, as well as the person's age and general health. Surgery is often the primary treatment. Although amputation is sometimes necessary, pre- or postoperative chemotherapy has often made it possible to spare the limb. When possible, surgeons avoid amputation by removing only the cancerous section of the bone and replacing it with a prosthesis.

Hormone therapy is another choice of treatment for secondary bone cancer. A number of hormone therapies are available; the drug most commonly used first is the antiestrogen drug TAMOXIFEN. If a patient is already taking tamoxifen when secondary bone cancer develops, other hormone drugs, known as AROMATASE INHIBITORS, may be considered.

If the secondary bone cancer does not respond to hormone treatment (or has stopped responding to it), patients may be offered chemotherapy. A number of chemotherapy drugs, given either alone or in combination, are used to treat secondary bone cancer. Secondary bone cancer can be slow to respond to chemotherapy, and patients may need several cycles at three or four weekly intervals before any benefit can be seen.

When radiation treatment is given, it is designed only to improve the patient's quality of life by improving mobility, decreasing pain, and preventing possible fractures. Radiation for secondary bone cancer can be given as a single dose, or as divided doses over a few days to lessen the risk of side effects.

Bisphosphonates are drugs that target the parts of the skeleton where there is high bone turnover, which in the case of secondary bone cancer are the areas where the osteoclasts have become overactive. They do not treat the cancer itself but may help slow the breakdown of the bone by restricting osteoclasts' action. They can be given either in tablet form or through a drip into a vein. They work by reducing high calcium levels in the blood, reducing pain that has not responded well to painkillers or is too widespread for local radiation, decreasing the risk of bone fractures, and possibly delaying the spread of the secondary bone cancer.

bone marrow The soft, fatty substance filling the cavities of the bones contains immature blood cells called STEM CELLS. Stem cells produce

- White blood cells (leukocytes), which fight infection
- Red blood cells (erythrocytes), which carry oxygen to and remove waste products from organs and tissues
- Platelets (thrombocytes), which enable the blood to clot

Most chemotherapy drugs for breast cancer affects the bone marrow, resulting in a temporary decrease in the number of cells in the blood. Different chemotherapy regimens affect different stem cells; some cause ANEMIA (low red cells), NEUTROPENIA (low white cells) and THROMBOCYTOPENIA (low platelets).

bone marrow aspiration A procedure in which a needle is inserted into the center of a bone, usually the hip, to remove a small amount of BONE MARROW for microscopic examination. Bone marrow is the spongy substance on the inside of the bone in which blood cells are manufactured.

After the test, there is some pain or soreness at the site. The sample is analyzed for iron stores, red blood cell and white blood cell production and maturation, cancer cells, and number of megakaryocytes (cells that produce platelets).

A bone marrow aspiration is used to determine the cause of an abnormal blood test.

bone marrow biopsy See BONE MARROW ASPIRATION.

bone marrow metastasis   Cancer that has spread from a primary tumor, such as one in the breast, to the BONE MARROW.

bone marrow transplant   A procedure to replace BONE MARROW that has been destroyed by high doses of CHEMOTHERAPY drugs or radiation. Researchers are still evaluating the effectiveness of bone marrow transplants although at this point the majority of studies do not suggest this intensive treatment is useful in breast cancer.

Transplants may be autologous (an individual's own marrow saved before treatment), allogeneic (marrow donated by someone else), or syngeneic (marrow donated by an identical twin).

Bone marrow transplants are used as part of chemotherapy or RADIATION THERAPY treatments. In this procedure, a patient's marrow is removed and stored so that a much higher dosage of drugs or radiation can be given, which would otherwise damage the bone marrow. After the treatment is finished, the healthy marrow is then replaced.

In the 1980s and 1990s many thought that this would be a useful treatment and that higher doses of treatment must be better. However, many large studies showed no benefit. Bone marrow transplants are only very rarely used to treat breast cancer now.

bone scan   An imaging technique that can be used to identify BREAST CANCER that has spread to the bones. The technique uses radiation to create images of bone on a computer screen or film, identifying areas where cells are unusually active, either breaking down or repairing bone. These areas of activity (called hot spots) can then be located by a camera. Hot spots do not necessarily indicate that there is cancer in a bone; bones can break down and repair themselves for other reasons, such as infections, arthritis or Paget's disease.

If a bone scan shows hot spots, plain X-rays are usually ordered. During the test, a small amount of radioactive material is injected into a blood vessel and travels over the next three to four hours through the bloodstream; it collects in the bones and is detected by a scanner. Other than the needle stick, a bone scan is painless.

Unless there are symptoms suggesting that breast cancer has spread to the bone (such as new pains or changes in blood tests results), a bone scan is not necessary except in cases of advanced cancer.

brachytherapy   A procedure in which radioactive material sealed in needles, seeds, wires, or catheters is placed directly into or near a malignant tumor. The procedure is also called internal radiation, implant radiation, or interstitial radiation therapy. Another version of this treatment, called high-dose-rate remote brachytherapy (or high-dose-rate remote RADIATION THERAPY or remote brachytherapy), is a type of internal radiation treatment in which the radioactive source is removed between treatments.

The term *brachytherapy* is derived from the ancient Greek words for "short distance." Brachytherapy has been used for more than a century to treat a number of cancers, including breast cancer. Its advantage is that it takes days rather than weeks. The disadvantage is that little long-term data exist on results. Standard radiation treatment is still external beam to the whole breast with a boost to the tumor site.

Henri Becquerel discovered natural radioactivity in 1896 when he discovered that uranium produced a black spot on photographic plates that had not been exposed to sunlight. Two years later, Marie and Pierre Curie, working in Becquerel's laboratory, extracted polonium from a ton of uranium ore. Later the same year, they extracted radium. In 1901, Pierre Curie came up with the idea of inserting a small radium tube into a tumor, a procedure that signaled the birth of brachytherapy. Two years later, Alexander Graham Bell made a similar suggestion (completely independently) in a letter to the editor of *Archives Roentgen Ray*. With these early experiences, scientists found that inserting radioactive materials into tumors caused cancers to shrink.

In the early 20th century, major brachytherapy research was carried out at the Curie Institute in Paris and at Memorial Hospital in New York. The advent of high-voltage teletherapy for deeper tumors and the problems associated with radiation exposure from high-energy radionuclides led to a decline in the use of brachytherapy toward the middle of the 20th century. However, over the past 30 years, scientists have again become interested in the use of brachytherapy.

New approaches involving synthetic radioisotopes and remote afterloading techniques have reduced radiation exposure hazards. In addition, newer types of imaging scans (computed tomography scan, magnetic resonance imaging, ultrasound) and sophisticated computers have made it easier to position the radiation for the best doses.

Brachytherapy has been proved to be effective and safe and provides an alternative to surgical removal of the breast while reducing the risk of certain long-term side effects.

There are several different types of seeds that are used in brachytherapy:

- Palladium (Pd-103) seeds produce radiation more rapidly and over a short period. Some researchers think that palladium seeds are best suited to treat faster-growing, more aggressive tumors.
- Iodine (I-125) seeds are usually recommended for use in the treatment of slow-growing tumors.
- Echogenic seeds have a specific feature that helps the doctor place the seeds within the cancerous tissue.

Even though very sensitive Geiger counters could detect radiation in the body of someone with radioactive seeds, the person would not be considered radioactive. Despite the low risk, some doctors recommend that close contact between the patient and pregnant women or small children be avoided for some period after the initial procedure.

In 2002 the U.S. Food and Drug Administration (FDA) approved Proxima Therapeutics' MAMMOSITE, a device designed specifically for breast brachytherapy. There are no long-term data on local recurrence, which is one reason why some women with a small, early breast tumor instead choose a more disfiguring MASTECTOMY.

MammoSite consists of a spaghettilike catheter with an inflatable balloon that is implanted at the tumor site when the tumor is removed. Later, a radioactive seed is inserted through the catheter, and a targeted dose of radiation is emitted through the balloon. Once the patient is given enough radiation, the catheter is removed. With this method, the radiation therapy is restricted to the tissues most likely to harbor residual cancer cells. The entire treatment takes five days.

One study suggests that five years after treatment, women who have had brachytherapy do as well as women who have had external radiation. But some doctors worry about brachytherapy because unlike external radiation, it does not affect cancer cells that may lurk in other parts of the breast. Because many have this concern, and because Proxima submitted no data proving MammoSite therapy is as effective long term as regular radiation, the FDA ordered Proxima to state that MammoSite is not a replacement for the whole-breast radiation that today's cancer guidelines call for after a lumpectomy.

Although doctors can use an FDA-approved medical device any way they want, the FDA requirement seems to leave potential users in something of a quandary. However, experts note that since 25 percent of lumpectomy patients do not receive radiation at all, some women may be more inclined to try MammoSite rather than nothing.

See also the AMERICAN BRACHYTHERAPY SOCIETY.

brain metastasis   The spread of cancer cells from the primary site through the bloodstream to the brain. When the original tumor occurred in the breast, the metastasis may be described as recurrent breast cancer, a secondary tumor, or secondary brain cancer.

When breast cancer has spread to the brain, it cannot be cured, so any treatment aims to control the symptoms to improve the patient's quality of life. Steroids are used to reduce the inflammation and pressure around the brain tumor and to relieve symptoms such as headache and NAUSEA. They are often prescribed before any assessments to confirm the diagnosis of a secondary brain tumor. Steroids for secondary brain cancer are given at first in high doses, and then reduced once other treatments such as radiation are administered. Some of the more common side effects of steroids in high doses are indigestion (when they are taken on an empty stomach), thrush (candidiasis) in the mouth, increased appetite and weight gain, and muscle weakness and sleeplessness (when they are taken later in the day).

RADIATION THERAPY is the most commonly used treatment for secondary brain cancer. It is given to the whole brain in daily dosages over about five days. FATIGUE, a common side effect of radiotherapy, is especially noticeable when the treatment is given to the brain. HAIR LOSS is another common side effect.

Surgery is rarely possible for secondary brain cancer because there are usually a number of small tumors rather than a single area that can be removed.

BRCA1 gene   See BREAST CANCER SUSCEPTIBILITY GENES.

BRCA2 gene   See BREAST CANCER SUSCEPTIBILITY GENES.

breakthrough pain   Intense increases in pain that occur rapidly even when painkillers are being used. Breakthrough pain can occur spontaneously or in relation to a specific activity. It is treated with short-acting pain medicines.

breast anatomy   The breast is a mammary gland that produces milk. Each breast has 15 to 20 sections called lobes, which contain many smaller lobules that end in dozens of tiny milk-secreting bulbs embedded in fatty tissue. The lobes, lobules, and bulbs are all linked by thin tubes called ducts. These ducts lead to the nipple, located in the center of a dark area of skin called the AREOLA. During breast-feeding, milk travels from the lobules into the ducts. There are no muscles in the breast, but muscles lie under each breast and cover the ribs. Each breast also contains blood vessels and vessels carrying colorless fluid called lymph, which lead to small bean-shaped organs called LYMPH NODES. Clusters of lymph nodes are found near the breast in the axilla (under the arm), above the collarbone, and in the chest. Lymph nodes are also found in many other parts of the body.

Breast and Cervical Cancer Mortality Prevention Act of 1990   A law that authorizes the U.S. Centers for Disease Control and Prevention to provide critical breast and cervical cancer screening services to underserved women, including older women, women who have a low income, and women of racial and ethnic minority groups.

breast cancer   One of the most common types of cancer among women in the United States, second only to skin cancer. It is diagnosed in more than 180,000 women and 1,500 men each year in the United States. The classic sign of breast cancer is a lump in the breast or (if the tumor has spread to the lymph nodes) under the arm.

Scientists are making progress in their fight against breast cancer, death rate is falling due to earlier diagnosis, and better treatments, and quality of life for patients is improving.

The breast is an organ that can have different types of cancers, including lobular, ductal, or inflammatory breast cancer.

Risk Factors

The exact causes of breast cancer are not known, but studies show that the risk of breast cancer increases as a woman gets older. This disease is uncommon in women under age 35; most breast cancers occur in women over age 50, and the risk is especially high for women over age 60. Breast cancer also occurs more often in Caucasian women than African-American or Asian women. Research has shown that the following factors increase a woman's chance of having breast cancer:

Race   Breast cancer occurs more often in Caucasian women than in African-American or Asian-American women.

Age   The most important factor in the risk for breast cancer is a woman's age. The older a woman is, the greater her probability of having breast cancer. A woman's chance of having breast cancer by age 30 is one in 2,525; by age 40 it is one in 217; by age 50, one in 50; by age 60, one in 24; by age 70, one in 14; by age 80, one in 10.

Personal history   Women who have had cancer in one breast face an increased risk of having it in the opposite breast.

Family history   A woman's risk for development of breast cancer increases if her mother, sister, or daughter had breast cancer, especially at a young age.

Breast changes   Atypical hyperplasia or LOBULAR CARCINOMA IN SITU may increase a woman's risk for development of cancers.

Genetic alterations Changes in certain genes (*BRCA1*, *BRCA2*, and others) increase the risk of breast cancer.

Estrogen Evidence suggests that the longer a woman is exposed to estrogen (whether made by her body, taken as a drug, or delivered by a patch), the more likely she is to have breast cancer. For example, risk is somewhat increased among women who began menstruation at an early age (before age 12), experienced menopause late (after age 55), never had children or had the first child after about age 30, or took hormone replacement therapy for long periods. Each of these factors increases the amount of time a woman's body is exposed to estrogen.

Diethylstilbestrol (DES) Between the early 1940s and 1971 this synthetic form of estrogen was used during pregnancy to prevent certain complications. Women who took DES are at a slightly higher risk for breast cancer, but this does not appear to be the case for their daughters who were exposed to DES before birth.

Radiation therapy Women whose breasts were exposed to radiation during radiation therapy before they reached age 30, especially those who were treated with radiation for HODGKIN'S DISEASE, are at an increased risk for breast cancer. Studies show that the younger a woman was when she received her treatment, the higher her risk for developing breast cancer later in life.

Alcohol Some studies suggest that women who have three or more drinks per day have twice the usual risk of developing breast cancer. One to two eight-ounce drinks a day is not associated with an increased risk for breast cancer. Taking a folate supplement can help lower the risk for breast cancer when a woman drinks alcohol.

Obesity Studies suggest that breast cancer is increasing in postmenopausal women who are overweight. There is no increased risk in obese premenopausal women.

Most women who develop breast cancer have none of the risk factors listed, other than the risk of growing older. Scientists are conducting research into the causes of breast cancer to learn more about risk factors and ways of preventing this disease.

Prevention

Women should talk with their doctor about factors that can affect their chance of getting breast cancer. Some risk factors, such as FAMILY HISTORY, genetic patterns, and age of menstruation and childbirth, cannot be altered. But others are a matter of choice. Choosing to breast-feed a child, eating a healthy diet, maintaining healthy weight, getting plenty of exercise, taking TAMOXIFEN, and avoiding ALCOHOL all may affect a woman's chances of developing of the disease. In addition, women at risk for inheriting a BREAST CANCER SUSCEPTIBILITY GENE can consider preventive surgery or more frequent MAMMOGRAMS and exams.

Exercise Recent studies suggest that regular EXERCISE may decrease the risk in younger women and decrease the chance of cancer recurrence in women who have breast cancer. Other studies suggest that women who have cancer who exercise live longer than those who do not.

Diet Some evidence suggests a link between DIET and breast cancer. Ongoing studies are looking at ways to prevent breast cancer through changes in diet or with dietary supplements, but it is not yet known whether specific dietary changes can actually prevent breast cancer. What someone eats may not be as important as how much.

BRCA *genes* Research also has led to the identification of mutations in certain genes that increase the risk of development of breast cancer. Women who have a strong family history of breast cancer may choose to have a blood test to see whether they have inherited a change in the *BRCA1* or *BRCA2* gene. If they have inherited the gene, some women choose prophylactic (preventive) surgery or medications to lower their risk or have more frequent mammograms and exams.

Preventive drugs Scientists are looking for drugs that may prevent the development of breast cancer. In one large study, the drug tamoxifen reduced the number of new cases of breast cancer among women at an increased risk for the disease. Doctors are now studying how another drug called raloxifene compares to tamoxifen.

Prophylactic mastectomy Some women at very high risk for breast cancer choose to have one or both breasts removed *before* disease occurs. Although this surgery does not completely eliminate the risk (some tiny bits of breast tissue always remain), it does lower the risk considerably, and in women with *BRCA* genes, improves survival. Some people consider this a controversial and radical step to avoid breast cancer; however, some women who are at high risk believe it is worthwhile. Insurance companies may or may not cover the surgery.

Symptoms

Early breast cancer usually does not cause pain or any other symptoms, but as it grows it can cause the following changes:

- A lump or thickening in or near the breast or in the underarm area
- A change in the size or shape of the breast
- Nipple discharge or tenderness
- Inversion of the nipple into the breast
- Ridges or pitting of the breast (the skin resembles the skin of an orange)
- A change in the appearance or texture of the skin of the breast, areola, or nipple

Mammograms and Breast Exams

Women should have regularly scheduled screening mammograms and clinical breast exams. A screening mammogram is the best tool available for finding breast cancer early and can often detect a breast lump before it can be felt. A mammogram can show small deposits of calcium (called microcalcifications) that may be an early sign of cancer, or precancerous change.

The AMERICAN CANCER SOCIETY recommends that women in their forties or older get screening mammograms every year. Women who are at increased risk for breast cancer should seek medical advice about when to begin having mammograms and how often to be screened. (For example, a doctor may recommend that a woman at increased risk begin screening before age 40 or change her screening intervals.) The following strong risk factors may be used for yearly screening at an earlier age (30 to 35):

- Previous breast cancer
- *BRCA1* or *BRCA2* mutations
- Mother, sister, or daughter who has a history of breast cancer

- ATYPICAL HYPERPLASIA found on any previous breast BIOPSY
- Two or more previous breast biopsies, even if the results were benign

If an area of the breast looks suspicious on the screening mammogram, additional mammograms may be needed. Depending on the results, the doctor may advise the woman to have a biopsy. Although mammograms are the best way to find breast abnormalities early, they are not perfect. A mammogram may miss some cancers that are present (false negative result) or may point to cancer when tissue is actually benign (false positive result). In addition, detecting a tumor early does not guarantee that a woman's life will be saved, because some fast-growing breast cancers may already have spread to other parts of the body before being detected. Nevertheless, studies show that mammograms reduce the risk of dying of breast cancer. Clinical breast exam is recommended every three years in women 20 to 40, and yearly after that.

Some women perform monthly breast self-exams to check for any changes in their breasts, although they are no longer recommended. When doing a breast self-exam, it is important to remember that each woman's breasts are different, and that changes can occur because of aging, the menstrual cycle, pregnancy, menopause, or use of birth control pills or other hormones. It is normal for the breasts to feel a little lumpy and uneven, especially immediately before or during a menstrual period. Women older than age 40 should be aware that even if they examine their own breasts each month, they still need to have regularly scheduled screening mammograms and clinical breast exams by a health professional.

Diagnosis

Diagnosis of breast cancer includes a careful physical exam, personal and family medical history, together with one or more of the following breast exams:

- *Clinical breast exam:* The doctor should carefully feel the breast and the tissue around it. Benign lumps often feel different from cancerous ones; the doctor can examine the size and texture of the lump and determine whether the lump moves easily.

- *Mammography:* (See previous discussion.)
- *Ultrasonography:* Using high-frequency sound waves, ultrasounds can show whether a lump is a fluid-filled cyst (not cancer) or a solid mass (which may or may not be cancer). This exam may be used along with mammography.

On the basis of these exams, the doctor may decide that no further tests are needed and no treatment is necessary. In such cases, the doctor may need to check the woman regularly to watch for any changes. However, in some cases the doctor needs more information and schedules a biopsy of fluid or tissue removed from the breast. For further evaluation a woman's doctor may refer her to a surgeon or oncologist who has experience with breast diseases.

Several types of biopsy exist, including a FINE NEEDLE ASPIRATION, a needle biopsy, or a surgical biopsy. In a *fine needle aspiration,* the doctor inserts a thin needle to remove fluid or cells from a breast lump. If the fluid is clear, it may not need to be checked by a lab. In a *needle biopsy,* the doctor removes tissue with a needle from a lump that looks suspicious on a mammogram but that cannot be felt. Tissue removed in a needle biopsy goes to a lab to be checked for cancer cells by a pathologist.

In an *incisional biopsy,* the surgeon cuts out a sample of a lump or suspicious area; in an *excisional biopsy,* the surgeon removes all of a lump or suspicious area and an area of healthy tissue around the edges. A pathologist then examines the tissue under a microscope to check for cancer cells.

Types of Breast Cancer

Most breast cancer occurs in the milk ducts of the breast (the tubes that carry breast milk to the nipple). This type of breast cancer is called DUCTAL CARCINOMA. A second, less common form of breast cancer occurs in the lobules, where breast milk is made; it is called LOBULAR CARCINOMA. Other less common forms of breast cancer are inflammatory, medullary, mucinous, and tubular breast cancer and Paget's disease. Breast cancers are also classified as *in situ* or *invasive.*

The pathologist can tell from a biopsy whether a cancer is present, what kind of cancer it is, and whether it is in situ or invasive. *In situ* means "in

place." Ductal and lobular carcinomas that have not spread outside the duct or lobule are called in situ cancers. They are often referred to as precancerous conditions because they can either develop into or raise the risk of invasive cancer.

Ductal or lobular carcinomas that have spread into surrounding breast tissue are called invasive. They should be distinguished from a metastasis. An invasive breast cancer has simply spread into other neighboring breast tissue, whereas a metastasic breast cancer has broken away from the primary tumor and spread to other organs of the body through either the bloodstream or the lymphatic system.

Most breast cancers can be detected early if screening guidelines are followed properly. Early detection usually means that the breast cancer has not had time to spread to other organs.

Invasive ductal carcinoma   The most common type of breast cancer is ductal carcinoma, which begins in the cells lining the ducts of the breast. Ductal carcinoma accounts for 85 percent of all breast cancers. These cancers may spread to lymph nodes or other organs, although if the cancer is less than 1 centimeter in diameter, spread is unlikely.

Cells that grow only within the duct tube (called intraductal cells) continue along the duct system, which eventually leads to the nipple. Between 15 and 20 percent of breast cancers are found at this stage. They can remain in this preinvasive stage for some time. Usually these lesions do not cause symptoms, except an occasional bloody discharge from the nipple. Occasionally, these intraductal cancer cells may appear as small flecks of calcium on a mammogram.

Ductal carcinoma in situ (DCIS)   Also called "intraductal carcinoma," DCIS refers to abnormal cells that are growing in the lining of a duct. With this type of precancer, the abnormal cells have not spread beyond the duct to invade the surrounding breast tissue and so they do not spread to lymph nodes or other organs.

However, women with untreated DCIS are at an increased risk of invasive breast cancer, as over time DCIS may become invasive. The treatment of DCIS is the same as for invasive cancer—either lumpectomy and radiation or mastectomy. Underarm lymph nodes are not usually removed. Women who have DCIS may want to consider taking tamoxifen to reduce the risk of developing invasive breast cancer.

Invasive lobular carcinoma   Lobular carcinoma in situ (LCIS) refers to abnormal cells in the lining of a lobule. This is not a cancer. The presence of these cells is a sign that a woman has an increased risk of developing breast cancer in either breast. This risk of cancer is increased for both breasts. Some women who have LCIS may take tamoxifen, which can reduce the risk of development of breast cancer; others may choose not to have treatment but simply return to the doctor regularly for checkups. Occasionally, women who have LCIS may decide to have preventive surgery to remove both breasts to try to prevent development of cancer, a technique called prophylactic mastectomy. (In most cases, in this situation removal of underarm lymph nodes is not necessary.) Because LCIS is a marker of breast cancer risk and not a true cancer, there is no need for surgery or radiation.

This type of breast cancer begins in the lobules, and then spreads through the basement membrane into the surrounding breast tissue. This type of cancer can spread beyond the breast to other parts of the body. About 10 to 15 percent of invasive breast cancers are invasive lobular carcinomas.

These tumors feel like thickened areas of the breast instead of lumps, apparently because the malignant cells grow around the breast's ducts and lobules. The typical outlook for this type of cancer is similar to that of IDC, and treatment is the same.

Inflammatory breast cancer   This is an uncommon type of locally advanced breast cancer in which the breast looks red and swollen (or inflamed) because cancer cells block the lymph vessels in the skin of the breast. The skin of the breast may also show a pitted appearance called *peau d'orange* (French for "the skin of an orange"). Inflammatory breast cancer accounts for about 1 percent of invasive breast cancers. This type of cancer is quite likely to spread to lymph nodes, and may be diagnosed with swollen lymph nodes but no tumor in the breast.

Inflammatory breast cancer generally grows rapidly, and the cancer cells often spread to other parts of the body.

The name for this type of breast cancer was chosen many years ago by doctors who thought the breast tissue was inflamed. In fact, the skin changes typical of this type of cancer are not due to inflammation but rather to spread of cancer cells within the lymphatic channels of the skin.

A biopsy can confirm the diagnosis of inflammatory breast cancer.

Because this type of cancer is very aggressive, surgical removal (even MASTECTOMY) does not control it locally. Therefore, aggressive CHEMOTHERAPY is usually given as a first step to dramatically shrink the cancer and return the skin to a normal appearance; hormonal therapy also may be used. Surgery and/or RADIATION THERAPY is then used to remove or destroy the cancer in the breast.

Stages of Breast Cancer

In most cases, the most important factor is the stage of the disease, which is based on the size of the tumor and whether the cancer has spread. In general, the smaller the tumor, the better; doctors consider breast cancer tumors less than two centimeters to be "small."

Stage 0: This is sometimes called noninvasive carcinoma or carcinoma in situ.

Stage I: This is an early stage of breast cancer in which the cancer has spread beyond the lobe or duct and invaded nearby breast tissue. Stage I means that the tumor is no more than about one centimeter across and cancer cells have not spread beyond the breast.

Stage II: This is still considered an early stage of breast cancer. The cancer has spread beyond the lobe or duct and invaded nearby breast tissue. In this stage, either the tumor in the breast is less than one centimeter across and the cancer has spread to the lymph nodes under the arm, or the tumor is between one and two centimeters (with or without spread to the lymph nodes under the arm); or the tumor is larger than two centimeters but has not spread to the lymph nodes under the arm.

Stage III: This is also called locally advanced cancer. In this stage, the tumor in the breast is large (more than two centimeters across) and the cancer has spread to the underarm lymph nodes, or the cancer is extensive in the underarm lymph nodes, or the cancer has spread to lymph nodes near the breastbone or to other tissues near the breast.

Stage IV: This is metastatic cancer in which the malignancy has spread beyond the breast and underarm lymph nodes to other parts of the body.

Recurrent: This means the disease has returned in spite of the initial treatment. Most recurrences appear within the first two or three years after treatment, but breast cancer can recur many years later. Cancer that returns only in the area of the surgery is called a local recurrence. If the disease returns in another part of the body, the distant recurrence is called metastatic breast cancer. The patient may have one type of treatment or a combination of treatments for recurrent cancer.

Other Tests

Some tests are done on the breast tissue itself: Estrogen and progesterone receptors (ER + PR) are evaluated, and the tissue is often checked for the presence of the HER-2-neu gene. If ER/PR are positive, the cancer can be treated with hormones; if HER-2-neu is present, more intensive chemotherapy may be indicated. The doctor may also order special exams of the bones, liver, or lungs, because breast cancer may spread to these areas. These are usually done if a patient has advanced breast cancer or if a patient with earlier breast cancer has any symptoms.

Treatment

Breast cancer may be treated with local or body-wide therapy. Some patients have both kinds of treatment. Local therapy is used to remove or destroy breast cancer in a specific area. Surgery and radiation therapy are local treatments. They are used to treat the disease in the breast. When breast cancer has spread to other parts of the body, such as the lung or bone, local therapy with radiation may be used to control cancer in those specific areas.

Systemic treatments are used to destroy or control cancer throughout the body. Chemotherapy, hormonal therapy, and biological therapy are systemic treatments. Some patients have systemic therapy to shrink the tumor before local therapy is performed. Others have systemic therapy to prevent the cancer from recurring or to treat cancer that has spread.

Surgery Surgery may include MASTECTOMY or breast-conserving treatment with LUMPECTOMY followed by radiation. They are equally effective in most cases. The surgeon will explain each type of surgery and help a woman decide how to proceed. Surgery causes short-term pain and tenderness in the area of the operation, so women may need to talk with their doctor about pain management. The skin over the surgical area may be tight, and the muscles of the arm and shoulder may feel stiff. Because nerves may be injured or cut during surgery, a woman may have numbness and tingling in the chest, underarm, shoulder, and upper arm (POSTMASTECTOMY PAIN SYNDROME). These sensations usually end within a few weeks or months, but some women have permanent numbness.

Breast-conserving therapy An operation to remove the cancer but not the breast is called breast-sparing surgery or breast-conserving surgery. *Lumpectomy* and *segmental mastectomy* (also called partial mastectomy) are types of breast-sparing surgery. After breast-sparing surgery, most women receive radiation therapy to destroy cancer cells that remain in the area.

Lumpectomy In a lumpectomy, the surgeon removes the breast cancer and some normal tissue around it. (Sometimes an excisional biopsy serves as a lumpectomy.) Often, some of the lymph nodes under the arm are removed.

In *segmental mastectomy,* the surgeon removes the cancer and a large area of normal breast tissue around it. Occasionally, some of the lining over the chest muscles below the tumor is removed as well.

Mastectomy Mastectomy is an operation to remove the breast (or as much of the breast as possible). BREAST RECONSTRUCTION is often an option, performed either at the same time as the mastectomy or in a later surgery. Women considering reconstruction should discuss this with a plastic surgeon before having a mastectomy.

Simple (or total) mastectomy is the removal of the whole breast without removal of lymph nodes.

In a *modified radical mastectomy,* the whole breast, most of the lymph nodes under the arm, and often the lining over the chest muscles are removed. The smaller of the two chest muscles is also taken out to help in removing the lymph nodes.

Radical mastectomy is the removal of the breast as well as the surrounding lymph nodes, muscles, fatty tissue, and skin. Formerly considered the standard for women with breast cancer, it is rarely used today. In rare cases, radical mastectomy may be suggested if the cancer has spread to the chest muscles.

Axillary lymph node dissection In most cases, the surgeon also removes lymph nodes under the arm to help determine whether cancer cells have entered the lymphatic system. This is called an axillary lymph node dissection.

Removing many of the lymph nodes under the arm slows the flow of lymph; that slowing may cause fluid buildup in the arm and hand, causing swelling (LYMPHEDEMA). To prevent this, women need to protect the arm and hand on the treated side from injury or pressure, even years after surgery. Women should not have blood pressure taken or injections given on the affected side, and they should contact the doctor if an infection develops in that arm or hand. Doctors can explain how women should handle any cuts, scratches, insect bites, or other injuries to the arm or hand.

A *sentinel–lymph node biopsy* is offered at some cancer centers. Researchers are hoping that this procedure may reduce the number of lymph nodes that must be removed during breast cancer surgery. Before surgery, the doctor injects a radioactive substance or blue dye near the tumor; the substance then flows through the lymphatic system to the first lymph nodes where cancer cells are likely to have spread (the sentinel nodes). This injection can be momentarily quite painful, but the burning lasts for only a few minutes. The doctor looks for the dye in the nodes or uses a scanner to locate the radioactive substance in these sentinel nodes. The surgeon makes a small incision and removes only the nodes that have radioactive substance or blue dye. A pathologist checks the sentinel lymph nodes for cancer cells; if no cancer cells are detected, removing additional nodes may not be necessary. If sentinel lymph node biopsy proves to be as effective as the standard axillary lymph node dissection, the new procedure could prevent the risk of lymphedema.

Radiation therapy Women who have had a lumpectomy usually receive radiation therapy after the surgical wound has healed to kill any remaining cancer cells. The radiation may be directed at the breast by an external machine or may occur from radioactive material in thin plastic tubes that are placed directly into the breast (BRACHYTHERAPY). Some women have both kinds of radiation therapy.

In women who have had a mastectomy, radiation to the chest wall is used if there is extensive lymph node involvement, if the cancer is large. Patients getting external radiation therapy usually go to the hospital five days a week for several weeks. For implant radiation, a woman stays in the hospital for several days while the implants remain in place; they are removed before the woman goes home.

Radiation therapy is sometimes also used before surgery, to destroy cancer cells and shrink tumors. It may be given alone or with chemotherapy or hormonal therapy. This approach is most often used in cases in which the breast tumor is large or not easily removed by surgery.

After several radiation therapy treatments, women are likely to become extremely tired. This feeling may continue for a while after treatment is over. Resting is important, but research has suggested that trying to stay reasonably active can help fend off fatigue.

It is also common for the skin in the treated area to become red, dry, tender, and itchy, and the breast may temporarily feel heavy and hard. Toward the end of treatment, the skin may become moist; exposing this area to air as much as possible helps the skin heal. These effects of radiation therapy on the skin are temporary, and the area gradually heals after treatment ends. However, there may be a permanent change in the color of the skin.

Systemic treatment Treatment of the body to prevent cancer recurrence. *Chemotherapy* is the use of drugs to kill cancer cells. CHEMOTHERAPY is usually given by IV and when used after surgery is used for a definite period of time—three to six months. Side effects are determined by which drugs are used.

Hormonal therapy Hormonal therapy blocks the estrogen needed by some cancers to grow. Its side effects depend on the kind of drug or treatment.

The drug tamoxifen is the most common hormonal treatment. It blocks the cancer cells' use of estrogen but does not stop estrogen production. Tamoxifen may cause hot flashes, vaginal discharge or irritation, nausea, and irregular periods. Women who are still menstruating may become pregnant more easily when taking tamoxifen.

Serious side effects of tamoxifen are rare; they include blood clots in the veins, a slightly higher risk of stroke, and cancer of the uterine lining. Any unusual vaginal bleeding should be reported to the doctor.

Young women whose ovaries are removed to deprive cancer cells of estrogen experience menopause immediately, and the symptoms are likely to be more severe than those associated with natural menopause. This treatment is common in Europe but still experimental in the United States.

Biological therapy Biological therapy is a treatment designed to enhance the body's natural defenses against cancer. For example, TRASTUZUMAB (Herceptin) is a monoclonal antibody that targets breast cancer cells that have too much of a protein known as human epidermal growth factor receptor-2 (HER-2). By blocking HER-2, Herceptin slows or stops the growth of these cells. Herceptin may be administered alone or with chemotherapy. This is used in women whose cancers are HER-2-neu positive and have spread to other organs.

The side effects of biological therapy depend on the types of substances used. Rashes or swelling at the injection site are common, and flulike symptoms also may occur. Herceptin may cause these and other side effects, but these effects generally become less severe after the first treatment. Less commonly, Herceptin can also cause damage to the heart that can lead to heart failure. It can also affect the lungs, causing breathing problems that require immediate medical attention. For these reasons, women are checked carefully for heart and lung problems before Herceptin is prescribed.

Treatment Options

A woman's treatment options depend on a number of factors. These factors include her age and menopausal status, her general health, the size and location of the tumor and the stage of the cancer, the results of lab tests, and the size of her breast. Certain features of the tumor cells (such as whether they depend on hormones to grow) are also considered before settling on a particular treatment.

Women who have early stage breast cancer (stages 0 through II) may have breast-sparing surgery followed by radiation therapy to the breast, or they may have a mastectomy, with or without breast reconstruction. Sometimes radiation therapy is also given after mastectomy. Breast-sparing surgery and mastectomy are equally effective. The choice depends mostly on the size and location of the tumor, the size of the woman's breast, certain features of the cancer, and the woman's preference about preserving her breast.

With either approach, lymph nodes under the arm usually are removed. Many women who have stage I and most who have stage II breast cancer have chemotherapy and/or hormonal therapy after primary treatment with surgery, or surgery and radiation therapy. This added treatment is called ADJUVANT THERAPY.

Chemotherapy also may be given to shrink a tumor before surgery, a technique called neoadjuvant therapy. Chemotherapy is given to try to destroy any remaining cancer cells and prevent the cancer from recurring, or coming back, in the breast or elsewhere. It also shrinks the cancer.

Patients who have stage III breast cancer usually have both local treatment to remove or destroy the cancer in the breast and chemotherapy or hormonal therapy to prevent the disease from spreading. The local treatment may include surgery and/or radiation therapy to the breast and underarm. Chemotherapy may also be given before local therapy to shrink the tumor.

Women who have stage IV breast cancer receive chemotherapy and/or hormonal therapy to destroy cancer cells and control the disease. Occasionally they have surgery or radiation therapy to control the cancer in the breast. Radiation may also be useful to control tumors in other parts of the body.

Rehabilitation

Rehabilitation is an important part of breast cancer treatment. All women recover differently, depending on the extent of the disease, type of treatment, and other factors.

Exercising the arm and shoulder after surgery can help a woman regain motion and strength in these areas and can also reduce pain and stiffness in the neck and back. Carefully planned exercises should be started as soon as the doctor says the woman is ready, often within a day or so after surgery. Exercising begins slowly and gently and can even be done in bed. Gradually, exercising can be more active, and regular exercise becomes part of a woman's normal routine. (Women who have a mastectomy followed by immediate breast reconstruction need special exercises, which the doctor or nurse explains.)

Often, lymphedema after surgery can be prevented or reduced by certain exercises and by resting with the arm propped up on a pillow. If lymphedema occurs, the doctor may suggest exercises and other ways to deal with this problem. For example, some women who have lymphedema wear an elastic sleeve or use an elastic cuff to improve lymph circulation. The doctor also may suggest other approaches, such as medication, manual lymph drainage, or use of a machine that gently compresses the arm.

Regular follow-up exams are important after breast cancer treatment. A woman who has had cancer in one breast should immediately report to her doctor any changes in the treated area or in the other breast. Because a woman who has had cancer in one breast is at risk of having the disease in the opposite breast, mammograms are an important part of follow-up care.

breast cancer, international rates of BREAST CANCER rates are the highest in industrialized countries. It is estimated that 1.2 million new diagnoses and 500,000 deaths from breast cancer will occur worldwide in 2004.

Since 1980, breast cancer rates worldwide have increased by 26 percent. In the United States, one in eight women will develop breast cancer in her lifetime; in the United Kingdom, it is one in 10 to 12; and in Australia one in 14. One in 24 women in Hong Kong has the disease each year—and this rate is expected to rise 20 percent over the next five years. In Japan, the incidence of breast cancer doubled between 1960 and the 1980s—although it remains lower than for the United States, Western Europe, Australia and New Zealand, and North Africa.

Many researchers have begun to investigate the possibility that the dominant causes of breast cancer around the world are environment and DIET. Yet overall rates in Japan and some Mediterranean countries remain low despite industrialization.

While breast cancer incidence is increasing, death rates in some countries are declining. In fact, the countries with the highest number of new cases annually have seen the greatest decline in mortality rate—the United States, Canada, Austria, Germany, the United Kingdom, Australia, and Sweden. At the same time, those countries that have lower incidence rates are experiencing an increasing mortality rate.

Breast Cancer Fund A national nonprofit organization founded in 1992 that supports research, education, patient support, and advocacy projects. Funds are raised through highly visible efforts such as Expedition Inspiration, a mountain climb by a team of BREAST CANCER survivors. The fund identifies the environmental and other preventable causes of the disease and is an advocate for their elimination. For contact information, see Appendix I.

breast cancer genes See BREAST CANCER SUSCEPTIBILITY GENES.

breast cancer in men Male BREAST CANCER is a disease in which malignant cells form in the tissues of the breast. Men at any age may develop breast cancer, but it is usually detected in men between 60 and 70 years of age. Male breast cancer makes up less than 1 percent of all cases of breast cancer. However, it appears to be increasing among men at an alarming rate. The AMERICAN CANCER SOCIETY estimates that 1,450 American men would be diagnosed with breast cancer in 2004.

The following types of breast cancer are found in men:

- *Ductal carcinoma in situ:* Abnormal cells that are found in the lining of a duct; also called intraductal carcinoma

- *Infiltrating ductal carcinoma:* Cancer that has spread beyond the cells lining ducts in the breast. Most men who have breast cancer have this type
- *Inflammatory breast cancer:* A type of cancer in which the breast looks red and swollen and feels warm
- *Paget's disease:* A tumor that has grown from ducts beneath the nipple onto the surface of the nipple

Causes

Risk factors for breast cancer in men may include the following:

- Exposure to radiation as during the treatment of HODGKIN'S DISEASE
- Presence of a disease related to high levels of estrogen in the body, such as Klinefelter's syndrome
- Several female relatives who have breast cancer, especially relatives who have an alteration in the *BRCA2* gene. Male breast cancer is sometimes caused by inherited gene mutations.

Diagnosis

Tests that examine the breasts (such as MAMMOGRAMS and ULTRASOUND) are used to detect and diagnose breast cancer in men as they are in women. Any man who notices changes or lumps in the breast should see a doctor. A biopsy can check for cancer.

Treatment and Prognosis

Survival rate for men with breast cancer is similar to survival rate for women with breast cancer when the stage at diagnosis is the same.

Breast cancer in men is treated the same as breast cancer in women. The treatment options and prognosis depend on whether the tumor cells are in the breast only or have spread to other places in the body; the type of breast cancer; certain characteristics of the cancer cells; whether the cancer is ̤east; and the patient's age and

̤

ention Trial (BCPT) A clinithe NATIONAL CANCER INSTITUTE

and conducted by the NATIONAL SURGICAL ADJUVANT BREAST AND BOWEL PROJECT. The study was designed to determine whether TAMOXIFEN could prevent breast cancer in women who are at an increased risk of development of this disease. The study began recruiting participants in April 1992 and closed enrollment in September 1997.

BCPT involved 13,388 premenopausal and postmenopausal women at more than 300 centers across the United States and Canada and was one of the largest breast cancer prevention studies to date. Results reported in the September 16, 1998, *Journal of the National Cancer Institute* showed there were 49 percent fewer diagnoses of invasive breast cancer in women who took tamoxifen than in women who took an inactive substance. Women on tamoxifen also had half the diagnoses of noninvasive breast tumors, such as ductal or LOBULAR CARCINOMA IN SITU. Three women in the tamoxifen group and six women in the placebo group died of breast cancer.

Most of the side effects associated with tamoxifen were temporary, and included HOT FLASHES, leg cramps and vaginal dryness. However, there were some long-term risks, including rare serious health problems: uterine cancer, blood clots in the lung, and stroke. Because of these risks, women who are using tamoxifen should be monitored by their doctors for any sign of serious side effects.

All participants have been asked to undergo regular follow-up examinations. BCPT participants who were randomized to the tamoxifen group and had not completed five years of tamoxifen therapy when the study ended were given the opportunity to continue on therapy.

Postmenopausal women who had been taking the placebo were invited to participate in another trial, the STUDY OF TAMOXIFEN AND RALOXIFENE.

breast cancer risk factors No one knows why BREAST CANCER develops in some women and not in others. But research has shown that the following factors affect a woman's chance of having breast cancer:

- *Race:* Breast cancer occurs more often in Caucasian than African-American or Asian-American women.

- *Age:* The most important factor in the risk for breast cancer is a woman's AGE. The older a woman is, the greater her probability of getting breast cancer. A woman's chance of having breast cancer by age 30 is one in 2,525; by age 40 it is one in 217; by age 50, one in 50; by age 60, one in 24; by age 70, one in 14; by age 80, one in 10.
- *Personal history:* Women who have had cancer in one breast face an increased risk of getting it in the opposite breast.
- *Family history:* A woman's risk for breast cancer development increases if her mother, sister, or daughter has had breast cancer, especially at a young age.
- *Breast changes:* Atypical hyperplasia or LOBULAR CARCINOMA IN SITU may increase a woman's risk for developing cancers.
- *Genetic alterations:* Changes in certain genes (*BRCA1/BRCA2* and others) increase the risk of breast cancer.
- *Estrogen:* Evidence suggests that the longer a woman is exposed to ESTROGEN (whether made by her body, taken as a drug, or delivered by a patch), the more likely she is to have breast cancer. For example, risk is somewhat increased among women who began menstruation at an early age (before 12), experienced menopause late (after age 55), never had children or had the first child after about age 30, or took HORMONE REPLACEMENT THERAPY for a long period. Each of these factors increases the amount of time a woman's body is exposed to estrogen.
- *Early menstruation/late menopause:* (See "estrogen" above.)
- *No children/childbirth late in life:* (See "estrogen" above.)
- *Diethylstilbestrol (DES):* Between the early 1940s and 1971 this synthetic form of estrogen was used during pregnancy to prevent certain complications. Women who took DES are at a slightly higher risk for breast cancer. This does not appear to be the case for their daughters who were exposed to DES before birth.
- *Breast density:* Breast cancers nearly always develop in lobular or ductal tissue, which appears dense on MAMMOGRAMS, and not in fatty tissue. In addition, when breast tissue is dense, seeing abnormal areas on a mammogram is more difficult.
- *Radiation therapy:* Women whose breasts were exposed to radiation during RADIATION THERAPY before age 30, especially those who were treated with radiation for Hodgkin's disease, are at an increased risk for development of breast cancer. Studies show that the younger a woman was when she received radiation treatment, the higher her risk for breast cancer later in life.
- *Alcohol:* Some studies suggest that women who have three or more drinks per day have twice the usual risk of development of breast cancer. Taking a folate supplement can help lower the risk for breast cancer when a woman drinks ALCOHOL.
- *Obesity*

Most women who develop breast cancer have none of the risk factors listed, other than the risk that accompanies growing older. Most women who have known risk factors do not have breast cancer. Scientists are conducting research into the causes of breast cancer to learn more about risk factors and ways of preventing the disease.

Scientists at the NATIONAL CANCER INSTITUTE have developed a computer program called the Breast Cancer Risk Assessment Tool, which can help estimate a woman's chances of development of breast cancer on the basis of several recognized risk factors. The Breast Cancer Risk Assessment Tool also provides information on TAMOXIFEN.

Doctors generally suggest that high-risk women be closely monitored and have regular medical checkups so that, if breast cancer develops, it is likely to be detected at an early stage. These women may also consider participating in prevention studies, taking tamoxifen, or undergoing preventive mastectomy. The decision is an individual one. For any medical procedure or intervention, both the benefits and the risks of the therapy must be considered. The balance of these factors varies, depending on a woman's personal and family health history and her appraisal of the benefits and risks. Women who are considering taking steps to reduce the risk of breast cancer should discuss their personal risk factors with their doctor.

breast cancer screening   Screening for breast cancer should be focused on the women who will benefit the most, according to new guidelines from the AMERICAN CANCER SOCIETY (ACS) published in May 2003. The guidelines are largely the same guidelines released in 1997; a few key changes signal some important new thinking about cancer screening in general.

In particular, the guidelines downplay the importance of screening in those for whom the benefit is small—for example, women below age 40 and women who have a short life expectancy due to other medical problems. They also emphasize more aggressive screening for those women who are at high risk.

The ACS strengthens its support for the recommendation that women should start MAMMOGRAMS at age 40. Although there has been considerable controversy about breast cancer screening for women between the ages of 40 and 50, several important panels and advocacy groups have stood by the recommendation to begin screening at age 40, because recent studies have shown that screening in this age group saves lives.

On the other hand, the ACS says that having a breast exam every three years is adequate for women younger than age 40. Breast cancer is very uncommon in this age group, and neither breast exams nor mammograms are good at detecting cancers in younger women.

More important, the ACS is no longer recommending that women perform BREAST SELF-EXAMS. In part, this change is based on recent studies that failed to show that regular breast self-exams saved lives.

Although not clearly endorsing any particular technology, the ACS is cautiously recommending that women at high risk—for example, women who have a strong family history of breast cancer—consider new technology such as breast ULTRASOUND or MAGNETIC RESONANCE IMAGING. For the first time, the American Cancer Society is suggesting that cancer screening can be stopped for some women, particularly those who have a limited life expectancy due to advanced age or serious underlying medical problems.

For most women, the new guidelines will mean few changes. If a woman is between the ages of 40 and 75, she should see her doctor every year for a breast exam and mammogram.

Less than one in 250 women will develop breast cancer by the time she reaches age 40. Unless a woman younger than 40 has a strong family history of breast cancer, screening should be low on her list of priorities. It is also important to remember that in young women, an abnormal lump detected by a breast exam or mammogram is much less likely to be cancer than a false positive finding.

If a woman is older than age 75 or has serious health problems such as heart disease or a different type of cancer, she should discuss with her doctor whether it makes sense to discontinue regular breast exams and mammograms. Since these screening tests are intended to detect the earliest stages of breast cancer—and breast cancer takes years or even decades to grow and spread—screening may have little to offer in terms of protecting her health or extending her life. However, if she is in good health, continued mammography makes sense.

When the next set of American Cancer Society guidelines are published in 2009, it is unlikely that they will include major changes for most women. On the other hand, there may be some changes in the recommendations for women at higher than average risk. In particular, results of studies on the role of new technology, such as ultrasound, magnetic resonance imaging, and digital mammography, as well as more information about genetic testing, should be available at that time.

breast cancer statistics   Breast cancer is the most common form of cancer among women in the United States. In a period of 50 years, a woman's lifetime risk of breast cancer nearly tripled. In the 1940s, a woman's lifetime risk of breast cancer was one in 22; current risk is one in eight.

In 2004, an estimated 215,990 women in the United States were diagnosed with invasive breast cancer, and 59,390 were diagnosed with DUCTAL CARCINOMA IN SITU, a noninvasive cancer contained in the milk ducts. An estimated 40,110 died of breast cancer in 2004.

About 3 million American women are living with breast cancer; 2 million have been diagnosed with the disease, and 1 million have the disease but do not yet know it.

The incidence of breast cancer has been rising since the 1980s, whereas the mortality rate has finally started to decline. Much of the increase in the reported incidence since the 1980s is associated with increased screening by physical examination and mammography. However, screening detects but does not account for this increased incidence. Breast cancer occurs among both women and men but is much more rare among men (only about 1,500 cases in the United States per year).

breast cancer susceptibility genes   Genes linked to development of hereditary BREAST CANCER, including *BRCA1* and *BRCA2, P-TEN, CHK2,* and *p53* genes. Genes are small pieces of DNA, the material that acts as a master blueprint for all the cells in the body. A person's genes determine such things as hair or eye color, height, skin color. Any mistakes in a gene that interfere with its job can lead to disease.

BRCA1/BRCA2

BRCA1 and *BRCA2* are the abbreviations for two TUMOR SUPPRESSOR GENES (BReast CAncer 1 and BReast CAncer 2) that normally help to suppress cell growth. A woman who inherits either gene in an altered form has a higher risk of breast, colon, or ovarian cancer. Mutations in these genes may also elevate risk for prostate or colon cancer in men. Experts believe that the inherited alterations in the *BRCA1* and *BRCA2* genes are responsible for nearly all cases of familial ovarian cancer and about half of all cases of familial breast cancer.

Each year, about 5 to 10 percent of the more than 192,000 American women with breast cancers have a hereditary form of the disease. By 1997, more than 200 mutations had been identified in the two *BRCA* genes alone.

The likelihood that breast and/or ovarian cancer is associated with *BRCA1* or *BRCA2* is highest in families who have

- A history of multiple cases of breast cancer
- Cases of both breast and ovarian cancers
- One or more family members who have two primary cancers (original tumors at different sites)

- An Ashkenazi (Eastern European) Jewish background

However, not every woman in such families carries an alteration in *BRCA1* or *BRCA2,* and not every cancer in such families is linked to alterations in these genes.

All women have two copies of *BRCA1* on chromosome 17 and *BRCA2* on chromosome 13. When functioning properly, these genes are thought to help suppress the growth of cancerous cells. People inherit one copy of each of their genes from their mother and a second copy of each gene from their father. If one parent has a defective *BRCA1* or *BRCA2* gene, there is a 50 percent chance the child may inherit this defective copy and a 50 percent chance the child may inherit the normal copy. If a person inherits a defective *BRCA1* or *BRCA2* gene, then each of that person's children likewise has a 50 percent chance of inheriting it.

The *BRCA1* and *BRCA2* genes produce a chemical substance that helps the body prevent cancer. Most women have two normal copies of both the *BRCA1* and *BRCA2* genes, both of which produce this cancer-preventing substance. However, some women have a genetic defect in one copy of either of their two *BRCA1* and *BRCA2* genes, which means they do not produce a normal amount of this cancer-fighting substance. These women are at very high risk of breast or ovarian cancer. According to estimates of lifetime risk, about 13.2 percent (132 in 1,000 individuals) of women in the general population will develop breast cancer, compared with estimates of 36 to 85 percent (360 to 850 in 1,000) of women who have an altered *BRCA1* or *BRCA2* gene. This means that women who have an altered *BRCA1* or *BRCA2* gene are three to seven times more likely to develop breast cancer than women without alterations in those genes.

Lifetime risk estimates of ovarian cancer for women in the general population indicate that 1.7 percent (17 in 1,000) have ovarian cancer, compared with 16 to 60 percent (160 to 600 in 1,000) of women who have altered *BRCA1* or *BRCA2* genes.

Women who have an inherited alteration in one of these genes have an increased risk of developing ovarian or breast cancer at a young age (before menopause) and often have multiple close family members who have the disease. These women also may have a higher probability of development of COLON CANCER.

BRCA *genes and other cancers* Two studies released in 2002 suggested that people who inherit *BRCA1* mutations are at an increased risk not only of breast and ovarian cancer but of a number of other cancers as well. However, the absolute magnitude of the increase in risk of these other cancers is small. Mutations in the *BRCA1* tumor suppressor gene have been associated with a marked increase in the risk of breast and ovarian cancer. They found small but statistically significant increases in the risk of colon, liver, pancreatic, uterine, stomach, and cervical cancers among female *BRCA1* mutation carriers, compared with the general population.

In male *BRCA1* mutation carriers, there was a slightly elevated risk of prostate cancer. However, this increase was seen only in men younger than age 65.

Men and BRCA genes Men who have an altered *BRCA1* or *BRCA2* gene also have an increased risk of breast cancer (primarily if the alteration is in *BRCA2*), and possibly prostate cancer. Alterations in the *BRCA2* gene have also been associated with an increased risk of lymphoma, melanoma, and cancers of the pancreas, gallbladder, bile duct, and stomach in some men and women.

BRCA *pattern differences* Some evidence suggests that there are slight differences in patterns of cancer between people with *BRCA1* alterations and people with *BRCA2* alterations, and even between people who have different alterations in the same gene. For example, one study found that alterations in a certain part of the *BRCA2* gene were associated with a higher risk for ovarian cancer in women, and a lower risk for prostate cancer in men, than alterations in other areas of *BRCA2*.

Most research related to *BRCA1* and *BRCA2* has been done on large families with many affected individuals. Estimates of breast and ovarian cancer risk associated with *BRCA1* and *BRCA2* alterations have been calculated from studies of these families. Because family members share a proportion of their genes and, often, their environment, it is possible that the large number of cancer cases seen in these families may be partly due to other genetic or environmental factors. Therefore, risk estimates that are based on families with many affected members may not accurately reflect the levels of risk in the general population.

Racial risk Specific gene alterations have been identified in different ethnic groups. In Ashkenazi Jewish families, about 2.3 percent (23 in 1,000 persons) have an altered *BRCA1* or *BRCA2* gene. This percentage is about five times higher than that found in the general population. Among people who have alterations in *BRCA1* or *BRCA2*, three particular alterations have been found to be most common in the Ashkenazi Jewish population. It is not known whether the increased frequency of these alterations is responsible for the increased risk of breast cancer in Jewish populations compared with that in non-Jewish populations.

Other ethnic and geographic populations, such as Norwegian, Dutch, and Icelandic people, also have a higher rate of certain genetic alterations in *BRCA1* and *BRCA2*. Information about genetic differences between ethnic groups may help healthcare providers determine the most appropriate genetic test to select.

Genetic Testing

Doctors can test for alterations in a person's *BRCA1* or *BRCA2* gene by using a simple blood test. The cost for genetic testing can range from several hundred to several thousand dollars, and not all insurance policies cover the test. To protect their privacy, some people may choose to pay for the test even when their insurer would be willing to cover the cost. It may be several weeks or months before test results are available.

In a family with a history of breast and/or ovarian cancer, it is most informative first to test a family member who has the disease. If that person is found to have an altered *BRCA1* or *BRCA2* gene, the specific change is referred to as a known mutation. Other family members can then be tested to see whether they also carry that specific alteration. In this scenario, a positive test result indicates that a person has inherited a known mutation in *BRCA1* or *BRCA2* and has an increased risk of development of certain cancers. However, a positive result provides information only about a person's risk of development of cancer—it cannot tell whether cancer will actually develop.

Other genetic changes In addition to classic *BRCA1* and *BRCA2* mutations associated with cancer, there are other changes in these genes that are not well understood. One study found that 10 percent of women who underwent *BRCA1* and *BRCA2* testing had an ambiguous genetic change.

Because everyone may have genetic alterations that do not increase the risk of disease, it is not clear whether a specific change affects a person's risk of developing cancer. As more research is conducted and more people are tested for *BRCA1* and *BRCA2* alterations, scientists will learn more about these genetic changes and cancer risk.

If the test result is positive If a patient tests positive for altered *BRCA1* or *BRCA2* genes, there are several possible approaches to take. Careful monitoring for symptoms of cancer may lead to diagnosis of disease at an early stage, when treatment is more effective. Surveillance methods for breast cancer may include mammography and a clinical breast exam. MRI is also being investigated in these high-risk women. For ovarian cancer, surveillance methods may include transvaginal ultrasound, CA-125 blood testing, and clinical exams.

Preventive surgery Patients may also choose prophylactic surgery, in which the doctor removes as much of the at-risk tissue as possible in order to reduce the chance of development of cancer. Preventive MASTECTOMY (removal of healthy breasts) and preventive salpingo-oophorectomy (removal of healthy fallopian tubes and ovaries) are not guarantees against developing these cancers, but these procedures reduce risk dramatically. However, not all at-risk tissue can be removed surgically, and rarely women have had breast cancer, ovarian cancer, or a type of cancer similar to ovarian cancer even after prophylactic surgery.

Exercise Those who have an altered gene may also choose to lower breast cancer risk by exercising regularly and limiting ALCOHOL consumption. Research results on the benefits of these actions are based on studies in the general population; the effect of these actions for people who have *BRCA1* or *BRCA2* alterations are not yet known.

Tamoxifen Some patients may consider use of preventive drugs such as TAMOXIFEN, which has been shown to lower the risk of invasive breast cancer by 49 percent in women at increased risk

for development of the disease. However, few studies have been done to see whether tamoxifen is effective for women who have *BRCA1* or *BRCA2* mutations. One study found that tamoxifen reduced the incidence of breast cancer by 62 percent in women who had alterations in *BRCA2*, but the results showed no reduction in breast cancer incidence with tamoxifen use among women who had *BRCA1* alterations, perhaps because many breast cancers associated with *BRCA1* are estrogen-receptor negative.

Testing risk Test results may have a direct impact on a person's emotions, social relationships, finances, and medical choices. People who receive a positive test result may feel anxious, depressed, or angry and may choose to use preventive measures that have serious long-term implications and uncertain effectiveness.

On the other hand, people who have a negative result may feel guilty because they have avoided a disease that affects a family member. They may also be falsely reassured that they have no chance of developing cancer, even though people who have a negative result have the same cancer risk as the general population. Because genetic testing can reveal information about more than one family member, the emotions caused by test results can create tension within families.

Test results can affect personal choices, such as marriage and childbearing. Issues surrounding the privacy and confidentiality of genetic test results also create problems.

Genetic discrimination Genetic discrimination occurs when people are treated differently by their insurance company or employer because they have a gene alteration that increases their risk of a disease. People who undergo genetic testing to find out whether they have an altered *BRCA1* or *BRCA2* gene may be at risk for genetic discrimination. A positive genetic test result may affect a person's health insurance coverage. For example, a person who has a positive result may be denied coverage for medical expenses related to the genetic condition, may be dropped from a current health plan, or may be unable to qualify for new insurance. Some insurers view the affected individual as a potential cancer patient whose medical treatment would be costly to the insurance company. To date, no health insurance issues have been a problem. However, patients having genetic tests may want to get life insurance first.

The Health Insurance Portability and Accountability Act (HIPAA) of 1996 provides some protection for people who have employer-based health insurance, because it prohibits group health plans from using genetic information as a basis for denying coverage if a person does not currently have a disease. However, the act does not prohibit employers from refusing to offer health coverage as part of their benefits or prevent insurance companies from requesting genetic information.

In 2000, the Department of Health and Human Services released a regulation called the HIPAA National Standards to Protect Patients' Personal Medical Records. This regulation covers medical records maintained by health-care providers, health plans, and health-care clearinghouses. Although the standards do not relate specifically to genetic information, they provide the first comprehensive federal protection for the privacy of health information.

A person who tests positive for a *BRCA1* or *BRCA2* alteration may experience genetic discrimination in the workplace if an employer learns about the test result. Although there are currently no federal laws specific to such genetic discrimination, some protection is offered through the Americans with Disabilities Act of 1990. In 1995, the Equal Employment Opportunity Commission expanded the definition of *disabled* to include individuals who carry genes that put them at higher risk for genetic disorders. The extent of this protection, however, has not yet been tested in the courts. Several states also have laws that address genetic discrimination by employers and health insurance companies. The degree of discrimination protection varies from state to state. Therefore, the decisions that people make about genetic testing while living in one state may have repercussions in the future if they move to another area.

P-TEN

A mutation in the *P-TEN* gene (also called *MMAC1*), found on chromosome 10, plays a role in several different types of cancers. *P-TEN* is considered to be a tumor suppressor gene, as are *BRCA1* and *BRCA2*. A *P-TEN* mutation can increase a woman's risk of development of breast cancer. It is believed to cause

COWDEN DISEASE, an unusual skin disease that produces increases risk of thyroid and breast cancer. In 4 to 75 percent of women who have Cowden disease, breast cancer eventually develops.

BP1 *Gene*

The *BP1* gene may help spur breast cancer and is active in many patients who have a specific type of leukemia. Experts suspect that when the gene is switched on, it interferes with cell regulation in a way that helps cancerous cells survive.

Scientists discovered that in breast cancer tissue from 46 patients, *BP1* was active in 89 percent of the tumors from black women but only 57 percent of white women's tumors. Moreover, *BP1* was found to be active in 100 percent of estrogen-receptor-negative tumors and 75 percent of estrogen-receptor-positive tumors.

However, it is not clear just what role *BP1* plays in overall cancer development, since *BP1* activity was also found in two benign breast tumors and in one sample of normal breast tissue.

DBC2 *Gene*

Scientists at Cold Spring Harbor Laboratory in New York and the University of Washington in 2002 discovered a tumor suppressor gene that is missing or inactive in as many as 60 percent of breast cancers and that is also altered in lung cancer. The discovery of the gene, called *DBC2* (for *deleted in breast cancer*), is highly significant because *DBC2* is among the first tumor suppressor genes to be clearly associated with sporadic breast cancer, which accounts for more than 90 percent of breast cancers.

The researchers showed that production of the *DBC2* protein in breast cancer cells kills the cancer cells or stops them from growing. Researchers discovered that the *DBC2* gene was turned off in almost 60 percent of breast cancer tumors; in contrast, all samples from normal breast tissue had functioning versions of the *DBC2* gene. When scientists placed a functional version of the gene into a breast cancer cell, the breast cancer stopped growing. This led researchers to conclude that *DBC2* clearly has some suppressive function in breast cancer.

Currently, no genetic tests can help identify women at increased risk for sporadic breast cancer, but the identification of genes like *DBC2* may improve prospects for such tests—and for new treatments. Since the activation of *DBC2* stops the growth of breast cancer cells, experts hope that they can use molecules that participate in this previously unknown biological pathway to treat breast cancer. It could one day be possible to use the gene itself directly in breast cancer, as a form of gene therapy. In 1997, the same research group at Cold Spring Harbor Laboratory identified one of the only other tumor suppressor genes (called *P-TEN*) to be clearly associated with sporadic cancer. In 1990, the same research group at the University of Washington discovered the first gene linked to hereditary breast cancer, called *BRCA1*.

BASE *Gene*

This recently discovered gene and the protein it encodes may lead to new weapons in the war against breast cancer. The protein *BASE* (an acronym for *breast cancer and salivary gland expression*) is secreted only by breast cancer and salivary gland cells, making it a potential target for therapies and diagnostic tests. Experts hope that genes that encode proteins such as this might be used to diagnose cancer early or to see how patients are responding to treatment. They are also considered a possible target for some kind of immunotherapy.

Experts found the gene and its associated protein through an exhaustive search through DNA associated with breast tumors. First, the researchers created a library of more than 15,000 genes taken from breast cancer cells, prostate cancer cells, and normal breast cells. Then they removed all the genes that are also expressed in essential tissue, such as the brain, the liver, the lungs, and the kidneys. That left about 3,000 to 4,000 genes to study. To narrow the search even further, the researchers focused on genes that showed up multiple times. One of those was the gene that encodes *BASE*, which was found in about 30 percent to 40 percent of breast cancers. The normal breast makes very little if any of the protein, but certain kinds of breast cancer make quite a lot.

Researchers hope that they will be able to use the new information to devise a breast cancer screening test that measures the level of *BASE* in the blood. This could help diagnose breast cancer in the way that prostate-specific antigen (PSA) levels are used to diagnose prostate cancer. Scientists may also be able to use *BASE* as a target for a vaccine.

Because it is not made in essential tissues, creating a vaccine that would destroy the cells that make it may be possible.

ZNF217 *Gene*

Multiple copies of this gene remove natural restrictions on cell growth and thereby increase the probability of malignancy, according to a study jointly conducted by researchers with the Lawrence Berkeley National Laboratory and the University of California at San Francisco (UCSF).

The scientists suspect that over the course of evolution, the human body has developed molecular mechanisms to count and limit the number of times breast cells divide as a means of limiting the growth of abnormal cells. When expressed inappropriately, *ZNF217* appears to interfere with these mechanisms, so that the affected cells continue dividing and accumulating additional changes necessary for malignancy.

Normal cells contain two copies of *ZNF217*, which are located on human chromosome 20. More than two copies are present in many different types of tumors, including some 40 percent of human breast cancer cell lines. The results of this study support the theory that overactivity of the *ZNF217* gene contributes to the development of breast cancer by promoting cell "immortality."

Cells are said to be immortal when they grow past the point at which they are supposed to die. It appears that simple overexpression of the *ZNF217* gene itself allows cells to continue growing when they would otherwise stop. However, continued growth allows the cells to accumulate additional changes that may favor malignancy.

The Berkeley Lab–UCSF researchers began searching for possible oncogenes in a specific area of chromosome 20 that was known to be amplified in a large number of human breast cancers. They identified *ZNF217* as a gene in this region of the genome whose level of expression consistently matched the levels of amplification found in breast tumors. *ZNF217* was relatively inactive in normal breast cells but highly active in a number of breast cancer cell lines.

Scientists determined the role of the *ZNF217* gene in breast cancer progression by inserting it into normal breast cells. Introducing extra copies of *ZNF217* into cultures of normal human mammary epithelial cells caused those breast cells to become immortal. The cells took on other characteristics as well that were similar to changes observed in cultures of breast cells exposed to chemical carcinogens. *ZNF217*-treated cells also displayed a new resistance to transforming growth factor beta (TGFb), a substance that normally stops the growth of many different types of cells.

Scientists hope that in the future, it may be possible to block *ZNF217*'s activity through the use of drugs designed to inhibit the production of specific disease-causing proteins, or through the use of some type of molecular inhibitor. However, much more work needs to be done before the means by which overexpression of *ZNF217* contributes to the development of breast cancer can be fully understood.

TSG101 *Gene*

Mutations in *TSG101* are associated with breast cancer in 15 percent of nonfamilial cases examined in one study. The *TSG101* gene was mapped to a region of chromosome 11 that had repeatedly been associated with a variety of cancers, particularly breast cancer.

Fanconi Anemia Genes

An error in any of the half dozen genes involved in Fanconi anemia, a rare childhood condition, can increase an individual's probability of developing breast cancer, according to investigators at Dana-Farber Cancer Institute and Children's Hospital.

Discovery of the new cancer-susceptibility genes grew out of more than 10 years of research into Fanconi anemia, a condition known to affect only 500 families in the United States. Children born with the condition usually have bone marrow failure early in life, leaving them unable to produce oxygen-carrying red blood cells. If they survive into young adulthood—often they need the help of a bone marrow transplant to do so—they are at risk for a variety of cancers. Most often they get leukemia, but they also may have tumors of the brain, head and neck, breast, colon, and other organs. In recent years, investigators have mapped out the chain of events by which the Fanconi genes are switched on. When a cell's DNA is damaged, five of the Fanconi genes team up to produce a pro-

tein complex that stimulates a sixth gene. That gene, dubbed D2, orders production of a protein found near *BRCA1*, whose job is to help repair damaged DNA. If *BRCA1* or its partner in DNA repair, *BRCA2*, is defective or not switched on properly, DNA damage can accumulate in cells, increasing their chance of malfunctioning and becoming cancerous. Proximity of the D2 protein to *BRCA1* suggested but did not prove that D2 activates *BRCA1*.

To find out whether D2 activated the *BRCA1* gene, researchers began to study a small group of children who have Fanconi anemia but do not have mutations in the six Fanconi genes. They drew blood samples from them and analyzed their cells for abnormalities in *BRCA1* and *BRCA2*. They found that whereas the *BRCA1* genes were normal, each patient had two flawed copies of *BRCA2*. This meant that each parent carried a copy of a flawed *BRCA2* gene and had transferred the mutated gene to the child. The finding proved that the chain of events that begins with the Fanconi anemia genes leads directly to *BRCA1* and *BRCA2*, which work together to repair damaged DNA. If *BRCA1* or *BRCA2* or any of the Fanconi genes is defective, the sequence of events is disrupted and DNA repair is blocked.

The chromosomal similarities between Fanconi anemia cells and breast cancer cells are so great that even a trained eye cannot distinguish them. Now that the link between mutations for Fanconi anemia and breast cancer has been established, doctors may soon be able to offer new tests for determining who is at risk for inherited breast cancer and potentially develop new drugs targeted at specific flawed genes.

breast conservation surgery   An operation to remove the cancer but not the breast is called breast-sparing surgery or breast-conserving surgery. Types of breast-conserving surgery include LUMPECTOMY (removal of the lump), quadrantectomy (removal of one-quarter of the breast), and segmental MASTECTOMY (removal of the cancer as well as some of the breast tissue around the tumor and the lining over the chest muscles below the tumor). After breast-sparing surgery, most women receive RADIATION THERAPY to destroy cancer cells that remain in the area.

breast density   The density of breast tissue is determined by the amount of connective tissue (which appears as light areas on a MAMMOGRAM) compared with amount of fatty tissue (which appears dark). Density is not related to firmness, nor can "density" be felt by touching the breast. Density is only detectable by viewing a mammogram of the breast. It is important because women with denser breasts may have an increased risk of breast cancer.

Because BREAST CANCER rarely develops in fatty tissue, cancer is more likely to occur in breasts with a lot of dense, non-fatty tissue. In addition, it is more difficult for doctors to detect abnormal areas in the breast on a mammogram if there is a lot of dense tissue.

Recently, an Australian twin study uncovered the fact that breast density is a genetically linked characteristic. Scientists are now trying to find the genes responsible for determining breast density, which could help define new subtypes of breast cancer and suggest better prevention strategies.

Although there is evidence that age and some lifestyle factors (such as having children) can alter breast density, there is still quite a difference in the distribution of breast density across women of the same age. The Australian study showed that genetic factors play a major role in explaining why women of the same age have different breast density and helps explain why having a family history of breast cancer is a risk factor for the disease. If there are many genes involved with breast density, it could be the combined effect of these genes, rather than a single mutation in just one "high-risk" gene such as *BRCA1* or *BRCA2,* that determines risk.

Health-care providers do not yet regularly use a woman's breast density to assess her breast cancer risk, however. This is partly due to the absence of an agreed-upon standard for assessing breast density; researchers are trying to use digital mammography techniques to standardize descriptions of breast density.

breast expander   A polyurethane flexible implant placed under the tissue and enlarged manually by inserting a fluid (usually saline solution).

See also BREAST RECONSTRUCTION; BREAST IMPLANTS.

breast-feeding and cancer   Breast-feeding may modestly reduce the risk of developing BREAST CANCER. More than half of 31 studies reported that women who breast-fed had a decreased risk of developing breast cancer (ranging from 10 percent to 64 percent) when compared to women who never breast-fed. The rest of the studies reported that breast-feeding had no influence on the risk of breast cancer.

The results of these studies may vary because of differences in the pattern of breast-feeding among women in different cultures, such as when solid foods are added, how often a child is fed, and the reasons for stopping breast-feeding. Also, some studies asked how long each child was breast-fed, whereas others asked for the total length of time all children were breast-fed. In addition, other reproductive factors, such as number of children and a woman's age at first birth, are very closely related to breast-feeding and may also influence breast cancer risk.

The longer that women breast-feed, the more they are protected from breast cancer; this effect is in addition to the protection gained from having children. A recent study pooled data from 47 separate studies from 30 different countries involving 50,000 women with breast cancer and nearly 100,000 women who did not have the disease. It showed that for every year a woman breast-feeds, her risk of breast cancer decreases by 4.3 percent—over and above the 7 percent risk reduction for each child she has.

Women from the developing world breast-fed for an average of about two years per child and averaged about six or seven children. By comparison, the average industrialized woman breast-fed for just two or three months per child and had about two or three children. In addition, these women do not usually breast-feed often enough to suppress their periods.

The results of this study help explain why breast cancer incidence is so high in developed countries. It is estimated that if a woman's reproductive habits from an industrialized country mirrored those of women in developing countries, her risk of breast cancer by the age of 70 would fall from 6.3 per 100 women to 2.7 per 100 women. Two-thirds of the decrease would be a result of longer breast-feeding and one-third a result of the greater number of children.

Scientists are still studying whether the age at which a woman first breast-feeds is important, as well as the effects of breast-feeding in women with a family history of breast cancer.

Finally, breast-feeding may be more effective in protecting against the development of pre-menopausal breast cancer than against post-menopausal breast cancer. In some studies in which no overall reduction in breast cancer risk associated with breast-feeding was detected, an analysis of the data by menopausal status revealed a slight protective effect of breast-feeding in pre-menopausal women. Many other studies that focused specifically on young women reported that the incidence of premenopausal breast cancer was lower among women who breast-fed.

Many researchers think that premenopausal breast cancer and postmenopausal breast cancer are different diseases. However, it is not clear why breast-feeding may be more protective against pre-menopausal breast cancer than postmenopausal breast cancer.

Length of Breast-feeding Period

Although a few studies report a decrease in the risk of breast cancer after only three or more months of breast-feeding, the evidence for risk reduction becomes more consistent the longer women breast-feed. The most consistent evidence of a rela-tionship between breast-feeding and a decreased risk of breast cancer has been reported in studies of Chinese women who breast-fed for long periods. In these studies, women who breast-fed for a total of six years or more (all children combined) over the course of their life had up to a 63 percent decrease in breast cancer incidence compared to women who never breast-fed.

Breast-feeding Recommendations

The American Academy of Pediatrics recommends that women begin breast-feeding within the first hour after birth, if possible. For most women, exclusive breast-feeding is recommended for about the first six months; breast-feeding should con-tinue for at least 12 months thereafter. Experts note that if women breast-fed each of their chil-

dren for just an extra six months, doing so could prevent 5 percent of breast cancers each year among them.

Patients with Breast Cancer and Breast-feeding

Since there are relatively few cases of breast cancer in premenopausal women, there are very few stud-ies that have looked at the effects on breast-feeding of treatment for breast cancer. The ability to breast-feed after treatment for breast cancer depends on the individual and on the treatment she received. Surgery and radiation may interfere with a woman's ability to breast-feed on the affected side. In some cases, women reported that there seemed to be less milk produced in the irradiated breast. However, they were able to breast-feed from the untreated breast. Other women have reported that they were able to breast-feed from both the treated and the untreated breasts.

Although lumps are common in the breasts of women who are breast-feeding, every lump should be evaluated. Although physical changes in the breasts of women who are pregnant or breast-feeding may hide a lump, women who are breast-feeding should still examine their breasts for changes or abnormalities. The best time to exam-ine the breasts is immediately after a feeding. Women who need any kind of treatment for breast cancer, including surgery, chemotherapy, or radia-tion, should talk with their health-care providers if breast-feeding is a concern.

How Breast-feeding Lessens Risk

There are several ways that breast-feeding may influence the risk of development of breast cancer. First, breast-feeding may cause hormonal changes such as a decrease in the level of estrogen. Studies have clearly shown that lower levels of estrogen decrease a woman's risk of breast cancer develop-ment. In addition, breast-feeding may suppress ovulation. According to some studies, women who have fewer ovulatory cycles over the course of their reproductive life may have a decreased risk of breast cancer.

In addition, breast-feeding may remove possible carcinogens stored in the adipose tissue of the breast or cause physical changes in the cells that line the mammary ducts. These changes may make the cells more resistant to mutations that can lead to cancer.

Breast-feeding and the Baby's Risk

There is some preliminary evidence that there may be a slight decrease in the risk of development of breast cancer among women who were breast-fed as infants. This protection may be due to the hormones and immune factors present in breast milk, or to the fewer calories consumed by breast-fed babies and the slower weight gain among them.

However, in some preliminary studies, no association was found between being breast-fed as an infant and having breast cancer later in life. In addition, one study reported that there was no difference in the risk of breast cancer among women who had been breast-fed by a mother who eventually had the disease (over and above the family history risk).

breast fluid Fluid present in ducts within the breast that may be present in many nonpregnant women who are not breast-feeding. The presence of abnormal cells in breast fluid may predict a doubled risk of BREAST CANCER, according to a recent study. Women from whom no fluid could be drawn, the study showed, had the lowest risk of breast cancer, and those with normal cells in the fluid were at about a 60 percent higher risk. The fluids were obtained by use of a manual breast pump that mimicked the suction force of a nursing infant.

The study suggests, but does not prove, that when a woman who is not pregnant or nursing produces fluid, that fluid may be an indication of increased risk. Scientists think that some women have some fluid in their breast ducts all of the time. They do not understand why it is possible to obtain fluid from some women and not from others. It could be, scientists suspect, that the fluid signals that there are changes under way in the breast.

Some scientists believe breast fluid status should be considered for inclusion on the list of factors that doctors now evaluate when predicting a woman's breast cancer risk.

See also BREAST CANCER RISK FACTORS.

breast implant A round or teardrop-shaped sac inserted into the body to reconstruct the shape or size of the breast removed during MASTECTOMY. An implant may be filled with saline water or synthetic material. Saline solution–filled breast implants are available for anyone who wants them.

Because some scientists are concerned about possible short- and long-term health problems associated with silicone-gel-filled breast implants, the U.S. Food and Drug Administration (FDA) has decided that breast implants filled with silicone gel may be used only in an FDA-approved clinical trial. A woman's surgeon can determine whether she is eligible and can make arrangements for her to join a silicone gel study, if desired.

See also BREAST EXPANDER; BREAST RECONSTRUCTION.

breast prosthesis An external artificial breast, made of latex, silicone gel, or foam, that can be worn by women who have had a MASTECTOMY. It usually takes four to six weeks after surgery before the chest wall heals.

A prosthesis closely resembles breast tissue in weight, movement, and drape. They are worn with a "mastectomy bra" (also called a surgical bra). These bras are designed with cup pockets to hold the breast form in place and are cut wider than others under the arm and across the chest. When a woman is correctly measured and fitted by a trained, professional fitter, the prosthesis should stay securely in place and match the shape and contour of the woman's body.

There are now hundreds of sizes and styles from which to choose that fit all body and skin types and thousands of dealers nationwide to help in the fitting process.

A properly fitted breast prosthesis is not used merely for cosmetic or psychological reasons, but for physical reasons as well. When a single breast is removed, the body may no longer be in balance and may compensate with slight curving of the spine and a dropped shoulder, changes that may lead to chronic lower back and neck pain.

Most weighted breast prostheses are made of silicone gel that has been "cured" in a manufacturing process and is not in a liquid state. Silicone in these prostheses cannot be absorbed through the skin and is completely safe.

Costs

Medical-grade prostheses tend to be expensive because they are made by hand and manufacturers follow several steps and procedures. They are considered to be medical devices and are therefore regulated by the U.S. Food and Drug Administration. Manufacturers carefully monitor the production and sale of these products through on-site quality assurance and warranty card information. Non-medical-grade prosthetics are not subject to the same inspection process and are often much less expensive, but their use is not covered by insurance, whereas medical-grade prosthetics usually are. They are also covered by Medicare and Medicaid, but coverage differs by state, so each woman should check for details with her local Social Security office.

breast reconstruction Almost every woman who chooses MASTECTOMY is eligible for the surgical reconstruction of the breast mound, which often can be done during surgery to remove the breast. Alternatively, breast reconstruction by a PLASTIC SURGEON can take place after recovery from the mastectomy.

There are several different ways that reconstruction can be performed, including BREAST IMPLANTS (usually saline solution) or creation of a surgical flap with tissue moved from another part of the woman's body. A woman's body type, her age, her general health, and the type of cancer treatment she will have all determine the type of reconstruction method.

A woman can begin discussing reconstruction as soon as she has been diagnosed with cancer. Ideally, the surgical ONCOLOGIST and the plastic surgeon work together to develop a strategy for reconstruction.

After evaluating the woman's health, the plastic surgeon explains the reconstructive options. Reduction or augmentation of the other breast may be considered so the two breasts match. The surgeon should also explain the anesthesia, the facility where the surgery will be performed, and the costs. In most cases, health insurance policies cover most or all of the cost of postmastectomy reconstruction.

Breast Implants

A breast implant is a silicone shell filled with a salt-water saline solution. Because of concerns that there was not enough information demonstrating the safety of silicone-gel-filled breast implants, the U.S. Food and Drug Administration (FDA) has determined that gel-filled implants should be available only to women who are participating in approved studies. Women interested in having silicone implants should talk with their doctor about the FDA's findings and the availability of silicone implants. The alternative saline solution–filled implant, a silicone shell filled with saltwater, continues to be available on an unrestricted basis.

In a one-stage procedure, the surgical oncologist performs the mastectomy and the plastic surgeon places an implant. In a two-stage procedure, at the time of mastectomy the skin is removed, leaving the chest wall flat. A tissue expander is placed under the skin, and over the ensuing months the implant is inflated with saline, stretching the chest skin. When it is stretched enough, the expander is removed and the permanent implant is placed. With either of these procedures, the surgery lasts between one and three hours, and normal activity can begin in between two to four weeks.

Sometimes, reconstruction is delayed if a woman has not decided at the time of mastectomy whether or not to have reconstruction, or if the woman needs radiation after mastectomy. Typically, radiating implants is avoided.

Flap Reconstruction

An alternative approach to implant reconstruction involves creation of a skin flap using tissue taken from other parts of the body, such as the back or abdomen. Surgeons are also experimenting with using buttock tissue.

In one type of flap surgery, the tissue flap remains attached to its original site (usually the abdomen), retaining its blood supply. The flap, consisting of the skin, fat, and muscle with its blood supply, is tunneled beneath the skin to the chest, creating a pocket for an implant or, in some cases, creating the breast mound itself without need for an implant.

Alternatively, in a TRAM flap procedure (short for TRANSVERSE RECTUS ABDOMINIS MYOCUTANEOUS

FLAP), the surgeon creates a breast mound using tissue removed from another part of the body—usually the abdomen.

Regardless of whether the tissue is tunneled beneath the skin as an attached flap or transplanted to the chest, this type of surgery is more

---

MANDATED INSURANCE COVERAGE FOR BREAST RECONSTRUCTION

Laws enacted in the following states require insurance coverage for postmastectomy reconstruction when the policy includes coverage for mastectomy.

Arizona—Covers surgical services for breast reconstruction and at least two external postoperative prostheses.

Arkansas—Enacted in 1997; covers prosthetic devices and reconstructive surgery.

California—Enacted in 1978; covers prosthetic devices or reconstructive surgery related to mastectomy, including restoration of symmetry; law was amended in 1991 to include coverage for pre-1980 mastectomies.

Connecticut—Enacted in 1987; covers at least a yearly benefit of $500 for reconstructive surgery, $300 for prosthesis, and $300 for surgical removal of each breast due to tumor.

Florida—Covers initial prosthetic device and reconstructive surgery incident to mastectomy; 1997 amendment specifies that surgery be in a manner chosen by the treating physician and that surgery to reestablish symmetry of the breasts be covered.

Illinois—Enacted in 1981; covers initial prosthetic device and reconstructive surgery incident to post-1981 mastectomies.

Indiana—Enacted in 1997; covers prosthetic devices and reconstructive surgery after mastectomy.

Kentucky—Enacted in 1998; covers all stages of breast reconstruction surgery after mastectomy to treat breast cancer.

Louisiana—Enacted in 1997; covers reconstructive surgery after mastectomy, including reconstruction of the other breast to produce a symmetrical appearance.

Maine—Enacted in 1995; covers both breast on which surgery was performed and other breast if patient elects reconstruction, in the manner chosen by the patient and physician.

Maryland—Enacted in 1996; requires coverage for reconstructive surgery resulting from a mastectomy, including surgery performed on a nondiseased breast to establish symmetry.

Michigan—Enacted in 1989; covers breast cancer rehabilitative services, delivered on an inpatient or outpatient basis, including reconstructive plastic surgery and physical therapy.

Minnesota—Enacted in 1980; covers all reconstructive surgery incidental to or following injury, sickness, or other diseases of the involved part, or due to congenital defect of a child.

Missouri—Enacted in 1997; covers prosthetic devices and reconstructive surgery necessary to achieve symmetry.

Montana—Enacted in 1997; covers reconstructive surgery after mastectomy resulting from breast cancer, including all stages of one reconstructive surgery on the nondiseased breast to establish symmetry and costs of any prostheses.

Nevada—Enacted in 1983; covers at least two prosthetic devices and reconstructive surgery incident to mastectomy; amended in 1989 to cover surgery to reestablish symmetry.

New Hampshire—Enacted in 1997; covers breast reconstruction, including surgery and reconstruction of the opposite breast to produce a symmetrical appearance, in the manner chosen by the patient and physician.

New Jersey—Enacted in 1985; covers reconstructive breast surgery, including cost of prostheses; amended in 1997 to extend coverage to reconstructive surgery to achieve and restore symmetry.

New York—Enacted in 1997; covers breast reconstruction after mastectomy, including reconstruction of a healthy breast required to achieve reasonable symmetry, in the manner determined appropriate by the attending physician and patient.

North Carolina—Enacted in 1997; covers reconstructive breast surgery, including reconstructive surgery on a nondiseased breast to establish symmetry.

Oklahoma—Enacted in 1997; covers reconstructive breast surgery performed as a result of a partial or total mastectomy, including all stages of reconstructive surgery performed on a nondiseased breast to establish symmetry.

Pennsylvania—Enacted in 1997; covers prosthetic devices and breast reconstruction, including surgery on the opposite breast to achieve symmetry, within six years of the mastectomy date.

Rhode Island—Enacted in 1996; covers prosthetic devices and reconstructive surgery which must be performed within 18 months, to restore and achieve symmetry incident to a mastectomy.

South Carolina—Enacted in 1998; covers prosthetic devices and breast reconstruction, including the nondiseased breast, if determined medically necessary by the patient's attending physician with the approval of the insurer.

Tennessee—Enacted in 1997; covers both the breast on which surgery is performed and the other breast if patient elects reconstruction, in the manner chosen by the patient and physician.

Texas—Enacted in 1997; covers breast reconstruction, including procedures to restore and achieve symmetry.

Virginia—Enacted in 1998; covers reconstructive breast surgery in mastectomy cases and surgery performed to reestablish breast symmetry.

Washington—Enacted in 1983; covers reconstructive breast surgery if mastectomy resulted from disease, illness, or injury; amended in 1996 to include surgery to reestablish symmetry.

Wisconsin—Enacted in 1997; covers breast reconstruction of the affected tissue incident to mastectomy and specifies that such surgery is not cosmetic.

complex than skin expansion. Scars are left at both the tissue donor site and the reconstructed breast, and recovery takes longer than recovery after an implant. On the other hand, when the breast is reconstructed entirely with a woman's own tissue, the results are generally more natural, and there are no concerns about a silicone implant. In some cases, the woman may have the added benefit of an improved abdominal contour (a "tummy tuck").

Many surgeons recommend an additional operation to enlarge, reduce, or lift the opposite breast to match the reconstructed breast. This procedure may leave scars on an otherwise normal breast.

Depending on the extent of the surgery, a woman is usually released from the hospital in two to five days. Many reconstruction options require surgical drains to remove excess fluids from surgical sites immediately after the operation, but these drains are removed within the first week or two after surgery. Most stitches are removed in a week to 10 days.

Recovery from a combined mastectomy and reconstruction or from a flap reconstruction alone it may take up to six weeks. If implants are used without flaps, and reconstruction is done apart from the mastectomy, recovery time may be briefer.

Reconstruction cannot restore normal sensation to the breast, but in time, some feeling may return. Most scars fade substantially over time (although it may take as long as one to two years), but they never disappear entirely.

In general, patients should refrain from any overhead lifting, strenuous sports, and sexual activity for three to six weeks after reconstruction. Chances are the reconstructed breast may feel firmer and look rounder or flatter than the natural breast. It may not have the same contour as the breast before mastectomy. For most mastectomy patients, however, breast reconstruction dramatically improves their appearance and quality of life after surgery.

Risks

There are risks associated with any surgery. In general, the usual problems of surgery are relatively uncommon. They may include bleeding, fluid collection, excessive scar tissue, or problems with anesthesia. Women who smoke, in particular, may have a harder time recovering, since nicotine can delay healing, resulting in conspicuous scars and prolonged recovery.

Occasionally, complications are severe enough to require a second operation. If an implant is used, there is a remote possibility of infection, usually within the first two weeks after surgery. In some of these cases, the implant may need to be removed for several months until the infection clears. A new implant can be inserted later.

The most common problem with implant reconstruction is scarring—called capsular contracture—which occurs if the scar (or capsule) around the implant begins to tighten. This squeezing of the soft implant can make the breast feel hard. Capsular contracture can be treated in several ways and sometimes requires either removal or "scoring" of the scar tissue, or removal or replacement of the implant.

Reconstruction has no known effect on the recurrence of disease in the breast; nor does it generally interfere with chemotherapy. However, capsular contraction is more common if the tissue is irradiated, so if post-mastectomy radiation is planned, reconstruction is often delayed.

breast self-exam (BSE) A procedure in which a woman examines her breasts thoroughly to detect any changes or suspicious lumps. For many years experts recommended that women examine their own breasts each month; in the spring of 2003 the AMERICAN CANCER SOCIETY announced it no longer recommends that women perform breast self-exams. In part, this change is based on recent studies that failed to show that regular breast self-exams saved lives. Since finding a lump on a self-exam can dramatically increase a woman's anxiety level, some experts think the exam actually does more harm than good. If a woman does not perform breast self-exams, she probably should not start; if she does examine her breasts regularly, experts now say she can consider stopping. Women at high risk should consult with their doctors; BSE may be more useful with these women.

Should women still choose to examine their own breasts, exams should be practiced at the end of the menstrual period or seven days after the start of the period and be performed monthly at the same time. When doing a breast self-exam, it is important to remember that all women's breasts are different and that changes can occur because of aging, the menstrual cycle, pregnancy, menopause, or use of birth control pills or other hormones. It is normal for the breasts to feel a little lumpy and uneven, especially immediately before or during a menstrual period. Women older than age 40 should be aware that even if they examine their own breasts each month, they still need to have regularly scheduled screening mammograms and clinical breast exams by a health professional.

How to Perform a Breast Self-Exam

In the wake of its new recommendations against the requirement for BSEs, the American Cancer Society also changed its recommended procedure for doing a BSE. These changes represent an extensive review of the medical literature and input from an expert advisory group.

There is evidence that the woman's position (lying down), area felt, pattern of coverage of the breast, and use of different amounts of pressure increase the sensitivity of BSE.

The American Cancer Society recommends the following method for BSE:

1. The woman should lie down and place her right arm behind her head. (The exam is done while lying down because in this position, the breast tissue spreads evenly over the chest wall and it is as thin as possible, making it much easier to feel all the breast tissue.)
2. Next, the woman should use the finger pads of her three middle fingers on her left hand to feel for lumps in the right breast. Overlapping dime-sized circular motions of the finger pads should be used to feel the breast tissue.
3. The woman should use three different levels of pressure to feel all the breast tissue. Light pressure is needed to feel the tissue closest to the skin; medium pressure to feel a little deeper; and firm pressure to feel the tissue closest to the chest and ribs. A firm ridge in the lower curve of each breast is normal. If a woman is not sure how hard to press, she should talk with a doctor or nurse. Each pressure level should be used to feel the breast tissue before moving on to the next spot.

4. Next, the woman should move around the breast in an up-and-down pattern starting at an imaginary line drawn straight down the side from the underarm and moving across the breast to the middle of the chest bone (sternum or breastbone). The entire breast area should be checked, moving down until only the ribs are felt, and up to the neck or collar bone. Evidence suggests that the up-and-down pattern (or the vertical pattern) is the most effective way to cover the entire breast and not miss any breast tissue.
5. The exam should be repeated on the left breast, using the finger pads of the right hand.
6. Finally, while standing in front of a mirror with hands pressing firmly down on the hips, the woman should look at her breasts for any changes of size, shape, contour, or dimpling. (Pressing down on the hips contracts the chest wall muscles and enhances any breast changes.)
7. Each underarm should be examined while sitting up or standing and with the arm only slightly raised, to easily feel in this area. Raising the arm straight up tightens the tissue in this area and makes it very difficult to examine.

During a monthly breast self-exam, the appearance of any of the following symptoms should be called to the immediate attention of a trained medical professional:

- Lumps, hard knot, or thickening in any part of the breast
- Unusual swelling, warmth, redness, or darkening that does not recede
- Change in the size or shape of your breast
- Dimpling or puckering of the skin of the breast
- An itchy, scaly sore or rash on the nipple
- Pulling in of the nipple or other parts of the breast
- Nipple discharge that starts suddenly
- Pain in one spot that does not vary with the monthly cycle

Brief Pain Inventory   A questionnaire used to measure pain.

CA 15-3 A marker in the blood for malignant tumors that may be measurable in some patients who have recurrent BREAST CANCER. Levels are rarely elevated in early-stage breast cancer.

CA 15-3 has been evaluated for its ability to determine diagnosis and prognosis, monitor therapy, and predict recurrence of breast cancer after primary treatment of breast cancer. Although many studies have shown that the incidence of high levels of CA 15-3 in the blood increases with more advanced stages of disease, until there is better evidence of clinical benefit, experts say that present data are insufficient to recommend routine use of the CA 15-3 test.

Nine percent of women with stage I, and 19 percent of women with stage II, breast cancer have high CA 15-3 levels. The incidence of abnormal values increases to 38 percent and 75 percent for patients at stages III and IV, respectively. However, low CA 15-3 levels do not mean that breast cancer has *not* spread, and a given CA 15-3 level cannot be used to determine the stage of disease.

When CA 15-3 is evaluated before surgery for patients who have primary breast cancer, levels have not correlated with prognosis. Still, very high CA 15-3 levels tend to indicate advanced disease, and a value five to 10 times normal could alert a physician that the patient's cancer may have spread and CAT scans and bone scans should be considered to make sure the liver, lungs and bones are healthy.

Cancers of the ovary, lung, and prostate may also raise CA 15-3 levels, as may certain noncancerous conditions, such as benign breast or ovarian disease, endometriosis, pelvic inflammatory disease, hepatitis, pregnancy, and breast-feeding.

CA 27-29 A tumor marker, similar to CA 15-3, found in the blood of most patients with breast cancer.

CA 27-29 levels also can rise in the presence of cancers of the liver, colon, stomach, kidney, lung, ovary, pancreas, and uterus. Higher levels also occur in certain nonmalignant conditions, such as pregnancy, ovarian CYSTS, benign breast disease, kidney disease, and liver disease.

As with other markers, routine use of this blood test for women with a history of breast cancer is not recommended. However, if a woman has worrisome symptoms (shortness of breath, bone pain, or weight loss), CA 27-29 in conjunction with scans may help determine if the breast cancer has returned. CA 27-29 also can be used to follow response to therapy.

CA 125 A tumor marker sometimes found in an increased amount in the blood that may suggest the presence of ovarian cancer.

However, CA 125 levels may also be elevated by cancers of the pancreas, liver, lung, and digestive tract. Noncancerous conditions that can cause elevated CA 125 levels include endometriosis, pelvic inflammatory disease, peritonitis, pancreatitis and liver disease, and any condition that inflames the tissue surrounding the lungs and chest cavity. Normal menstruation and pregnancy can also cause an increase in the level of CA 125.

cachexia The loss of body weight and muscle mass common among patients with cancer.

caffeine A mild stimulant found in coffee, tea, chocolate, and many soft drinks, in addition to many over-the-counter medications. Several large-scale studies investigating the link between caffeine and cancer risk have been inconclusive, but research by the NATIONAL CANCER INSTITUTE suggests that caffeine is not related to BREAST CANCER.

calcification Deposits of calcium in the tissues. Macrocalcifications are large deposits of calcium that are usually not related to cancer. On the other hand, microcalcifications are specks of calcium that may be found in an area of rapidly dividing cells, which may be a sign of cancer when many are grouped together. Calcification in the breast can be seen on a MAMMOGRAM but cannot be detected by physical examination. Calcifications may occur with both benign and malignant changes, so when they are found on a mammogram the radiologist may decide to just watch them by repeating the mammogram in six to 12 months, or may recommend a biopsy. Most biopsies of calcifications will be benign.

calcium See DAIRY FOODS.

calcium channel blockers Drugs used to treat high blood pressure and heart disease. Some calcium channel blockers have been linked to an increased risk of BREAST CANCER in older women. In one study, postmenopausal women who took calcium channel blockers had twice the risk of developing breast cancer than other women. However, there was no link between other high blood pressure drugs and breast cancer risk. The study primarily looked at short-acting calcium channel blockers and not the longer-acting variety used by most Americans. Longer-acting varieties have a slower absorption rate and are taken only once a day.

The National Institutes of Health urged patients not to stop using them without consulting their physician. Officials note that the dangers of uncontrolled high blood pressure may outweigh any possible cancer risk. They also stress that these are preliminary findings from an observational study with a small number of cases. The findings do not establish a causal relationship between calcium blocker use and breast cancer.

Other observational analyses also have indicated a link between short-acting calcium channel block-

ers and cancer risk in older persons. Studies in the August 24, 1996, issue of *The Lancet* and the July 1996 issue of the *American Journal of Hypertension* found a significantly greater risk of cancer from short-acting calcium channel blockers than from other high blood pressure drugs such as beta-blockers and angiotensin-converting enzyme (ACE) inhibitors. Short-acting calcium channel blockers also have been linked with an increased risk of death of heart attack. This evidence led the NHLBI to warn physicians in September 1995 that one particular calcium channel blocker—short-acting nifedipine—should be prescribed only with great caution because of the increased risk of death from its use.

Ongoing, randomized, controlled clinical studies of this issue are continuing, including the government sponsored ALLHAT (Antihypertensive and Lipid-Lowering Treatment to Prevent Heart Attack Trial). ALLHAT includes only a longer-acting calcium channel blocker.

cancer A general term used to describe more than 100 different types of uncontrolled growth of abnormal cells. A cancer cell divides and reproduces abnormally. It invades and destroys surrounding tissue, leaves the original site, and travels via lymph or blood systems to other parts of the body, where it begins new cancerous tumors—a process referred to as metastasis.

Cancer Care, Inc. A national nonprofit agency founded in 1944 that offers free emotional support, information, financial assistance, and practical help to patients and their families. Services are provided by oncology social workers and are available in person, over the telephone, and through the agency's Web site.

As the oldest and largest national nonprofit agency devoted to offering professional services, Cancer Care has helped more than 2 million people nationwide through its toll-free counseling line and teleconference programs, office-based services, and Internet support. All services are provided free and are available to people of any age, with any type of cancer, at any stage of the disease.

A section of the Cancer Care Web site and some publications are available in Spanish, and staff can respond to calls and e-mails in Spanish. For contact information, see Appendix I.

CancerFax A service sponsored by the NATIONAL CANCER INSTITUTE (NCI) that provides summaries of cancer information (in English or Spanish), via fax machines. NCI fact sheets on various cancer topics, as well as other NCI information, are also available through CancerFax. CancerFax does not provide listings of clinical trials.

CancerFax can be accessed 24 hours a day, seven days a week, by anyone in the United States by dialing (800) 624-2511 from a touch-tone phone or from the telephone on a fax machine and following the recorded instructions. Anyone who is calling from outside the United States may use the local number (301-402-5874). For a fact sheet that explains how to use CancerFax, consumers may call the CANCER INFORMATION SERVICE at (800) 4-CANCER.

Cancer Genetics Network A national network of centers specializing in the study of inherited predisposition to cancer. It supports collaborative investigations on the genetic basis of cancer susceptibility, ways to integrate this new knowledge into medical practice, and methods to address the psychosocial, ethical, legal, and public health issues.

The network includes the following:

• Carolina–Georgia Cancer Genetics Network Center (Duke University Medical Center, Emory University, and the University of North Carolina/Chapel Hill)
• Georgetown University Medical Center's Cancer Genetics Network Center (Georgetown University Lombardi Cancer Center, Washington, D.C.)
• Mid-Atlantic Cancer Genetics Network Center (Johns Hopkins University and the Greater Baltimore Medical Center)
• Northwest Cancer Genetics Network (Fred Hutchinson Cancer Research Center in Seattle and University of Washington School of Medicine in Seattle)
• Rocky Mountain Cancer Genetics Coalition (University of Utah, University of New Mexico, and University of Colorado)

• Texas Cancer Genetics Consortium (M. D. Anderson Cancer Center, Health Science Center at San Antonio, Southwestern Medical Center at Dallas, and Baylor College of Medicine)
• University of Pennsylvania Cancer Genetics Network
• UCI–UCSD Cancer Genetics Network Center (University of California/Irvine and University of California/San Diego)
• Informatics Technology Group (provides supporting information)

Cancer Hope Network A nonprofit organization that provides support to cancer patients and their families by matching them with trained volunteers who have had and recovered from a similar cancer experience. Matches are based on the type and stage of cancer, treatments, side effects, and other factors such as age and gender.

This program was based on the belief that matching cancer patients with someone who had recovered from a similar experience could make a real difference in their own fight. It is available to all cancer patients and their families from anywhere in the United States at no cost. After patients contact the organization and discuss their situation, they are matched with an appropriate volunteer who has recovered from the same cancer.

Patients may contact the group at any point, but ideally they should be matched with a volunteer before treatment, to give them a chance to discuss any fears and questions about treatment. However, the program benefits patients at all stages of their cancer experience.

Volunteers are former patients who have survived a cancer experience and who want to help others as they deal with the disease; they have been off treatment for at least one year and have gone through extensive training before their first patient visit. For contact information, see Appendix I.

Cancer Information and Counseling Line A toll-free telephone service operated by professional counselors who provide up-to-date medical information, emotional support through short-term counseling, and resource referrals to callers nationwide between the hours of 8:30 A.M. and 5 P.M. MST. Individuals may also submit questions about cancer and request resources via e-mail. For contact information, see Appendix I.

Cancer Information Service   A service sponsored by the NATIONAL CANCER INSTITUTE to interpret research findings for the public and to provide personalized responses to specific questions about cancer. Consumers can reach the Cancer Information Service (CIS) by calling (1-800-422-6237) or by visiting the Web site (http://cis.nci.nih.gov).

Cancer Legal Resource Center   An organization that provides information on cancer-related legal issues to people with cancer and others impacted by the disease. A joint program of Loyola Law School and the Western Law Center for Disability Rights, the center offers outreach to cancer support groups, cancer survivors, and caregivers. It also provides speakers for outreach programs at hospitals, community centers, and cancer organizations and for employers.

The center also connects patients with volunteer attorneys and other professionals who can furnish additional legal information. It trains law students to appreciate and understand the legal needs of people who are battling cancer and of cancer survivors. The organization works with major cancer centers in Los Angeles but accepts calls from the greater Los Angeles area, Orange County, and outside California. For contact information, see Appendix I.

CancerMail   CancerMail is a service of the NATIONAL CANCER INSTITUTE that provides comprehensive cancer information summaries and other related information via e-mail. To obtain a contents list, consumers can send an e-mail to cancermail@cips.nci.nih.gov with the word *help* in the body of the message. CancerMail responds by sending a contents list via e-mail. Instructions for ordering documents through e-mail are also provided.

CancerNet   A Web site that provides cancer information from the NATIONAL CANCER INSTITUTE. Topics covered include treatment options, clinical trials, reduction of cancer risk, and means of coping

with cancer. Information on support groups, financial assistance, and educational materials are also available. The Web site address for CancerNet is http://cancernet.nci.nih.gov.

Cancer Research Foundation of America   (CRFA) A nonprofit group that seeks to prevent cancer by funding research and providing educational materials on early detection and nutrition. The group focuses on cancers that can be prevented through lifestyle changes or early detection followed by prompt treatment, including cancers of the breast, cervix, colon/rectum, lung, prostate, skin, and testicles.

When CRFA began its work in 1987, prevention was not regarded as a major strategy in the war against cancer. Scientists focused on discovering new cancer treatments rather than thinking about ways to prevent the disease from developing.

Today, prevention research is recognized as essential to the fight against cancer. Now that scientists better understand how tumors develop, they are learning ways that people can reduce their cancer risks. Since its inception, the foundation has provided funding to more than 200 scientists at more than 100 leading academic institutions across the country. For contact information, see Appendix I.

Cancer Survivors Network   A telephone- and Internet-based service for cancer survivors, their families, caregivers, and friends. The telephone component gives survivors and families access to prerecorded discussions. The Web site offers live on-line chat sessions, virtual support groups, prerecorded talk shows, and personal stories. Cancer Survivors Network is supported by the AMERICAN CANCER SOCIETY. For contact information, see Appendix I.

cancerTrials   A Web site sponsored by the NATIONAL CANCER INSTITUTE that provides information and news about cancer research. The primary mission of cancerTrials is to help people consider clinical trials as an option when making cancer care decisions. The site can be accessed at http://cancertrials.nci.nih.gov.

candidiasis A condition in which a yeast (*Candida albicans*) grows out of control in moist skin areas of the body. Also called thrush or moniliasis, the condition usually affects the mouth, but it can appear under the breasts or in the groin; rarely, it may spread throughout the body.

The yeast that causes candidiasis naturally grows in both the vagina and the mouth, where it is usually kept under control by bacteria present in the body. However, the yeast may grow if the bacteria are destroyed by an antibiotic or a person is taking drugs that affect the immune system, such as cancer CHEMOTHERAPY.

Symptoms

Infection of the mouth causes white-colored raised patches that usually do not cause pain or itching. However, the yeast overgrowth affects the taste buds. In skin folds or with diaper rash, it forms an itchy red rash with flaky white patches and may burn or sting.

Treatment

Topical or oral antifungal drugs usually clear up the infection, but it may recur. Compresses with Burow solution, plenty of air, and infrared heat lamps to dry the affected parts may help.

Eating yogurt (eight ounces daily) with active *Lactobacillus acidophilus* reduces the colonization of the vagina and mouth and may decrease recurrent yeast infections.

capecitabine See XELODA.

capsaicin A component of cayenne and red pepper used on the skin to treat peripheral nerve pain, such as that in POSTMASTECTOMY PAIN SYNDROME.

carcinoembryonic antigen (CEA) A class of antigen normally found in everyone's blood in small amount that may appear at higher levels in people who have certain types of cancer, including BREAST CANCER. CEA was originally isolated from colon tumors, and is commonly used to follow patients with that disease.

However, this is not a test specific for cancer, because high CEA levels can also occur in non-cancerous conditions such as inflammatory bowel disease, pancreatitis, and liver disease. Tobacco use can also contribute to higher-than-normal levels of CEA.

carcinoma The most common type of cancer, it may arise from any organ: skin, breast, lung, colon, pancreas, and many others. Cancers other than carcinomas include the rare SARCOMA (which begins in connective tissue), lymphomas (cancers of the lymph system), and leukemias (cancers of the blood).

carcinoma in situ An early stage of cancer development, when malignant cells have not invaded surrounding tissue. This is usually highly curable with surgery.

carotenoid A substance, found in yellow and orange fruits and vegetables and in dark-green, leafy vegetables, that may reduce the risk of developing cancer. The most widespread pigments in the natural world, carotenoids play an important role in the colorful appearance of many plants and animals, including red peppers, tomatoes, paprika, flamingos, canaries, ladybugs, and salmon.

The color-producing properties of carotenoids are so powerful that many manufactured products, such as soft drinks, use carotenoids as coloring (although in such low concentrations that they do not produce much nutritional benefit). The most common individual carotenoid found naturally is BETA-CAROTENE, a yellow-orange pigment that lends its color to carrots, sweet potatoes, and other fruits and vegetables. Beta-carotene is a provitamin A carotenoid; that means that it is a type of carotenoid that the body can easily convert into vitamin A. In recent years, studies have linked lower levels of carotenoids with a decreased risk of several different kinds of cancer.

Beta-carotene pills, lutein pills, and other carotenoids can be found at health food stores and supermarkets alongside other supplements. However, experts caution that scientists still do not really understand how carotenoids work as preventative agents. Although studies indicate that a diet rich in fruits and vegetables may decrease risk of a wide variety of cancers, scientists still do not know precisely how carotenoids reduce cancer risk and how they may interact with other agents. In addition, studies on the effects of carotenoids supplementing the diet with ambiguous results. For example, one study focusing on the use of supplements of beta-carotene and alpha-tocopherol (a form of vitamin E), published in the *New England Journal of Medicine* in 1994, found that smokers who received beta-carotene supplements had an 18 percent higher incidence of lung cancer and an 8 percent higher mortality rate than did smokers who received placebo.

causes of breast cancer   Scientists have identified many factors that contribute to the development of BREAST CANCER, including AGE, FAMILY HISTORY, defective genes (*BRCA1/BRCA2*), ALCOHOL, DIET, and excessive ESTROGEN exposure (including early onset of menstruation and no pregnancies), and obesity. Avoiding these risk factors whenever possible could have a significant effect on an individual's chance of getting breast cancer.

See also CARCINOGENS.

cellulitis   Infection that occurs in soft tissues. A woman who has lymph nodes removed during surgery for breast cancer has an increased risk for cellulitis in the arm on that side. Cellulitis causes pain, swelling, redness and warmth. The infection must be treated immediately with antibiotics. Episodes of cellulitis predispose a patient to LYM-PHEDEMA.

c-erbB-2   Another name for the ONCOGENE called *HER-2/NEU.*

chemotherapy   The use of drugs to control cancer by interfering with the growth or production of malignant cells. Chemotherapy for BREAST CANCER is usually a combination of drugs that may be given in a pill or by injection, usually in cycles followed by a period of time for recovery, followed by another course of drugs. Treatment time when given as adjuvant chemotherapy after surgery may range between three to six months.

Commonly used drug combinations in the adjuvant treatment of breast cancer are CA (cyclophosphamide and ADRIAMYCIN), CA with a TAXANE (taxol or taxotere), CAF (Cytoxan, Adriamycin and fluorouracil), and CMF (Cytoxan, methotrexate and fluorouracil).

Chemotherapy treatment is also given to treat metastatic disease. There are many chemotherapy drugs used to treat that illness. Side effects of chemotherapy vary—some regimens are intense and others are easily tolerated, but they are all given as outpatient treatments, and side effects are generally well managed.

When given to treat metastatic disease, it is important to understand that the major goal is to improve quality of life. There may be some increase in life expectancy with chemotherapy, but the aim is to keep symptoms from cancer at a minimum and the symptoms caused by the chemotherapy at a minimum as well.

History

The first drugs used as chemotherapy agents were not used to treat cancer but as part of chemical warfare. During mustard gas experiments after World War I and during World War II, a large number of soldiers were accidentally exposed to the gas. They were subsequently discovered to have unusually low white blood counts. It did not take scientists long to realize that a drug that damaged rapidly growing white blood cells might also damage rapidly growing malignant cells. Several patients with lymphoma during the 1940s were thus injected with mustard gas, and they experienced a remarkable (albeit temporary) improvement.

Types of Chemotherapy

Chemotherapy drugs are divided into different types, depending on how they work and what parts of the cell cycle they affect. Chemotherapy types typically used to treat breast cancer include

- ALKYLATING AGENTS
- ANTIMETABOLITES
- ANTITUMOR ANTIBIOTICS
- Mitotic inhibitors

Nolvadex (tamoxifen citrate): Approved in 1998 to reduce the incidence of breast cancer in women at high risk, it received additional approval in 2000 for use in women who have ductal carcinoma in situ (DCIS). After breast surgery and radiation, Nolvadex is indicated to reduce the risk of invasive breast cancer.

Taxol (paclitaxel): Taxol received approval in 1999 for adjuvant treatment of node-positive breast cancer given in sequence with standard doxorubicin-containing combination chemotherapy. In studies, there was an overall favorable effect on disease-free and overall survival rates in the total population of patients who had receptor-positive and receptor-negative tumors, but the benefit has been specifically demonstrated only in patients who have estrogen- and progesterone-receptor-negative tumors.

Taxotere (docetaxel): This drug was first approved in 1996 for the treatment of locally advanced breast cancer that has progressed or relapsed during anthracycline-based treatment. It received additional approval in 2001 for treating patients whose breast cancer has spread throughout the body (metastatic breast cancer), despite treatment with an anthracycline chemotherapy such as Adriamycin and doxorubicin.

Xeloda (capecitabine): This drug received accelerated approval in 1998 for treatment of metastatic breast cancer resistant to both paclitaxel and anthracycline-based chemotherapy or for patients resistant to paclitaxel for whom anthracycline therapy may be contraindicated. It subsequently was approved in 2001 for treating patients with metastatic breast cancer whose disease has progressed after treatment with an anthracycline-based therapy (such as Adriamycin and doxorubicin).

How It Works

Chemotherapy drugs interfere with the ability of cancer cells throughout the body to divide and reproduce themselves. Whereas normal cells typically divide in very controlled ways, malignant cells grow and reproduce in a rapid, haphazard way. Chemotherapy drugs are taken up by rapidly dividing cells—which in addition to cancerous cells include some healthy cells that normally divide quickly, such as those in the lining of the mouth, the bone marrow, the hair follicles, and the digestive system. However, whereas healthy cells can repair the damage caused by chemotherapy, cancer cells cannot—and so they eventually die.

Chemotherapy drugs damage cancer cells in different ways. If a combination of drugs is used, each drug is chosen because of its individual effects. Chemotherapy must be carefully planned so that it destroys more and more of the cancer cells during the course of treatment, but does not destroy the normal cells and tissues. With some types of cancer, chemotherapy can destroy all the cancer cells and cure the disease.

Adjuvant therapy To reduce the chance of cancer returning, chemotherapy may be given after surgery, when all the visible cancer has been removed, or after RADIATION THERAPY, so that if any cancer cells remain that are too small to see, they can be destroyed. Chemotherapy is designed to kill any tiny cancer cells that may have been left behind. Chemotherapy in this setting is given to increase the number of patients who are cured of their disease.

Neoadjuvant therapy Chemotherapy also can be given before surgery to shrink a tumor and make it easier to remove. This is usually given to people whose cancer cannot be removed easily during an operation.

Chemotherapy in metastatic disease Chemotherapy is also used to treat patients whose breast cancer has spread, as a way of increasing life and improving the quality of life. In this case, side effects become extremely important, since patients will be taking chemotherapy for most of the rest of their lives, and they need to be able to live a near-normal life. The goal in this case is to minimize the side effects of chemotherapy and minimize the symptoms caused by the cancer.

There are many more drugs available for treatment of metastatic disease than for adjuvant chemotherapy. However, not all patients respond to one particular type of chemotherapy, and even if there is a response, at some point the vast majority of breast cancers become resistant to the chemotherapy and the drugs need to be stopped or changed.

High-Dose Chemotherapy

For some types of cancer that have a high risk of recurrence, a course of very-high-dose chemotherapy is given after an initial dosage of standard chemotherapy. As very high doses of chemotherapy normally destroy the bone marrow, the bone marrow is replaced after chemotherapy. This is done by using stem cells that have been collected from the bone marrow or blood before high-dose chemotherapy. Bone marrow transplants are no more effective than standard chemotherapy, so they are no longer commonly used.

How it is given Chemotherapy may be administered in different ways, depending on the type of cancer and the particular chemotherapy drugs used. It is most often given in pill or liquid form by mouth or intravenously. It may sometimes be given intramuscularly, subcutaneously (under the skin), intra-arterially (into the artery), intrathecally (into the central nervous system through the cerebrospinal fluid), intrapleurally (into the chest cavity), intraperitoneally (into the abdomen), intravesically (into the bladder), or intralesionally (into the tumor itself).

Intravenous Chemotherapy for breast cancer is often given by injection into a vein, a procedure that generally takes from half an hour to a few hours, or sometimes up to a few days.

Ports If it is difficult for the nurses to place an IV, semipermanent or permanent catheters can be inserted into the veins. A PICC line is a slender plastic tube called a catheter that is threaded into a large vein in the arm and on into the large vein near the heart. It is taped in place on the patient's arm, covered with a dressing, and left for weeks to months.

A PORT is a catheter placed under the skin in the upper arm or chest with a catheter running through the veins toward the heart. The port is completely under the skin and can be left in place for many months.

PICCs and ports are generally very safe, placed by a radiologist or surgeon, and require little care (PICC) or no care (port). They do, however, need to be flushed every few days (PICC) or once a month (port). Occasionally these lines may cause blood clots or infections.

Frequency

How often and how long a patient gets chemotherapy depend on the type of cancer, the treatment goals, the particular drugs used, and the patient's body's response to treatment. Chemotherapy is often given in cycles of treatment periods with rest periods in between, to give the body a chance to recover. Adjuvant chemotherapy is given for a definite period of time; given for metastatic disease, duration depends on response and side effects.

Chemotherapy on the Job

Most people can continue working while receiving chemotherapy, although they may need to change their work schedule if the drugs make them feel tired or sick. Federal and state laws require employers to let patients work a flexible schedule to meet treatment needs. Social workers and the staff of congressional or state representatives can provide information on state and federal laws that guarantee patient protections.

Side Effects

Different chemotherapy drugs cause a variety of side effects that may vary from person to person and treatment to treatment. Almost all side effects are short term and gradually disappear once the treatment has stopped. The main areas of the body that may be affected by chemotherapy are those where normal cells rapidly divide and grow, such as the lining of the mouth, digestive system, skin, hair, and bone marrow.

However, sometimes chemotherapy can cause permanent changes or damage to the heart, lungs, nerves, kidneys, reproductive organs, or other organs. Certain types of chemotherapy may have delayed effects (such as the occurrence of a second type of cancer) that do not appear until many years later. Patients need to balance their concerns about permanent effects with the immediate threat of cancer.

Great progress has been made in preventing and treating some of chemotherapy's common as well as rare serious side effects. Many new drugs and treatment methods destroy cancer more effectively while doing less harm to the body's healthy cells.

Fatigue, infection, and unusual bleeding are all very common side effects, because chemotherapy lowers the number of blood cells produced by the bone marrow—white blood cells that are essential for fighting infections, red blood cells that carry oxygen, and platelets that help clot the blood and prevent bleeding.

Fatigue This is a very common side effect of chemotherapy that patients report as being quite different from normal tiredness. FATIGUE caused by chemotherapy can begin suddenly and may be experienced as lack of energy, weakness, and a complete inability to work or think. Moreover, it seems unrelated to activity and does not improve with rest.

Fatigue associated with chemotherapy is related to low blood cell counts, stress, depression, poor appetite, lack of exercise, and many other factors. Chemotherapy can interfere with the bone marrow's ability to make red blood cells, which carry oxygen to all parts of the body. When there are too few red blood cells, body tissues do not get enough oxygen to do their work and patients may become tired and lethargic. Because the amount of oxygen being carried around the body is lower, patients also may become breathless. These are all symptoms of anemia (low hemoglobin level in the blood). People who have anemia may also feel dizzy and light-headed and have aching muscles and joints. The tiredness fades gradually once the chemotherapy has ended, but some people find that they still feel tired a year or more afterward.

Oncologists order regular blood tests to measure hemoglobin during chemotherapy, and a blood transfusion can be given if the hemoglobin level falls too low. The extra red cells in the blood transfusion very quickly pick up the oxygen from the lungs and take it around the body; patients then feel more energetic, and the breathlessness improves. There are drugs that can be given to treat anemia; sometimes iron supplements are required. Some studies have also suggested that maintaining a moderate level of physical exercise (such as walking) can help prevent fatigue.

Nausea/vomiting Although many patients fear the NAUSEA and vomiting that have historically been reported as a side effect of chemotherapy, in fact drugs used today have made these side effects far less common.

Because of very effective antinausea medications, many women do not get sick at all during their treatment for breast cancer, and if they do get sick, illness is quite mild. It is particularly important that patients closely follow their physicians' guidelines regarding antinausea medication. This medication is usually given together with IV chemotherapy; patients can then take additional antinausea medication at home *before nausea begins.* Once nausea starts, controlling it is far more difficult. Low doses of steroids can be helpful in reducing nausea and vomiting.

Antinausea medications that are highly effective include lorazepam (Ativan), prochlorperazine (Compazine), promethazine (Anergan), metoclopramide (Reglan), dexamethasone (Decadron), ondansetron (Zofran), and granisetron (Kytril).

Chemotherapy drugs cause nausea and vomiting because they tend to irritate the stomach lining; irritation stimulates nerves in the vomiting center in the brain. Certain chemotherapy medications are more likely to cause nausea and vomiting, including the following:

- Carboplatin
- Carmustine
- Cisplatin
- Cyclophosphamide
- Cytarabine
- Dacarbazine
- Dactinomycin
- Doxorubicin
- Etoposide
- Lomustine
- Mechlorethamine
- Melphalan
- Methotrexate
- Plicamycin
- Procarbazine
- Streptozocin

The reaction to chemotherapy varies from person to person and from drug to drug. If patients are going to feel sick, the symptoms usually begin a few minutes to several hours after chemotherapy, depending on the drugs given. The sickness may last for a few hours or for several days. Some people never vomit or feel nauseous. Others feel mildly nauseated most of the time; some become severely nauseated for a limited time during or after a treatment. Certain risk factors that influence severity of nausea include the person's previous experience with motion sickness, youth (older patients have less nausea), alcohol use, and bad experiences with nausea and vomiting.

To prevent problems, women should

- Avoid big meals so the stomach does not feel too full. Eating small meals throughout the day is better than eating a few large meals.
- Drink liquids at least an hour before or after mealtime, instead of with meals.
- Eat and drink slowly.
- Avoid sweet, fried, or fatty foods.
- Eat foods cold or at room temperature to avoid strong smells. (Many women swear by cold white foods, such as cold chicken or ice cream.)
- Chew food well for easier digestion.
- Drink cool, clear, unsweetened fruit juices, such as apple or grape juice. Avoid carbonated beverages, which can burn sensitive throats.
- Suck on ice cubes.
- Try to avoid bothersome odors such as cooking smells, smoke, or perfume.
- Prepare and freeze meals in advance.
- Rest in a chair after eating but avoid lying flat for at least two hours after a meal.
- Breathe deeply and slowly during bouts of nausea.
- Use relaxation techniques.
- Avoid eating for at least a few hours before treatment, if nausea usually occurs during chemotherapy.

Appetite/weight change Patients who are receiving chemotherapy may lose their appetite and lose weight because of nausea and vomiting, and the drugs can also directly affect appetite by affecting the body's metabolism. In severe cases, loss of appetite can lead to CACHEXIA, a form of malnutrition. In general, appetite returns a few weeks after chemotherapy is completed. If loss of appetite is severe, doctors can prescribe medications that may improve the condition.

However, adjuvant chemotherapy often causes women to gain weight. Many factors contribute to this; often the nausea from chemotherapy is controlled by eating, metabolism may change, and many women stop exercising.

Bone marrow suppression Chemotherapy damages the blood-cell-producing tissues of the bone marrow, triggering a condition called bone marrow suppression. While chemotherapy targets rapidly-dividing cancerous cells, it also affects normal rapidly-dividing cells in the body, such as those produced in bone marrow tissues. Until the bone marrow recovers from the damage, the patient has abnormally low numbers of white blood cells, red blood cells, and platelets.

Instead, new blood cells are temporarily prevented from forming in the marrow.

Normally, blood cells are constantly replaced as they wear out (white blood cells last about six hours, platelets last about 10 days, and red blood cells last about four months). When chemotherapy is given, however, worn-out cells are not replaced, so blood counts begin to drop. However, blood cell counts do not drop as soon as chemotherapy is given, because the drugs do not affect cells circulating in the blood. The type of chemotherapy drug and the strength of the dose influence the effect on blood cells.

In general, white blood cells and platelets drop to their lowest level within one or two weeks after a dose of chemotherapy. Because red blood cells last longer, their levels drop more slowly. The side effects of low levels of various types of blood cells peak when the blood counts are lowest.

Low white blood cell count Because white blood cells fight infection, when a person's white cell count drops during chemotherapy, the patient becomes more vulnerable to infection. Neutrophils are the most common subtype of white blood cells, and they are an important defense against infection. The normal range of neutrophils is between 2,500 and 6,000 cells per cubic millimeter; a patient who has a neutrophil count of 1,000 or less is considered to be at risk for infection; and a patient whose count is less than 500 is considered to have a severely low count. Because the risk of infection is great, chemotherapy treatments are delayed if a person has a very low white blood count.

When counts are low during chemotherapy, an infection can begin in almost any part of the body, including the mouth, skin, lungs, urinary tract, rectum, or reproductive tract. Fever is an important first sign of infection; for this reason, patients are usually told to call their doctor or nurse if they have a fever of 100.5°F or above. Other signs of infection include sore throat, cough or shortness of breath, nasal congestion, shaking chills, burning during urination, and redness or swelling of the skin. If patients have an infection when their white blood cell levels are very low, they may need antibiotics.

Sometimes, drugs called hematopoietic growth factors can help the bone marrow make more white blood cells. Growth factors (also called COLONY-STIMULATING FACTORS) are sometimes given after chemotherapy treatment to stimulate the bone marrow to produce new white cells quickly, thereby reducing the risk of infection. The most common growth factors used to prevent low white blood cell counts are the short-acting granulocyte colony-stimulating factor (filgrastim [Neupogen]), and the long-acting Neulastin.

Most infections a woman with breast cancer may contract are caused by the bacteria normally found on the skin and in the intestines and genital tract. In some cases, the cause of an infection may not be known.

When the white count is lower than normal, patients can try to prevent infections by taking the following steps:

- Washing hands often during the day, especially before meals or after using the bathroom
- Cleaning the rectal area gently but thoroughly after each bowel movement
- Avoiding people who have communicable diseases (colds, flu, measles, or chicken pox)
- Avoiding crowds
- Avoiding people who have recently received immunizations, such as vaccines for polio, measles, mumps, and rubella (German measles)
- Avoiding nicks when using scissors, needles, or knives; use of an electric shaver instead of a razor can prevent breaks or cuts
- Using a soft toothbrush that will not cut gums
- Taking a warm (not hot) bath, shower, or sponge bath every day
- Cleaning cuts and scrapes immediately with warm water, soap, and an antiseptic

Low red blood count   A person who does not have enough red blood cells is anemic. Normally, blood has between 4.0 and 6.0 million red blood cells per cubic millimeter. Another measurement used is the hematocrit—the percentage of total blood volume occupied by red blood cells. A normal hematocrit range is between 36 percent and 42 percent.

Patients who have anemia feel tired, dizzy, and irritable and experience headaches, shortness of breath, and rapid breathing. Anemia caused by chemotherapy is usually temporary, but sometimes blood transfusions are needed until the bone marrow can begin producing red blood cells again. Alternatively, doctors may prescribe ERYTHROPOI-ETIN (Procrit or Aranesp), a growth factor that boosts production of red blood cells in the bone marrow.

Low platelet count   Anticancer drugs also can compromise the bone marrow's ability to make platelets, the blood cells that help stop bleeding by making blood clot. Low platelet count (called *thrombocytopenia*) may cause a patient to bruise easily, bleed longer than usual after a minor cut, have bleeding gums or nosebleeds, and experience severe internal bleeding. Low platelet counts are temporary, but they can cause serious blood loss if there is an injury. If counts are very low, a platelet transfusion can be given. Transfused platelets do not last long, but a platelet growth factor can be given as a drug for patients with severe thrombocytopenia.

Patients should report to their doctor any symptoms of unexpected bruising, small red spots under the skin, reddish or pinkish urine, black or bloody bowel movements, or bleeding from the gums or nose.

Diarrhea/constipation   DIARRHEA is caused by the damage to rapidly dividing cells in the lining of the digestive system. The amount and duration of diarrhea depend on the type, dosage, and duration of drugs the patient receives. Some of the chemotherapy drugs that cause diarrhea are 5-flu-orouracil, Xeloda, methotrexate, Adriamycin, and docetaxel.

Although many women may think of diarrhea as just an annoyance, in severe cases it can be life threatening and may lead to dehydration, malnutrition, or electrolyte imbalance. If diarrhea occurs, patients may need antidiarrheal medicine, and IV fluids. The chemotherapy dose may need to be changed; in severe cases patients may need to be hospitalized.

In addition, patients who have diarrhea should

- Eat smaller amounts of food but eat more often.
- Avoid high-fiber foods, such as whole grain breads and cereals, raw vegetables, beans, nuts, seeds, popcorn, and fresh and dried fruit.
- Eat low-fiber foods, such as white bread, white rice, noodles, creamed cereals, ripe bananas, canned or cooked fruit without skins, cottage, cheese, yogurt, eggs, mashed or baked potatoes without the skin, pureed vegetables, chicken or turkey without the skin, and fish.
- Avoid coffee, tea, alcohol, sweets, and fried, greasy, or highly spiced foods.
- Avoid milk and milk products (except yogurt);
- Eat more potassium-rich foods (bananas, oranges, potatoes, and peach and apricot nectars).
- Drink plenty of fluids to replace those lost through diarrhea. Mild clear liquids such as apple juice, water, weak tea, or clear broth are best. If diarrhea is severe, liquids such as Gatorade may be recommended.

Some chemotherapy drugs (such as vinblastine or vincristine) also can cause CONSTIPATION, as can other drugs the patient may be taking at the same time (especially narcotic pain and antinausea medications). Some patients may become constipated because they are less active or less well nourished than usual. Dehydration, decreased fluid intake, and depression can all cause constipation. Patients can drink warm or hot fluids to help loosen the bowels, eat high-fiber foods (such as whole wheat bread or fresh fruit). Some patients use a mixture of bran, applesauce, and prune juice to maintain fiber level. Exercise also helps.

Mouth sores   Good oral care is important during cancer treatment, because chemotherapy drugs can cause STOMATITIS and esophagitis—sores in the mouth and throat. In addition to being painful and affecting the appetite, these sores can become infected by the germs in the mouth. Because infec-tions can be hard to fight during chemotherapy and can lead to serious problems, taking every possible step to prevent them is important.

Sores in the throat and mouth usually occur about five to 10 days after treatment. Patients who have not been eating well since beginning chemotherapy are more likely to have mouth sores (either canker sores or the whole mouth may be affected). Mouth sores usually begin with dryness, followed by inflamed gums, mouth, and throat. The tongue may swell, and swallowing and eating may become painful and difficult.

If possible, patients should see a dentist before starting chemotherapy to have teeth cleaned and to take care of any problems, such as cavities, abscesses, gum disease, or poorly fitting dentures. Because chemotherapy can make cavities more likely, the dentist may suggest using a fluoride rinse or gel each day to help prevent decay. Cleaning the teeth regularly and gently with a soft toothbrush helps to keep the mouth clean. If the mouth is very sore, gels, creams, or pastes can be used to paint over the ulcers to reduce the soreness. Baby teething gels may help.

Chemotherapy may alter tastes, which can affect appetite and nutrition. Typically, normal taste returns after the chemotherapy treatment ends.

Hair loss   HAIR LOSS is one of the most common, and worrisome, side effects of chemotherapy. Although a few drugs used to treat breast cancer do not cause hair loss (or the amount of hair lost is slight), most do cause partial or complete reversible hair loss. Chemotherapy affects the rapidly dividing cells of the hair follicles, making hair brittle so that it may break off near the scalp or spontaneously release. This usually begins two to three weeks after the first chemotherapy treatment, although occasionally it can start within a few days.

The amount of hair lost depends on the type of drug or combination of drugs used, the dosage given, and the person's individual reaction to the drug. Body hair may be lost as well, especially if treatment lasts longer than a few months, and some drugs even trigger loss of the eyelashes and eyebrows. Hair lost as a result of chemotherapy almost always grows back once treatment is over.

Many women find that, at least temporarily, their hair grows back a different texture.

Women who have lost their hair during chemotherapy need to take special care of their scalp and any remaining hair. Patients should use mild shampoos, soft hairbrushes, and low heat when drying hair. During chemotherapy, patients should avoid using brush rollers to set hair and should not dye hair or have a permanent. Hair should be cut short, because a shorter style can make remaining hair look thicker and fuller; it also makes hair loss easier to manage if it occurs. Many patients shave their heads before losing hair. This makes the loss psychologically easier.

Once hair loss occurs, patients should use a sunscreen, sunblock, hat, or scarf to protect the scalp from the sun. Some women choose to wear turbans, scarves, caps, wigs, or hairpieces; others leave their head uncovered. Unlike some other side effects of chemotherapy, hair loss is not life threatening, but it can have a devastating psychological impact. Hair loss can cause depression, loss of self-esteem, and even grief reactions.

Experts recommend that women who want a wig should buy one before losing a lot of hair, so the wig is the right color and style. Some women prefer to buy a wig or hairpiece at a specialty shop just for cancer patients. Local chapters of the American Cancer Society and the social work department at many hospitals have more information on wig choices. A hairpiece needed because of cancer treatment is a tax-deductible expense and may be at least partially covered by health insurance.

Skin/nail changes   Some drugs can affect the skin, making it drier or slightly discolored. These changes may be worsened by swimming, especially in chlorinated water. The drugs may also make skin more sensitive to sunlight during and after treatment. Nails may grow more slowly, and white lines may appear. Nails also may become more brittle and flaky. Some types of chemotherapy (such as Taxotere) may cause an uncomfortable lifting up of the nail.

Nerves   Some chemotherapy drugs can affect the nerves in the hands and feet, causing tingling, numbness, or a sensation of pins and needles (peripheral neuropathy). In most cases, this feeling gradually fades after chemotherapy ends, but in severe ones nerves may be permanently damaged.

Nervous system   Some drugs can directly affect the central nervous system (the brain and spinal cord), causing feelings of anxiety and restlessness, dizziness, sleeplessness, headaches, or concentration and memory problems. Other drugs rarely can lead to a loss of the ability to hear high-pitched sound or cause a continuous noise in the ears known as tinnitus.

Vaccinations   Patients who are undergoing chemotherapy should not be given any live virus vaccinations, including vaccines against polio, measles, mumps, rubella (German measles), tuberculosis, yellow fever, or oral typhoid. Killed vaccines that do not pose problems for patients on chemotherapy include vaccinations against the flu, diphtheria, tetanus, meningococcus, hepatitis A or B, rabies, and Japanese encephalitis. However, the recently introduced nasal flu vaccine contains a live virus and should not be given to chemotherapy patients. A killed virus form of the polio and typhoid vaccines is available.

Radiation recall   Some people who have had radiation therapy experience a skin problem during chemotherapy known as radiation recall. In this condition the skin over an area that has received radiation turns red and may blister and peel.

Kidney/bladder problems   When breakdown products from some anticancer drugs are excreted through the kidneys, they can irritate the bladder or cause temporary or permanent damage to the bladder or kidneys. Some anticancer drugs turn the urine orange, red, green, or yellow or give it a strong or medicinelike odor for 24 to 72 hours. The color changes are harmless. Symptoms of kidney damage include headache, lower back pain, weakness, nausea, vomiting, fatigue, high blood pressure, change in urination pattern, urgent need to urinate, and swelling. Patients who have had kidney problems in the past are at higher risk for development of problems during chemotherapy. Patients should always drink plenty of fluids to ensure good urine flow and help prevent problems.

Flu symptoms   Flulike symptoms may bother some patients a few hours to a few days after chemotherapy is administered, especially if they are receiving biological therapy at the same time.

Aching muscles and joints, headache, fatigue, nausea, slight fever (less than 100°F), chills, and poor appetite may last one to three days. Infection (or the cancer itself) also can cause these symptoms.

Liver damage   Chemotherapy drugs are metabolized by the liver, which occasionally can become damaged during cancer treatment. However, this problem is temporary and usually improves once treatment is stopped. Symptoms of liver damage include jaundice (yellowed skin and eyes), fatigue, and pain in the lower right ribs or right upper abdomen.

Older patients and those who have had hepatitis are more likely to develop liver problems after chemotherapy, especially if the drugs include methotrexate, cyclophosphamide (Cytoxan), or doxorubicin (Adriamycin).

Heart problems   Heart damage from adjuvant breast cancer chemotherapy is rare and occurs in less than 1 or 2 percent of patients. Other rare side effects include symptoms of dry cough, ankle swelling, shortness of breath, puffiness, or erratic heartbeats. Patients at higher risk for heart damage include those who have had previous heart problems, high blood pressure, prior radiation to the chest and patients who smoke. Because of the small risk of heart damage, in some patients at risk, assessments are made before chemotherapy. In patients on herceptin, heart damage also may occur, although it is rare. Evaluations of heart function are done periodically during herceptin therapy.

Fluid retention   The body may retain fluid during chemotherapy, which may be caused by hormonal changes as a result of therapy or the cancer itself. Patients may need to avoid table salt and foods that contain a lot of salt. If the problem is severe, a doctor may prescribe a diuretic to help the body get rid of excess fluids.

Infertility   Some chemotherapy treatments may cause temporary or permanent infertility. During chemotherapy, a woman's menstrual periods may become irregular and stop, and hot flushes, dry skin, and vaginal dryness may occur. In many women, after treatment the ovaries start producing eggs again and menstruation returns to normal. Usually, the younger the woman, the more likely she is to become fertile again after treatment. Although chemotherapy may reduce fertility, it is still possible for a woman on chemotherapy to become pregnant during treatment. Pregnancy should be avoided during chemotherapy because the drugs may harm the baby. Therefore barrier methods of contraception (condoms or diaphragm) should be used during therapy. Birth control pills are avoided in women with a history of breast cancer.

Long-term problems   Although most side effects of chemotherapy stop once treatment ends, some patients experience long-term problems related to their treatment for breast cancer. These long-term effects depend on the type of drugs used and whether other treatments (such as radiation) were given.

Some drugs can permanently damage internal organs, such as the heart, reproductive system, or kidneys. Nerves also can be permanently damaged; symptoms may include numbness, tingling, or prickling sensations. These are seen more commonly with platinum drugs or taxanes.

It is also possible that some types of chemotherapy can lead to the development of a second type of cancer through damaged bone marrow; rarely, leukemia or myelodysplastic syndrome (a type of preleukemia) can develop.

Cost

The cost of chemotherapy varies with the kinds and dosages of drugs used, how long and how often they are administered, and whether they are given at home, in an office, or in the hospital. Most health insurance policies cover at least part of the cost of many kinds of chemotherapy. There are also organizations that help with the cost of chemotherapy and with transportation costs. Nurses and social workers have information about these organizations. In some states, Medicaid (which makes health-care services available for people with financial need) may help pay for certain treatments.

chemotherapy, high-dose   An aggressive and grueling treatment for breast cancer that uses dosages of chemotherapy so high that they destroy the patient's BONE MARROW. Recent studies suggest this treatment method offers little or no benefit over standard chemotherapy for women who have the risk of recurrence. The research could signal the end for the expensive and controversial treatment.

High-dose chemotherapy uses many times the normal level of anticancer drugs. Because the treatment kills the bone marrow, the patient must have a transplant of blood-forming stem cells collected from her own blood or bone marrow. The approach became widely used as ADJUVANT TREATMENT breast cancer when preliminary studies suggested it was better than the conventional chemotherapy offered to women after surgery.

But more rigorous studies in the 1990s found that the intensive treatment did not improve the outcome for women whose cancer had spread to other parts of the body. Because of those disappointing results, and the approach is seldom used now outside of medical studies.

childbirth and breast cancer   Women who have had many children have a lower risk of developing BREAST CANCER. Women who have never had children have a higher risk.

childhood events and breast cancer   BREAST CANCER is a disease that may develop and progress over the course of a woman's entire life, beginning in adolescence, when breast cells begin to divide rapidly. Since cells undergoing rapid division are more likely to be damaged by cancer-causing agents, environmental exposures before or during puberty may increase a woman's lifetime risk of development of breast cancer. Also, scientists are studying whether a healthy DIET and good EXERCISE habits in young girls may help to prevent the development of breast cancer later in life. Although it is possible that factors in early life affect the risk of breast cancer, there is very little solid information about what those factors might be and how they could be changed.

Estrogen and Breast Cancer

A woman's risk for breast cancer increases with her exposure to ESTROGEN. Menstruation raises estrogen levels. Therefore, the earlier a girl starts menstruating, the higher her lifetime risk for breast cancer.

Height, weight, diet, exercise, and FAMILY HISTORY may all influence age at menarche. There is a trend toward an earlier age at menarche among girls living in industrialized countries, and taller, heavier girls usually start menstruating earlier than shorter, lighter girls. In addition, the distribution of fat on a girl's body is related to the levels of hormones circulating in her body and may affect the age when she begins menstruating. Girls with fat around their hips may have an earlier menarche than girls with abdominal fat.

Height, weight, and the distribution of body fat are influenced by heredity. However, diet and exercise behavior that helps maintain healthy weight may prevent changes in hormone levels that could promote the development of breast cancer.

Although age at menarche is an established risk factor for breast cancer, doctors do not advise that anyone try to delay the onset of a girl's menstrual periods. The normal establishment of regular menstrual cycles is critical for reproduction. Delaying a girl's menarche by dieting, extreme weight loss, or vigorous and stressful exercise may affect her ability to have children later. Also, emphasis on dieting and weight may contribute to eating disorders such as anorexia and bulimia. Instead, an active lifestyle that allows normal development should be the goal during adolescence.

Childhood Diet

There is no strong evidence supporting an effect of childhood nutrition in the development of breast cancer.

Most studies that have been done to date did not take into account the effect of established risk factors for breast cancer, such as age at menarche or height and weight.

Few studies have assessed the influence of diet during childhood on the risk of development of breast cancer in adulthood. In studies that did, women were asked to remember what they ate as children—a difficult task for anyone.

Dietary Fat

There is conflicting evidence on whether a child's fat consumption through adolescence is a risk factor for the development of breast cancer. Two studies reported no association between fat intake during childhood and the development of breast cancer. Two other studies reported an increased breast cancer risk associated with the consumption of the fat in meat or fried meat.

Vegetarian Diet

Two studies did not show any association between a vegetarian diet during adolescence and the risk of breast cancer in adulthood. Two others demonstrated that girls who ate a vegetarian diet or lots of fiber (found in vegetables, fruits, and whole grains) had lower levels of circulating estrogens.

Exercise

Several studies have reported a decrease in breast cancer risk among women who got regular exercise as adolescents. Exercise may reduce breast cancer risk by decreasing estrogen level, weight, and insulin resistance; by strengthening the immune system; or by raising age at menarche. Athletes usually begin menstruating later than nonathletes. However, the effect of moderate exercise on age at menarche is less clear. Some researchers have reported that girls who are moderately active still have differences in hormone levels and a delay in the onset of menstruation when compared to inactive girls. Others have reported no effect of moderate physical activity on the age at menarche. Differences in the way the researchers assessed physical activity or problems with recall of earlier exercise practices may account for the differences in results. Later age at menarche in athletes may also be due to heredity.

Childhood Obesity

No studies have suggested that adolescent obesity is a risk factor for breast cancer; in fact, it appears that a heavier weight in adolescence may be protective. However, overweight adolescents are more likely to be overweight adults, and adult overweight is a risk factor for postmenopausal breast cancer. Therefore, it is important to establish a healthy lifestyle and healthy weight during adolescence.

Teenage Lifestyle Issues

Although few studies have examined SMOKING during adolescence, one Canadian study found that teenage girls almost double their lifetime risk of breast cancer if they start smoking within five years

of their first menstrual period. Some researchers think that carcinogens in cigarette smoke may cause more damage during adolescence, when the breast cells are rapidly dividing and are thus more vulnerable. Experts think this may be because during puberty, the cells that make up the breast are developing so fast that they are more susceptible to damage caused by the carcinogens in tobacco smoke. While this is not definite, there is clearly an increased risk of cervical cancer in smokers.

ALCOHOL consumption has been identified as a likely risk factor for breast cancer, but the influence of alcohol consumption in adolescence is not clear. Experts are not sure whether onset of drinking at an early age, lifetime alcohol consumption, or the intensity of drinking is most important. Encouraging teenagers not to drink may lessen their lifetime consumption of alcohol.

Studies of oral contraceptive use and breast cancer risk have focused on adult women who started taking BIRTH CONTROL PILLS in their 20s. Today, the Pill is a much more popular form of birth control among teenagers. A few studies have reported that there may be a tiny increase in risk associated with early use of oral contraceptives. However, benefits include avoiding pregnancy and normalizing menstrual cycles.

Radiation

Exposure of the breasts to radiation during adolescence increases the risk of breast cancer. Recent studies have demonstrated that teenagers who received radiation treatment for Hodgkin's disease or X-ray treatment for scoliosis had a higher risk of breast cancer. Today, doctors use a lower dosage of radiation, take X-rays of the spine from the back, and cover the breasts with a lead apron to decrease patient exposure to X-rays. However, women who had this radiation exposure as children or teens must be careful about screening mammography.

cigarettes See SMOKING.

cigars See SMOKING.

clear margins An area of tissue surrounding a tumor that is free of cancer cells. During BREAST CANCER surgery, the surgeon tries to remove the tumor and a wide margin of healthy tissue all around the malignancy. If no cancer cells are found near the edges of the sample, it is said to have "clear margins." After surgery, if the excised tissue is found by the lab to have cancer cells near the margin of healthy tissue, the surgeon often operates again in an attempt to remove a wider margin of healthy tissue around the original tumor.

clinical breast exam (CBE) A physical examination of the breasts to check for changes in the tissue, skin, or nipple performed by a trained health-care provider such as a doctor or nurse. Annual MAMMOGRAMS together with clinical breast exams are the best way to detect breast cancer early, when it can be treated most effectively. Experts recommend that all women age 20 and over should have a clinical breast exam every year; women age 40 and over also should have an annual mammogram.

A trained breast examiner can identify lumps the size of a pea, smaller than a woman can typically find, according to the National Cancer Institute. In addition, a trained examiner can find lumps in areas that are difficult for mammography to reveal, such as near the chest wall.

Many health professionals can perform clinical breast exams, including physicians, nurse practitioners, nurses, and physician assistants. Most women have an exam as part of their annual gynecological visit or routine annual physical exam.

Women who may be at higher risk for breast cancer or have a mother or sister who has been diagnosed with breast cancer should be particularly attentive about getting regular clinical breast exams.

The physician first looks at the woman's breasts to assess any changes in their size or shape. The visual exam should be conducted while the woman assumes various positions because breast tissue looks different in each one. The woman should sit, stand, lie down, raise her arms, let her arms dangle by her side, and press her arms against her hips. The clinician looks at the breasts and moves the finger pads across the breast area, varying the pressure in order to feel the tissues. The provider should also examine the areas around the breasts, which also contain breast tissue: under the arms, around the collarbone, across to the breast bone,

and down to the ribcage. This part of the exam should be conducted with the woman both lying on her back and seated upright on the examination table. A medical history, including information about the woman's menstrual cycle, symptoms, and FAMILY HISTORY of breast conditions, should also be taken.

If the CBE reveals something unusual, the patient may be referred for a diagnostic mammogram or another imaging scan. Diagnostic mammograms, are used to look at very specific areas inside the breast. In some cases, the provider may wait until the woman's next menstrual cycle is complete and reexamine her before conducting further tests.

clinical cancer centers A type of cancer center sponsored by the NATIONAL CANCER INSTITUTE that cares for patients and conducts programs in clinical and laboratory research, and may also have programs in other areas such as basic research or prevention, control, and population-based research. The centers focus on both laboratory research and clinical research within the same institutional framework, which is a distinguishing characteristic of many clinical cancer centers. For contact information for individual clinical cancer centers, see Appendix II.

clinical trial A research study that tries to answer specific questions about vaccines, new drugs, or new ways of using known treatments, including whether they are both safe and effective. Carefully conducted clinical trials are the fastest and safest way to find treatments that work.

For all types of trials, participants work with a research team that includes doctors, pharmacists, nurses, and scientists, who check the health of subjects at the beginning of the trial, give specific instructions for participation, and monitor participants carefully during and after the trial. Some clinical trials involve more tests and doctor visits than the participant would normally have for breast cancer.

To help someone decide whether or not to participate, scientists explain the study and provide an *informed consent* document that discusses the study's purpose, duration, required procedures, and key contacts. Risks and potential benefits are explained carefully and clearly, and then the participant decides whether or not to sign the document. Informed consent is not a contract—it is just a way to guarantee the patient understands all the pros and cons of the trial. The participant may withdraw from the trial at any time.

Well-designed clinical trials can help patients play an active role in their own health care, gain access to new treatments that are not yet widely available, obtain free expert medical care at leading hospitals, and help others by contributing to medical research.

Of course, there are risks in clinical trials. The treatment may have unpleasant, serious, or even life-threatening side effects. It may not be effective for the participant. The protocol may require more time and effort than standard treatment, including trips to the study site, hospital stays, or complex dosage requirements.

However, the ethical and legal codes that govern medical practice also apply to clinical trials. Most clinical research is also regulated by the government, with built-in safeguards to protect participants. The trial follows a carefully controlled study plan that details what researchers will do. As a clinical trial progresses, researchers report its results at scientific meetings, to medical journals, and to various government agencies.

Types of Clinical Trials

There are a variety of types of clinical trials, including those specializing in screening, prevention, diagnosis, treatment, and quality of life.

Screening trials test the best way to detect certain diseases or health conditions.
Prevention trials look for better ways to prevent disease in people who have never had the disease. These approaches may include medicines, vitamins, vaccines, minerals, or lifestyle changes.
Diagnostic trials are conducted to find better tests or procedures for diagnosing a particular disease or condition.
Treatment trials test new treatments, new combinations of drugs, or new types of surgery or radiation therapy.
Quality of life trials (or "supportive care" trials) explore ways to improve comfort and the quality of life for individuals with a chronic illness.

Phases of Clinical Trials

Clinical trials occur in four phases: PHASE I TRIALS test a new drug or treatment in a small group; PHASE II TRIALS expand the study to a larger group of people; PHASE III TRIALS expand the study to an even larger group of people; and PHASE IV TRIALS take place after the drug or treatment has been licensed and marketed.

Expanded Access Protocol

Most investigational drugs are administered during controlled clinical trials that assess their safety and efficacy. Sometimes patients do not qualify for these trials because of other health problems, age, or other factors. To help patients who may benefit from the drug but do not qualify for the trials, regulations allow manufacturers of investigational new drugs to apply for an "expanded access" protocol.

This allows people who have a life-threatening or serious disease to obtain a research drug. It also generates additional safety information about the drug. Expanded access protocols can be done only if scientists are actively studying the new treatment in well-controlled studies or all studies have been completed. There must be evidence that the drug may be an effective treatment for patients like those to be treated under the protocol. The drug cannot expose patients to unreasonable risks, given the severity of the disease to be treated. Expanded access protocols are generally managed by the drug company, with the investigational treatment administered at a doctor's office or hospital. (See Appendix IV.)

clodronate A type of BISPHOSPHONATE drug that may be effective in preventing the spread of BREAST CANCER to the bones and other parts of the body and may help prolong life for some patients.

Clodronate is used for treatment of bone tumors associated with other cancers because it appears to have a direct effect on osteoclasts (cells associated with bone wasting).

Clodronate does not kill cancer cells but appears to have a bone-bolstering effect. Scientists believe that effect offers a survival advantage. However, doctors are reluctant to routinely recommend bisphosphonates because in the United

States, clodronate is approved only in intravenous (IV) forms, not in pill form. Most doctors and patients are reluctant to consider triweekly IV pamidronate (the U.S.-approved bisphosphonate) for two years, the standard dosage found to be effective in clinical studies.

In one study, over two years of active treatment about half as many women who were on clodronate experienced cancer spread to the bone as women who were taking the placebo. But clodronate appeared to reduce the number of bone metastases only while women were actively taking the drug. During the total follow-up period (about five and one-half years), the differences in rate of bone metastases became too small to be considered important. There was no difference in the rate of metastases to other organs; about the same number of women in both groups had metastatic disease during the entire follow-up period. Nonetheless, there was a somewhat surprising, significant difference in survival rate: there were about one-fourth fewer deaths among those who took the clodronate.

Women who are interested in adding bisphosphonates to breast cancer treatment should discuss this option with their treating oncologists, because it is not promoted as a standard treatment.

cobalt 60   A radioactive form of the metal cobalt, which is used as a source of radiation to treat cancer.

coenzyme Q10 (ubiquinone, or ubidecarenone) A compound produced naturally in the body that helps cells produce energy needed for cell growth and maintenance. Coenzyme Q10 is found in most body tissues, especially in the heart, liver, kidneys, and pancreas; the lowest amounts are found in the lungs. It is also an antioxidant (a substance that protects cells from harmful chemicals called FREE RADICALS).

Coenzyme Q10 was first identified in 1957, but scientists did not consider its use as a potential cancer drug until 1961, when a deficiency of the enzyme was noted in the blood of cancer patients. Low blood levels of coenzyme Q10 have been found in patients with breast cancer, among other malignancies.

Animal studies have found that coenzyme Q10 stimulates the immune system and increases resistance to disease. In part because of this, researchers have theorized that coenzyme Q10 may be useful as an ADJUVANT TREATMENT for cancer.

No serious side effects have been reported, but some patients who used coenzyme Q10 experienced mild insomnia, higher levels of liver enzymes, rashes, nausea, and upper abdominal pain. Other reported side effects have included dizziness, visual sensitivity to light, irritability, headache, heartburn, and fatigue.

Patients should discuss with their health-care provider possible interactions between coenzyme Q10 and prescription drugs they may be taking. Certain drugs, such as those that are used to lower cholesterol or blood sugar level, may also reduce the effects of coenzyme Q10. Coenzyme Q10 may also alter the body's response to warfarin (a drug that prevents the blood from clotting) and insulin.

Coenzyme Q10 is used by the body as an antioxidant, which protects cells from free radicals, the highly reactive chemicals that can damage cells. Some conventional cancer therapies, such as chemotherapy and RADIATION THERAPY, are designed to kill cancer cells in part by triggering the formation of free radicals. Researchers are studying whether combining coenzyme Q10 with conventional therapies helps or hinders the fight against cancer. Several companies distribute coenzyme Q10 as a dietary supplement, which is regulated as a food, not a drug. This means that evaluation and approval by the U.S. Food and Drug Administration are not required before marketing, unless specific health claims are made about the supplement. Because dietary supplements are not formally reviewed for manufacturing consistency, there may be variations in the composition of the supplement from one batch to another.

colloid cancer   A very rare form of ductal BREAST CANCER (also known as mucinous cancer) that is formed by mucus-producing cancer cells. Colloid carcinoma has a slightly better prognosis and a slightly lower chance of spreading than do invasive lobular or invasive ductal cancer of the same size. It accounts for 5 percent or less of breast cancers.

colony-stimulating factor (CSF, or hematopoietic growth factor)

A substance that usually does not directly kill tumor cells, but that encourages BONE MARROW stem cells to divide and develop into white blood cells, platelets, and red blood cells. Doctors use CSFs to help patients who are having cancer treatment to boost their blood count.

Because CHEMOTHERAPY drugs can damage the body's ability to make white blood cells, red blood cells, and platelets, patients who receive these drugs have a higher risk of developing infections, becoming anemic, and bleeding more readily. By using CSFs to stimulate blood cell production, doctors can increase the dosages of anticancer drugs without increasing the risk of infection or the need for transfusion with blood products. As a result, researchers have found CSFs particularly useful when combined with high-dose chemotherapy.

Examples of CSFs and their use in cancer therapy include the following:

- GRANULOCYTE CSF (G-CSF) (filgrastim) and granulocyte-macrophage CSF (GM-CSF) (sargramostim) increase the number of white blood cells, reducing the risk of infection in patients who are receiving chemotherapy. They can also stimulate the production of stem cells in preparation for stem cell or BONE MARROW TRANSPLANTS.
- ERYTHROPOIETIN increases the number of red blood cells and reduces the need for red blood cell transfusions in patients who receive chemotherapy.
- Oprelvekin reduces the need for platelet transfusions in patients who are receiving chemotherapy.

Researchers are studying CSFs as a potential treatment of some types of leukemia, metastatic colorectal cancer, melanoma, lung cancer, and other types of cancer.

combination chemotherapy
Treatment in which two or more chemicals are used to maximize killing of tumor cells.

combined modality therapy
Use of two or more types of treatments to supplement each other. For instance, surgery, radiation, CHEMOTHERAPY, hormonal therapy, or immunotherapy may be used alternatively or together for maximum effectiveness.

Compazine (prochlorperazine)
A relatively inexpensive drug that is given either intravenously or orally to help control the episodes of NAUSEA and vomiting that occur more than 48 hours after administration of CHEMOTHERAPY. This drug belongs to a general class of drugs called phenothiazines. It works by blocking messages to the part of the brain that controls nausea and vomiting.

This drug can cause sleepiness, dry mouth, constipation, blurred vision, restlessness, weight gain, or increased heart rate. Rarely, it may cause jaundice, sensitivity to light, rash, or hives.

See also ANTINAUSEA MEDICATION.

complementary and alternative medicine
A broad group of healing philosophies and approaches (also referred to as integrative medicine) that may be used to treat breast cancer. *Complementary treatment* refers to therapy used in addition to conventional approaches; *alternative* indicates that a treatment is used *instead of* conventional medicine. Conventional treatments are those that are widely accepted and practiced by the mainstream medical community.

Depending on how they are used, some treatments can be considered either complementary or alternative. Unlike conventional treatments for breast cancer, complementary and alternative therapies often are not covered by insurance companies. Cancer patients considering complementary or alternative therapies should discuss this decision with their doctor, because the therapies may interfere with standard treatment or may be harmful when used with conventional treatment.

complete blood count
A laboratory test to determine the number of red blood cells, white blood cells, platelets; the hemoglobin level; and other components of a blood sample. A complete blood count is often used during chemotherapy to make sure a patient is healthy enough to receive treatment.

complete remission
The disappearance of all signs of cancer in response to treatment. Remission does not always mean the cancer has been cured.

comprehensive cancer center A type of special cancer institution sponsored by the NATIONAL CANCER INSTITUTE (NCI) that conducts programs in all three areas of research—basic research, clinical research, and prevention and control research—and interactive research linking these areas.

In 1990, there were 19 comprehensive cancer centers across the United States; today more than 40 cancer centers meet the NCI criteria for comprehensive status.

computed tomography scans Commonly called CT or CAT scans, these specialized X-ray studies can be used to evaluate the body for the spread of breast cancer. With abdominal CAT scans a drink is given to show the stomach; in all CAT scans IV contrast dye is given to highlight internal organs more clearly.

computer-aided detection (CAD) A diagnostic method that involves the use of computers to call suspicious areas on a MAMMOGRAM to the radiologist's attention. In 1998, the U.S. Food and Drug Administration approved a breast-imaging device that uses CAD technology; others are being developed.

A typical computer-aided detection device scans a mammogram with a laser beam and converts it into a digital signal that is processed by a computer. The image is then displayed on a video monitor, with suspicious areas highlighted for the radiologist to review. The radiologist can compare the digital image with the conventional mammogram to see whether any of the highlighted areas was missed on the initial review and require further evaluation.

Experts hope that CAD technology may improve the accuracy of screening mammography. Scientists are also studying how to incorporate CAD technology into digital MAMMOGRAPHY.

constipation The passage of painfully hard, infrequent, dry stools. CONSTIPATION affects a proportion of women who have BREAST CANCER and who are receiving CHEMOTHERAPY. Narcotic pain and antinausea medications also can lead to constipation, as can decreased fluid intake, lack of EXERCISE, and depression.

contrast digital mammography An enhanced method of MAMMOGRAPHY, combining contrast dye with DIGITAL MAMMOGRAPHY, that may allow for a better diagnosis of BREAST CANCER in dense breasts. Contrast digital mammography may make cancers stand out against dense breast tissue that were hidden when conventional film was used. The technique gives an enhanced view of new blood vessels created by a tumor. This technique is experimental.

Cooper's ligaments Flexible bands of tissue that pass from the chest muscle between the lobes of the breasts, providing shape and support to the breasts.

coping behavior Interventions focused on improving a woman's ability to cope with BREAST CANCER diagnosis, treatment, and recovery may have beneficial effects on emotional adjustment and possibly on her physiological processes. Several studies have suggested that stress, mental state, and coping style all work together to affect biological factors such as immune function and hormone levels, both of which play a role in cancer progression.

While stress, distress, depression, anxiety, and posttraumatic stress disorder (PTSD) all have been linked to an impaired immune function and hormone imbalances, healthy coping skills have been shown to improve these factors.

Symptoms of anxiety and depression affect 30 percent to 40 percent of women first diagnosed with breast cancer, and PTSD is estimated to affect 3 percent to 10 percent of these women. Virtually all patients with breast cancer experience some level of stress and distress.

The researchers define *coping* as the conscious effort to regulate cognitive, behavioral, emotional, and physiological responses to stress. They describe a woman who "actively copes" as someone who takes a direct and rational approach to dealing with a problem. "Passive coping" involves indirect approaches such as avoidance, withdrawal, and wishful thinking.

Studies have shown that people who adopt active coping strategies have better immune function and lower cortisol (stress hormone) levels; people who use passive coping strategies have the opposite findings.

Some researchers believe there is clear evidence that treatment can have positive effects on adjustment, and treatment of disease-related symptoms (such as pain or NAUSEA). A more limited body of research suggests that such interventions have a positive effect on immune function and cortisol levels. Likewise, there is some preliminary evidence that psychotherapeutic approaches can reduce recurrence and improve survival rates. Survival benefits of psychological treatment have not been clearly demonstrated, however.

Some researchers believe that both active coping and effective psychological treatment also can improve cancer treatment by ensuring that women more closely follow their cancer treatment regimens.

core biopsy   Removal (with a large needle) of a piece of tissue to be sent to a lab for microscopic analysis.

See also BIOPSY.

Cowden disease   A rare autosomal dominant condition appearing most often in women, characterized by a high risk of breast and thyroid cancer. Women who have Cowden disease have an estimated lifetime risk of 30 to 50 percent for breast cancer and about a 10 percent lifetime risk for thyroid cancer.

Cowden disease patients typically experience growths all over their body, which start as tiny wartlike bumps on the face, hands, feet, tongue, and lips. Women sometimes develop very severe benign FIBROCYSTIC BREAST CHANGES that begin in their teens. Because these benign tumors appear as large, hard lumps of connective tissue, many doctors unfamiliar with Cowden disease immediately suspect cancer.

Cowden disease may also increase a woman's risk of endometrial cancer. Therefore, women who have the *P-TEN* mutation who also have breast cancer may not be candidates for treatment with TAMOXIFEN, which itself can increase the risk of endometrial cancer.

Mutations in the *P-TEN* GENE on chromosome 10 have been implicated in Cowden disease. Genetic testing for *P-TEN* mutations is available both commercially and on a research basis.

cribriform   A pattern of cancer cell growth inside the breast duct that resembles mesh.

cruciferous vegetables   A family of vegetables that contain substances that may protect against breast cancer. These substances, INDOLES and isothiocyanates, are PHYTOCHEMICALS that have been found to block or reduce cell damage. Cruciferous vegetables include kale, collard greens, broccoli, cauliflower, cabbage, brussels sprouts, and turnips. These vegetables also may increase the blood-thinning effect of coumadin.

cryoablation   Freezing away of growths, such as BREAST CANCER tumors, by using extreme cold.

Cryoablation, which destroys cells by shattering their outer walls during freeze-and-thaw cycles, was first studied in the 1960s. It proved too risky for use deep inside the body because doctors could not see what they were aiming to freeze, and there were many complications. Although dermatologists and gynecologists continued to freeze away easy-to-see skin or cervical growths, other uses of cryoablation ceased.

Today the use of cryoablation to treat deep internal growths is making a slow comeback, thanks to improved medical imaging that allows doctors to see deep inside the body while they work. They can place a needle that emits freezing argon gas into a tumor or organ and watch until ice encases the lesion. It is approved to treat patients whose colorectal cancer has spread to the liver.

The federal government recently approved a cryoablation system to destroy FIBROADENOMAS (benign breast tumors) that is being used in a few centers. Currently this approach is investigational.

Patients considering any use of cryoablation should choose an experienced cryosurgeon because the technique requires extensive training and practice to prevent complications from freezing normal tissue.

cutaneous breast cancer   Cancer that has spread from the breast to the skin. After MASTECTOMY, local recurrences of breast cancer can occur on the skin of the chest wall.

cyclophosphamide   See CYTOXAN.

cyst   An accumulation of fluid in the breast that is usually benign. Lumps in the breast are often found to be harmless cysts. Although the exact causes of cysts are not known, they are known to change with hormonal variations, either during normal menstrual cycles or as the result of postmenopausal hormone replacement. Contrary to popular belief, caffeine has no proven effect on cysts.

Cysts do not become malignant or increase the risk of cancer. Most of the time, cysts may be left alone, although sometimes a physician may drain them with a small needle. Some cysts appear "complex" on ultrasound and may contain extra tissue. These cysts may be malignant and are often drained or biopsied. If a cyst is drained, it should disappear completely on exam.

See also FIBROCYSTIC BREAST CHANGES.

cystosarcoma phyllodes (CSP)   A rare type of breast tumor now called a phyllodes tumor (as it is not a sarcoma). It often appears in the breast of a young woman and usually looks and feels like a FIBROADENOMA. However, unlike benign fibroadenomas, these lesions grow quickly. The lesions do not spread to lymph nodes and do not involve the duct system of the breast. The malignant form is extremely rare but may spread to the lungs or other organs.

Treatment

Surgery to remove the lesion with very wide CLEAR MARGINS (no malignant cells along the edge of the tumor) is effective. Because so much normal tissue needs to be removed, MASTECTOMY is often done. Axillary lymph nodes are rarely removed because this type of tumor rarely spreads.

cytokines   A class of substances that are produced by cells of the immune system and can affect the immune response. Cytokines can also be produced in the laboratory by recombinant DNA technology and given to people to boost immune responses.

Examples of cytokines used in cancer treatment include interferon and interleukin, as well as Neupogen and erythropoeitin.

cytotoxic   An agent that can cause the death of cancer cells. The term usually refers to drugs used in CHEMOTHERAPY treatments.

cytotoxic T cells   White blood cells that can directly destroy specific cells. T cells can be separated from other blood cells, grown in the laboratory, and then administered to a patient to destroy tumor cells. Scientists are trying to harness this treatment to use against breast cancer. Certain CYTOKINES can also be given to a patient to help form cytotoxic T cells in his or her body.

Cytoxan (cyclophosphamide)   A type of CHEMO-THERAPY drug that belongs to a group of drugs called ALKYLATING AGENTS. This medication disrupts and destroys breast cancer cell growth. The medication is given either orally or intravenously (IV). The IV form does not usually cause hair loss, but the oral form may. Cytoxan is an effective drug for breast cancer and is part of almost every regimen of ADJUVANT TREATMENT.

Side Effects

Most commonly, Cytoxan causes hair loss, NAUSEA and vomiting, APPETITE LOSS, mouth or lip sores, DIARRHEA, decreased sperm production in men, and lower sperm count. It can lower BLOOD COUNT (white blood cells, red blood cells, and platelets), so the doctor checks blood counts before each treatment. Cytoxan can lower white blood cell count between one and two weeks after the drug has been given, thereby increasing the risk of infection. A decrease in platelet counts can increase the risk of bleeding.

Less common side effects include acne, fatigue, dark nail beds, and bloody urine. Rarely, lung problems or heart changes may be associated with high dosages.

dairy products It is unclear whether eating dairy foods affects a woman's risk of developing BREAST CANCER. Although many studies have examined the breast cancer risk of dairy foods in general and specific dairy foods in particular, the results have been conflicting.

In some studies, women who ate large amounts of dairy foods had lower breast cancer risk. Other studies showed higher breast cancer risk associated with eating dairy foods, and several studies showed no differences in risk. This problem is complicated by the fact that all of these studies had design limitations.

The results of existing studies do not give women enough information to choose individual dairy foods specifically to reduce breast cancer risk. But experts say that concern about cardiac health and risk of other cancers suggests that a choice of low-fat dairy products would be wise.

Several studies indicated the possibility of a small decrease in breast cancer risk associated with childhood and adolescent milk consumption. A small decrease in risk for breast cancer was associated with drinking whole milk daily during childhood. One study found no change in the risk of breast cancer associated with eating dairy foods as an adolescent. A second study found a decrease in the risk of both premenopausal and postmenopausal breast cancers associated with eating fat from milk, cheese, and yogurt as an adolescent. The American Academy of Pediatrics currently recommends that children above the age of two years drink milk containing 2 percent fat rather than whole milk.

Contaminants in Dairy Products

Some consumers are concerned about the effects of the use of hormones by dairy farmers to increase milk production. However, the U.S. Food and Drug Administration (FDA) has evaluated milk from hormone-treated animals and does not consider it to cause a health problem.

Pesticide residues in milk products are also an area of public concern. The FDA is responsible for milk product testing and regularly performs tests that can detect more than 350 different pesticides. Contamination of milk products with pesticide residues is rare, and when it is seen, it is typically below the tolerances set by the Environmental Protection Agency (EPA). For example, in 1998, 96 percent of dairy product samples had no detectable contamination, and all of the samples with detectable contamination had pesticide levels below EPA tolerances.

Recommendations

Although no conclusions about dairy products can be drawn, experts recommend that women concerned about breast cancer choose low-fat milk products; add vegetables, grains, and fruits to their diet; exercise regularly; and maintain a healthy weight.

DBC2 A newly discovered TUMOR SUPPRESSOR GENE. The gene, whose name is an acronym of *deleted in breast cancer,* was discovered by scientists at Cold Spring Harbor Laboratory in New York and the University of Washington. Their study was published in the *Proceedings of the National Academy of Sciences.* The discovery is significant because *DBC2* is among the first tumor suppressor genes to be associated with noninherited BREAST CANCER. Noninherited disease, in contrast to forms of cancer associated with a family history of the disease, accounts for more than 90 percent of all forms of breast and other cancers. The researchers showed that production of the DBC2 protein in breast cancer cells kills the cancer cells or stops them from growing.

In 1997, the same research group identified one of the only other tumor suppressor genes (called P-TEN GENES) to be clearly associated with noninherited cancer. In 1981, the same group discovered the first cancer-causing ONCOGENE (called RAS) in human cells.

In 1990, the same research group at the University of Washington discovered the first gene linked to hereditary breast cancer (*BRCA1*).

It is too soon to say whether DBC2 will be as important as the *BRCA* genes, but an understanding of the genetic code can help experts pinpoint the beginnings of breast cancer.

DCIS   See DUCTAL CARCINOMA IN SITU.

Decadron (dexamethasone)   A glucocorticoid steroid that is also a powerful antinausea medicine. It is prescribed for patients with BREAST CANCER who are undergoing CHEMOTHERAPY. It can be used alone or in combination with ondansetron (ZOFRAN) or granisetron (KYTRIL) to help control acute episodes of chemotherapy-induced NAUSEA or vomiting. It also can be used alone to improve appetite and to improve a person's general feeling of well-being.

The drug works by interfering with the pathways responsible for nausea and vomiting related to chemotherapy. The first dose is often given intravenously during chemotherapy. Doses in pill form are given for several days after chemotherapy. Pills should be taken with food or milk to protect the stomach from irritation.

Side Effects

Decadron may cause a change in how white blood cells move, causing an increase in the white blood cell count. It also may cause a temporary boost in blood sugar level.

As other steroids can, it can cause weight gain if used for prolonged periods. Other common side effects include fluid retention, depression, decreased potassium level, increased appetite, sleep problems, skin bruises, mood changes, and slowed wound healing.

deep inferior epigastric perforator flap (DIEP flap)   A new type of BREAST RECONSTRUCTION in which blood vessels, called deep inferior epigastric perfora-

tors, or DIEPs, together with the skin and fat connected to them, are removed from the lower abdomen and used to create a breast mound. Muscle is left in place. As many other reconstructive procedures, this is very involved surgery that may not be appropriate for all patients.

deodorants and breast cancer   Despite persistent rumors about a link between antiperspirants or deodorants and BREAST CANCER, no research supports any such link. The U.S. Food and Drug Administration, which regulates food, cosmetics, medicines, and medical devices, also does not have any evidence or research data to support the theory that ingredients in underarm antiperspirants or deodorants cause cancer.

In 2002, one study examined the personal hygiene habits of 813 women who had breast cancer and 793 women without the disease and found no link between cancer and body odor control cosmetics. Participants in the study who had breast cancer were no more likely to use antiperspirants or deodorants. This indicates that use of the personal products does not cause the disease.

The original rumor linking breast cancer with deodorants started more than 10 years ago, probably the result of a widely distributed anonymous e-mail.

DES   See DIETHYLSTILBESTROL.

dexamethasone   See DECADRON.

diabetes type 2   Postmenopausal women who have type 2 diabetes may have a minimally higher risk of development BREAST CANCER than other women. Data from the NURSES' HEALTH STUDY, involving more than 100,000 women, revealed a very small link between type 2 diabetes and breast cancer. Researchers are not sure what accounts for the increased risk.

Breast cancer incidence is higher in more affluent countries and among women with high socioeconomic status. Although delayed childbearing, earlier onset of menstruation, and higher alcohol consumption in high-socioeconomic status populations may explain part of this risk, a Western sedentary lifestyle and possibly a DIET high in refined carbohydrates, sugars, and animal fats also may play an important role. This lifestyle and diet often result in insulin resistance, a condition characterized by a decreased sensitivity to insulin. Insulin causes a rise in estrogen level and is also a growth-promoting hormone that affects both normal and malignant breast tissue. The effect of estrogen on the spread of hormone-dependent breast cancer may depend on the presence of insulin.

The data from the Nurses' Health Study provide the largest population, with the longest follow-up, in which the association between type 2 diabetes and breast cancer has been studied. The findings of a minimal association are consistent with several previous reports of a slightly elevated risk.

In 1998, about 16 million U.S. adults were diagnosed with type 2 diabetes, so even a slight increase in breast cancer risk in women with type 2 diabetes would be a public health concern. If type 2 diabetes plays a role in the development of breast cancer, interventions that improve insulin sensitivity, such as exercise and diet changes, may lower the incidence of breast cancer.

A woman can decrease her risk of type 2 diabetes by controlling her weight and exercising a few times a week.

diagnosis of breast cancer   BREAST CANCER is usually diagnosed by MAMMOGRAPHY or CLINICAL BREAST EXAM. Once the cancer is confirmed, other assessments are done to determine the extent of the cancer. These include further surgery, with examination of the tissue by a pathologist, together with a chest X-ray, blood tests, and sometimes a CAT scan or BONE SCAN. However, most findings on mammogram are not cancer; most biopsies are benign; and most lumps turn out to be harmless.

Breast Self-Exam (BSE)

The AMERICAN CANCER SOCIETY once recommended that all women examine their own breasts monthly. However, after research in 2003 revealed that BREAST SELF-EXAMINATIONS were not effective, the society changed its recommendations, noting that women in their 20s should be told about the benefits and limitations of BSE.

Today the society recommends that women should be aware of how their breasts normally feel and report any new breast changes to a health professional as soon as they are found. It is normal for

the breasts to feel a little lumpy or uneven. It is also common for a woman's breasts to be swollen and tender right before or during her menstrual period. It is not uncommon for cysts and cystic changes to fluctuate with birth control pill usage, menstrual cycles, and aging. However, if a woman feels anything hard or new, it is important for her to contact her doctor, even if a recent mammogram was negative.

For women over age 40, a monthly BSE is not a substitute for regularly scheduled screening mammograms and clinical breast exams by a health professional. The Cancer Society stresses that it is acceptable for women to choose not to do BSE or to do BSE occasionally.

Although there are some features of a mass that suggest whether it is likely to be benign or cancerous, women examining their own breasts should discuss any new lump with their health-care professionals. Experienced health-care professionals can examine the breast and determine whether the changes a woman notices are probably benign. They can determine when additional tests are appropriate to rule out a cancer and when follow-up exams are the best strategy. If there is any suspicion of cancer, the doctor will perform a biopsy.

Physical Exam

When a doctor is evaluating a woman for breast cancer, important parts of the exam include the clinical breast exam and evaluation of LYMPH NODES under the arms, the neck, and behind the collarbone, together with evaluation of the heart, lungs, and abdomen. It is also important for the doctor to know about any other medical problems and to ask about family history.

Clinical Breast Exam

A clinical breast examination by a health-care provider is recommended every three years for women under age 40, and yearly thereafter.

The doctor can tell a lot about a lump's size, its texture, and whether it moves easily by carefully feeling the lump and the tissue around it. Benign lumps often feel different from cancerous ones; the doctor can examine the size and texture of the lump and determine whether the lump moves easily, a sign that the lump is probably benign. If a lump is found, especially if a woman is premenopausal, the woman may be asked to return after the next menstrual cycle, because many benign lumps disappear.

Mammogram

A screening mammogram is the best tool available for finding breast cancer early, before symptoms appear. Screening mammograms are used to look for breast changes in women who have no signs of breast cancer.

Mammograms can often detect breast cancer before it can be felt and can reveal small deposits of calcium in the breast. Although most calcium deposits are benign, a cluster of very tiny specks of calcium (called MICROCALCIFICATIONS) may be an early sign of cancer.

More than 90 percent of all breast cancers are detected by mammogram. Most doctors agree with the current American Cancer Society recommendation of screening mammograms every year for women at age 40. However, this means that 10 percent of breast cancers are missed. It is more common to miss cancers in women with dense breasts—a condition seen more often in younger women.

A typical mammography screening includes two views of each breast (one from above and one from the side). Normally, the technician examines the X-ray pictures immediately to make sure pictures are clear. A physician then looks at the mammograms and if a mass, changes from earlier mammograms, abnormalities of the skin, or enlargement of the lymph nodes is found, further testing may be recommended. This could include an ultrasound of the breast, a biopsy or needle sampling, or consultation with a breast surgeon.

Limitations However, although mammography is the best screening tool available now, it is not a perfect test. Mammograms are the best way to find breast cancer early, but they do have some limitations. A mammogram may miss some cancers that are present (a false-negative result) or may find things that turn out not to be cancer (a false-positive result). Mammography may not help a woman who has a small but fast-growing tumor that has already spread at the time of detection. And mammography may pick up cancers or pre-cancers that then get treated, but might never have been evident had they been left alone. However,

this is not a reason to skip mammograms, which save lives.

Results of between 5 percent and 10 percent of mammograms are abnormal. Of those in younger women that are followed up with additional tests (another mammogram, FINE-NEEDLE ASPIRATION, ULTRASOUND, or BIOPSY) most are not cancer.

Under the MAMMOGRAPHY QUALITY STANDARDS ACT (MQSA), the U.S. Food and Drug Administration (FDA) sets high standards for mammography facilities, and the roughly 10,000 mammography facilities nationwide certified by the FDA are inspected annually. MQSA regulations require facilities to hire capable technicians, use high-quality equipment that produces clear images, and employ skilled radiologists to interpret the results. The rules also require that doctors and patients be fully and quickly informed of results so that any follow-up testing or treatment can begin immediately.

The names and locations of FDA-certified mammography facilities can be found by calling the CANCER INFORMATION SERVICE (1-800-4-CANCER). In addition, the FDA has included a list of all FDA-certified mammography facilities in the United States on its Internet home page (http://www.fda.gov/cdrh/faclist.html).

Ultrasounds

Using high-frequency sound waves, ultrasonography can often show whether a lump is solid or filled with fluid. If filled with fluid, with smooth outlines, it is a cyst, and no further tests may be needed and no treatment may be necessary. However, a solid lump may be malignant and a biopsy may be needed.

At times, fluid or tissue must be removed from the breast (a biopsy) to make a conclusive diagnosis. These additional tissue tests may include the following:

- *Fine-needle aspiration:* A thin needle is used to remove fluid from a breast lump to show whether a lump is a fluid-filled cyst (benign) or a solid mass (possibly malignant). Clear fluid removed from a cyst may not have to be checked by a lab.
- *Core-needle biopsy:* A needle with a larger diameter is used to remove small pieces of tissue from

the mass that can then be analyzed. These analyses can determine whether the mass is benign or cancerous and therefore whether further treatment is required.

- *Surgical biopsy:* The surgeon cuts out part or all of a lump or suspicious area. A pathologist examines the tissue under a microscope to check for cancer cells. An EXCISIONAL BIOPSY is a surgical procedure in which the entire lump area and some surrounding tissue are removed for examination. If the mass is very large, an INCISIONAL BIOPSY, in which only a portion of the area is removed and analyzed, is done.

Staging

When cancer is found, the pathologist can identify the type of cancer it is (whether it began in a duct or a lobule) and whether it has invaded nearby tissues in the breast. Special lab tests of the tissue help the doctor learn more about the cancer.

For example, estrogen- and progesterone-receptor tests can help predict whether the cancer is sensitive to hormones. A positive test result means hormones help the cancer grow and that the tumor is likely to respond to hormonal therapy, such as TAMOXIFEN. Other lab tests are sometimes done to help the doctor predict whether the cancer is likely to grow slowly or quickly. The doctor may order X-rays and blood tests, or special exams of the bones, liver, or lungs to see whether breast cancer may spread to these areas.

To find out whether the cancer has spread, doctors remove some underarm lymph nodes to test for cancer cells that have spread and to help make treatment decisions. Checking for cancer cells in the lymph nodes is also a way to determine how advanced the cancer is (STAGING of cancer). Breast cancer is rated from stage 0 to stage IV. Staging uses the diagnostic information to tell the cancer physician (oncologist) how widespread the disease is.

On the Horizon

New imaging technologies under development for breast cancer screening include magnetic resonance imaging, screening ultrasound, and PET scans. In addition to imaging technologies, National Cancer Institute–supported scientists are exploring methods to detect breast cancer by using simple tests of the blood, urine, or nipple aspirates and to detect genetic alterations that place women at increased risk for breast cancer.

In addition, the government is working with the Department of Defense, the Central Intelligence Agency (CIA), National Aeronautics and Space Administration (NASA), and other public and private entities to explore ways in which imaging technologies from other fields may be applied to the early detection of breast cancer. In particular, the computer technologies that have been used to improve spy satellites may help improve breast cancer detection as well. In October 1996, the government awarded $1.98 million to the University of Pennsylvania to conduct a multisite clinical trial of an imaging technology with the potential to improve the early detection of breast cancer. The technology was originally used by the intelligence community for missile guidance and target recognition.

diaphanography A near-infrared (NIR) light-imaging technique no longer used today that was introduced in the 1930s as an attempt to locate and identify BREAST CANCER. This type of imaging was a simple, low-cost, risk-free procedure, which, unlike X-ray MAMMOGRAPHY, did not use ionizing radiation. Unfortunately, the initial promise of NIR diaphanography was never realized, primarily due to the effect of intense light scattering. Scattering blurs the ability to find small, buried, light-absorbing tumors much in the same way that a cloud obscures the view of an airplane passing overhead.

diarrhea Passage of loose or watery stools, at least three times a day, that may or may not be painful. Often it is accompanied by gas, bloating, and cramps. Diarrhea occurs in some patients during CHEMOTHERAPY because the drugs damage the rapidly dividing cells in the gastrointestinal tract. The severity of diarrhea depends on the type and dosage of chemotherapy. Some drugs that cause diarrhea include 5-fluorouracil, methotrexate, and DOCETAXEL. It can be life threatening if it is severe enough to trigger dehydration and electrolyte imbalances.

One or two loose stools can be treated with Kaopectate and extra fluids. More severe diarrhea should be treated with fluids and electrolytes.

diet   Although many studies have established an association between diet and lifestyle factors and the risk of development of BREAST CANCER, little is known about the effect of diet and lifestyle on breast cancer survival. This information is important, however, to survivors of breast cancer who want to make choices to improve the length and quality of their life.

The effect of diet after cancer diagnosis is an area of research that calls for much more study.

It is uncertain whether aspects of diet before diagnosis affect breast cancer survival rate. Twelve studies have examined the effect of diet before breast cancer diagnosis on various aspects of survival in the disease; their results were not in agreement.

All of the studies examined fat consumption. Four studies reported no association between survival rate and dietary fat consumption before diagnosis. However, five studies reported that eating high levels of dietary fat was associated with an increase in the risk of death. The effect of fat on the risk of death of breast cancer and the risk of having breast cancer is an area of controversy, and more studies can be expected in the future.

Some of the studies also examined the vitamin content of foods consumed before cancer diagnosis. Women who ate foods with the highest levels of vitamin C and beta-carotene (vitamin A from vegetable sources) were found to have a decreased risk of death in two studies, but no association with risk was found in a third study. Vitamin E intake from food was reported to be associated with a decrease in risk of death in one study, was associated with an increase in risk in another, and had no association with risk in a third study. Clarification of the role of these vitamins in this context will require more study.

dietary fat   The relationship between the consumption of fat and the risk of BREAST CANCER is not clear. For years, some researchers have believed that fat intake is a primary culprit in the develop-

ment of breast cancer. However, this link has not yet been proved conclusively and is still considered to be highly controversial.

Some studies suggest that a high-fat diet may raise the concentration of hormones such as ESTROGEN, which has been linked to breast cancer. A diet that is high in fat may lead to obesity, which is an established risk factor for postmenopausal breast cancer (although obesity can be linked with breast cancer, and dietary fat consumption can be linked to obesity, it is still not possible to extrapolate that breast cancer can be caused by a high-fat diet). Other researchers think that a high-fat diet in childhood may lead to faster growth and an earlier onset of menstruation, another established risk factor for breast cancer. Still other scientists are studying the idea that high fat intake may alter the expression of genes involved in the growth of breast cancer. And some fats (such as olive oil and fish oil) may decrease the risk of breast cancer because they produce fewer cell-damaging free radicals.

The *Journal of the National Cancer Institute* published a University of Southern California report that concluded that lowering consumption of fat calories may reduce the risk of breast cancer. In countries that have a high incidence of breast cancer such as the United States, fat calories constitute about 34 percent of an individual's total calories. In countries that have a low incidence (such as China), fat contributes much less, about 15 to 20 percent of total calories. More than 95 studies using four different animal models of breast cancer found that dietary fat intake increased the development of breast tumors in lab animals, depending on the type of fat in the diet.

According to the AMERICAN CANCER SOCIETY Advisory Committee, the association between high-fat diets and breast cancer is weak. Therefore, the committee says, the best ways to reduce the risk of breast cancer are to drink less alcohol, eat a diet rich in fruits and vegetables, get plenty of exercise, and prevent obesity.

In 25 studies that looked at the effect of total fat intake on breast cancer risk by asking women with or without breast cancer about their dietary habits during the previous year, results were inconsistent. Only two of those studies reported that a high-fat diet was significantly associated with an increased risk of breast cancer. (However, several of the studies reported a modest but not significant increase in the incidence of breast cancer in women who had the highest levels of fat intake when compared to women at the lowest levels of fat intake.)

In cohort studies, a large group of women who do not have breast cancer report their usual dietary habits and are then recontacted years later to determine how many of them developed breast cancer. None of the cohort studies reported a significant increase in the risk of breast cancer associated with high fat intake, despite the fact that all of them were done in Western countries where the average total fat intake usually accounted for well above 30 percent of total calories consumed.

It is difficult to link dietary fat and breast cancer in humans because it is difficult to study the relationship between specific nutrients and breast cancer. Humans eat food, not individual nutrients, so it is a person's entire diet that may be what is most important. In addition, studies differ in design and in the way dietary fat intake is measured. In many studies, the range of fat intake in the population studied may be too narrow to allow conclusions to be drawn. For example, because so many American women eat high-fat diets, it may be that there are not enough women who eat a low enough level of fat to allow a difference in breast cancer rates to be determined. Moreover, studies of diet and breast cancer risk usually include information about current dietary habits only. These studies are not able to determine whether a high dietary fat intake during early childhood or adolescence influences breast cancer risk.

It also may not just be dietary fat that affects breast cancer. Instead, it could be that diet, exercise, and obesity influence breast cancer risk independently or together.

Kinds of Dietary Fat

A high-fat diet may have a less important as the *kind* of dietary fat consumed, such as saturated, monounsaturated, or polyunsaturated fat. Studies have found that both saturated fats and polyunsaturated fats (especially those containing omega-6 fatty acids found in vegetable oils) increase the growth of breast tumors in lab animals. In human studies of saturated and polyunsaturated fats, the results are mixed, and it is not possible to draw a conclusion. The results of the human studies may be different because the different types of fatty acids are found in many different kinds of foods and oils that may also have independent effects on breast cancer risk.

Saturated fatty acids are found in higher concentrations in foods such as meats and dairy products, in which the fat is solid at room temperature. Polyunsaturated fatty acids are found in higher concentrations in foods from plants, such as vegetable oils and food made from them in which the fat is liquid at room temperature. Monounsaturated fatty acids are found in highest concentrations in foods such as olive oil and canola oil. The different types of fatty acids may have different effects on the development of breast cancer.

Also, there may be differences in the structure of the saturated, monounsaturated, and polyunsaturated fatty acids in different types of foods and oils. For instance, sometimes when food is processed, vegetable oils become more saturated, as in the production of margarine, cookies, or snack foods.

Beneficial Fats

Although studies do not show conclusively that specific types of fats can prevent breast cancer, they do offer hope that there may be ways to change the diet that may reduce breast cancer risk.

Olive oil Several studies have suggested that olive oil and similar oils containing monounsaturated fats can reduce a woman's risk of breast cancer. In one recent six-year study conducted jointly by Swedish and American researchers, results suggest that monounsaturated fat found in olive, canola, and nut oils can reduce a woman's risk of breast cancer, whereas polyunsaturated fat (fish, corn, safflower, and sunflower oils) has the opposite effect.

The study, of 61,471 Swedish women between the ages of 40 and 76, correlated their breast cancer risk with the amount and type of fats in their diet. For each additional 10 grams of monounsaturated fat eaten, a woman's breast cancer risk was estimated to drop by 45 percent. In contrast, each extra five grams of polyunsaturated fat increased her breast cancer risk by 69 percent.

Animal studies have shown that monounsaturated oils lowered the risk of breast cancer, and studies from Spain, Greece, and Italy have shown high olive oil use correlated with low breast cancer risk.

Still, more research needs to be done to precisely measure the effects of increasing monounsaturated fat consumption before major dietary changes are recommended.

The possible relationship between the consumption of olive oil (which contains monounsaturated fat) and breast cancer risk has led to studies of monounsaturated fat. Meat and canola oil also contain monounsaturated fat. Most of the studies report no association between monounsaturated fat consumption and the risk of breast cancer; a few studies report that monounsaturated fat consumption increases the risk of breast cancer, whereas others report that it decreases the risk.

One possible reason for the discrepancy in results may be that there is something about olive oil specifically, and not its monounsaturated fat, that is influencing breast cancer risk. Olive oil also contains vitamins, flavonoids, and phenolic compounds that may help slow the development of breast cancer.

Fish oil   There is evidence from several animal studies that fish oils slow the development and decrease the growth of breast tumors, but nothing that suggests fish affects the development of breast cancer. Women who eat a lot of fish usually have a high omega-3/omega-6 ratio. In animal studies, a high omega-3/omega-6 ratio decreased the incidence, size, and growth of breast tumors.

Why Fat Is Important

Regardless of a possible link between fat and breast cancer, humans need to eat certain types of essential polyunsaturated fatty acids because they are not produced in the body but are necessary to help maintain cellular activities. Dietary fat functions as an energy source, makes food tender and flavorful, and is necessary for the absorption of fat-soluble vitamins A, D, and E. Fat stored in the body insulates it against temperature extremes and protects vital organs from trauma.

Fat Guidelines

National experts recommend that Americans consume less than 30 percent of their total calories from fat, less than 10 percent of total calories from saturated fat, and 1 to 2 percent of calories from linoleic acid (one of the essential polyunsaturated fatty acids). Under these guidelines, a diet of 2,000 calories would include fewer than 600 calories from fat (or 67 grams of fat). In addition to these specific guidelines on fat, women should eat a healthy diet of fruits, vegetables, and whole grains and remain physically active. For example, eating reduced-fat snack foods is not as healthy as eating more fruits, vegetables, and whole grains.

diethylstilbestrol (DES)   A potent synthetic form of ESTROGEN that was used by pregnant women between the early 1940s and 1971 to prevent miscarriage. Mothers who took DES during pregnancy have a slightly higher risk for BREAST CANCER. Daughters of mothers who took DES during pregnancy with them have a range of health problems, including a higher chance of a rare form of vaginal cancer. These women do not appear to have a higher risk for breast cancer.

differentiation   A term that refers to the maturity of the cancer cells in a BREAST CANCER tumor. Differentiated tumor cells resemble normal cells and tend to grow and spread at a slower rate than undifferentiated or poorly differentiated tumor cells, which lack the structure and function of normal cells and therefore tend to grow more quickly and grow uncontrollably.

digital mammography   A technique for recording X-ray images in computer code instead of on X-ray film, as conventional MAMMOGRAPHY does. The digital images are displayed on a computer monitor and can be enhanced before they are printed on film. Images can also be manipulated so that a radiologist can magnify or zoom in on any area.

The actual procedure for a MAMMOGRAM with a digital system, as far as a patient is concerned, is the same as for conventional mammography. However, from a diagnostic point of view, digital mammography may have some advantages over conventional mammography. The images can be stored and retrieved electronically; that capacity makes long-distance consultations with other mammography specialists easier. Because the images can be adjusted by the radiologist, subtle differences between tissues may be seen more easily. Moreover, the better accuracy of digital mammography may reduce the number of follow-up procedures and biopsies.

Despite these benefits, studies have not shown that digital mammography is more effective than conventional mammography in finding cancer.

The first digital mammography system received U.S. Food and Drug Administration (FDA) approval in 2000. Women who are considering digital mammography should talk with their doctor or contract a local FDA-certified mammography center to find out whether this technique is available at that location. Only facilities that have been certified to practice conventional mammography and have FDA approval for digital mammography may offer the digital system. A list of conventional mammography facilities is available by calling the CANCER INFORMATION SERVICE at 1-800-4-CANCER (1-800-422-6237) or by visiting the FDA Web site (http://www.accessdata.fda.gov/scripts/cdrh/cfdocs/cfmqsa/search.cfm).

See also COMPUTER-AIDED DETECTION.

disphosphonates See BISPHOSPHONATES.

docetaxel (Taxotere) Drug prepared from the needles of European yew trees. In the same family as TAXOL, it was approved in 1998 to treat locally advanced or metastatic (spreading) BREAST CANCER, which has progressed during anthracycline-based therapy or has relapsed during anthracycline-based ADJUVANT TREATMENT. Taxotere is a new type of chemical that inhibits cancer cell growth, interfering with cancer cell division and eventually killing the cell. About two out of three breast cancer subjects treated with CHEMOTHERAPY in the United States receive anthracyclines at some point in the treatment of their disease.

Side Effects
This drug may cause low white blood cell and platelet counts, fluid retention, and weight gain, HAIR LOSS, skin rash, hypersensitivity, NAUSEA, and DIARRHEA.

do not resuscitate order (DNR order) A legal directive by a physician that instructs hospital staff not to try to help a patient whose heart has stopped or who has stopped breathing. A patient can request a DNR order either by filling out an ADVANCE DIRECTIVE form or by telling the doctor that cardiopulmonary resuscitation should not be performed. DNR orders are accepted by doctors and hospitals in all states.

doubling time The time required for cells to double in number. BREAST CANCER has been shown to double in size every 23 to 209 days. It would take one cell, doubling every 100 days, eight to ten years to reach a size detectable by imaging techniques.

doxorubicin See ADRIAMYCIN.

ductal breast cancer See DUCTAL CARCINOMA.

ductal carcinoma The most common type of BREAST CANCER. This malignancy begins in the cells lining the ducts of the breast and accounts for 85 percent of all breast cancers.

Ductal carcinoma has a preinvasive stage known as DUCTAL CARCINOMA IN SITU. This type of breast cancer starts when a ductal cell begins to divide abnormally. The cells pile up and fill the ducts, but do not penetrate the boundary between the ducts and the underlying supportive tissue (called the basement membrane). They have not grown into other breast tissue and are considered preinvasive.

Between 15 and 20 percent of breast cancers are found at this point and can remain in this premalignant stage for some time. Most of the time, these lesions do not cause symptoms, except an occasional bloody NIPPLE DISCHARGE. These intraductal cancer cells may appear as small flecks of calcium on a MAMMOGRAM. These preinvasive cancers are treated surgically but because they do not spread, chemotherapy is never used.

DCIS is not life threatening at this stage, but the cells may continue to divide and move up and down the duct, eventually breaking through the basement membrane and invading breast tissue.

Once the cancer cell penetrates and invades into the underlying breast tissue, it becomes an invasive ductal cancer (IDC). As it grows, the ductal carcinoma becomes a larger, invasive tumor that may spread into the blood or lymphatic system. Breast cancers usually do not spread into the blood if the invasive tumor is smaller than one centimeter. Some invasive tumors never have this ability to spread. In general, small invasive ductal breast cancers have a good prognosis.

There are subtypes of invasive ductal cancers: tubular, medullary, mucinous and papillary cancers. Many of these have an excellent prognosis.

ductal carcinoma in situ (DCIS)   Also called intraductal carcinoma, this type of early BREAST CANCER (or precancer) consists of abnormal cells that are growing in the lining of a breast duct. The abnormal cells have not spread beyond the duct to invade the surrounding breast tissue, but women who have DCIS are at an increased risk of invasive breast cancer. If the cancer is detected at this stage, there is no risk of its spreading into the blood or lymph system.

Diagnosis

DCIS rarely causes a lump, but it usually appears on a mammogram as a sprinkling of calcifications. These calcifications are actually dead cancer cells that have calcified inside the ducts. (These calcium flakes are not related to calcium intake.) DCIS can range in virulence from low-grade, very slow-growing cancers to high-grade, faster-growing malignancies. However, any DCIS if left untreated has the potential to move into breast tissue and become invasive.

Treatment

Before MAMMOGRAPHY, DCIS was rarely diagnosed, so doctors are still trying to understand the best way to treat it. The ducts involved must be removed with a clear surrounding margin of cancer-free breast tissue. Underarm LYMPH NODES are not usually removed. In most cases, radiation is then given to decrease the chance of local recurrence. Sometimes the DCIS is small enough and low grade enough to be treated with lumpectomy alone. If DCIS is large or high grade, a mastectomy is recommended, which has a cure rate of almost 100 percent.

The question many women struggle with is whether to remove the entire breast for an almost 100 percent cure rate or have a local excision with radiation for a better cosmetic appearance, but a lower cure rate. (A local excision with radiation results in a 10 percent recurrence rate.)

Women who have DCIS may want to consider taking TAMOXIFEN to reduce the risk of development of invasive breast cancer.

See also DUCTAL CARCINOMA.

ductal cell   A cell from the duct of the breast.

ductal lavage   An investigational technique used to collect cells from milk ducts in the breast, where 95 percent of BREAST CANCER starts, so that the cells can be checked for cancer under a microscope.

The concept for the procedure was based on research indicating that breast cancer begins in the lining of the milk ducts, involving a series of molecular changes from normal to abnormal, and eventually to malignant. As long as abnormal cells are contained within the ducts or lobules, they are called "preinvasive," but once they invade surrounding tissues, they are considered INVASIVE BREAST CANCER.

The procedure can be done in a doctor's office or outpatient clinic and takes about an hour. To obtain the cells, the doctor applies an anesthetic cream to the nipple and then uses a suction device to draw fluid from the milk ducts to the nipple's surface. At this point, a hair-sized catheter is inserted into the nipple, followed by a small amount of anesthetic and then a small amount of saltwater into the duct. Fluid containing cells from the duct is withdrawn through the catheter and is then removed, along with breast cells. The cells are checked under a microscope to identify changes that may indicate cancer or changes that may increase the risk for breast cancer.

In one recent study published in the *Journal of the National Cancer Institute,* 507 high-risk women at 19 U.S. medical centers were tested with ductal lavage. The test found atypical cells in 24 percent of the women and malignant cells in two women, although all the women had had normal mammogram results in the year before they had ductal lavage. Such cells are not necessarily cancerous, but in women who are already at high risk the cells indicate that the breast cancer risk over the next decade is 18 times that of the average woman of the same age.

Most women in the study reported no more discomfort than they would feel during a mammogram.

Ductal lavage is not intended to replace MAMMOGRAPHY or a CLINICAL BREAST EXAM, but it can help women at high risk for breast cancer assess their risk. Although experts do not fully understand the relationship between atypical cells and breast cancer, atypical cells are considered to be an intermediate marker for breast cancer. If a woman learns she has some of these atypical cells, she may decide to be more aggressive in her risk-reduction treatment.

Ductal lavage is currently available at selected centers around the country.

However, experts warn that the test may not be practical for any but very-high-risk women, since it may detect many cellular abnormalities that never become cancerous. High-risk women include those who have certain genetic mutations or a family history of breast cancer, as well as women who have already had cancer in one breast and are worried about the other. They face a variety of choices, such as whether to have increased monitoring and mammograms, take the drug TAMOXIFEN, or have their breasts removed. The procedure is available at about 100 centers around the country and costs $400 to $700. However, it is not available everywhere and should not substitute for mammogram and clinical breast exam.

ductal papillomas Small noncancerous fingerlike growths in the mammary ducts that may cause a bloody NIPPLE DISCHARGE. These lesions are commonly found in women 45 to 50 years of age.

duct ectasia A widening and hardening of the milk duct in the breast, characterized by a thick green or black NIPPLE DISCHARGE, which usually affects women in their 40s and 50s. The nipple and surrounding tissue may be red and tender.

Duct ectasia is a benign condition but can sometimes be mistaken for cancer if a hard lump develops around the abnormal duct. Clear nipple discharge is often due to duct ectasia or a cyst.

Duct ectasia does not usually need treatment, though occasionally, the affected duct is surgically removed by an incision at the border of the AREOLA. The condition also improves with the application of heat or antibiotic drugs.

ductogram A diagnostic procedure (also called a galactogram) that employs a special type of contrast-enhanced MAMMOGRAPHY used for imaging the breast ducts. Ductography can help diagnose the cause of an abnormal NIPPLE DISCHARGE and is valuable in diagnosing INTRADUCTAL PAPILLOMAS.

The procedure takes between a half hour and an hour. Before the procedure, the nipple is usually cleaned and sterilized to remove dried discharge. The radiologist then presses the breast to elicit a fluid discharge. After identifying the discharging duct, the radiologist feeds a small hollow needle, (or cannula), into this area of the nipple. Usually only downward guidance is needed to insert the cannula into the patient's breast duct. Once the cannula has been gently fed down the duct, a small amount of contrast dye is injected into the breast through the cannula. A mammogram is then taken; the dye helps give a better view of the duct anatomical characteristics on the resulting images. After the procedure is completed, a bandage is placed over the nipple to prevent fluid or dye from staining the patient's clothes.

Some physicians coat the tip of the cannula with anesthetic gel and also dab it on the surface of the nipple. If the doctor is still unable to thread the cannula into the breast duct after three attempts, the procedure is typically postponed for one or two weeks.

A ductogram procedure can be mildly uncomfortable but is not usually painful. It is likely to be more uncomfortable when there is not a significant quantity of nipple discharge, making it difficult for the physician to find the opening of the discharging duct. This difficulty may require probing to find the right duct. If there is significant fluid discharge, the cannula insertion into the breast duct is usually much easier to perform and less uncomfortable for the patient.

The injecting of the dye is not painful but may cause a "full" sensation similar to the sensation that results when the breast fills with milk during breast-feeding.

In some cases, contrast dye may flow from the breast duct out into the surrounding breast tissue. If this occurs, the cannula is removed from the breast and the patient may be treated with a pain reliever if necessary. The procedure is usually rescheduled for a later date, typically one to two weeks later. To help minimize the likelihood of this occurring, ductography should be performed by radiologists who have significant experience using the procedure.

Most women can undergo ductography; the procedure may be more difficult to perform in those who have severe allergies to the contrast medium used during the procedure. In some cases, it may be possible to perform ductography by using a nonionic contrast dye, since little dye is actually absorbed during the procedure. Women who have had previous surgery that has completely disconnected the nipple pores from the underlying ducts may not be able to have ductography. Severe nipple retraction also makes the procedure difficult.

edrecolomab A type of MONOCLONAL ANTIBODY used in cancer detection or therapy. Monoclonal antibodies are laboratory-produced substances that can locate and bind to cancer cells.

eggs Eating eggs may possibly help young girls avoid BREAST CANCER later in life, according to a Harvard University study, whereas eating more butter was associated with a slight increased risk.

Although the researchers are not sure how egg consumption decreases breast cancer risk, they think the protection may be linked to the food's high levels of various nutrients, including amino acids, vitamins, and minerals. Most important are eggs' high levels of folate and vitamin D—nutrients that have been linked to reduced risk of breast cancer in other studies.

Because the study was based on women's recollections of their dietary habits of more than 40 years before, the authors admit to the possibility of serious flaws. However, many experts believe the study shows that what children eat may have a significant effect on their future risk of development of breast cancer.

In any case, experts conclude that it is important to make sure children eat healthy foods daily, including lots of vegetables, whole grains, beans, soy, fruits, and nonfat dairy products such as yogurt and milk.

See also DIET.

electrical impedance scanning Electrical impedance is a measurement of the speed at which electricity travels through something. Electrical impedance scanning capitalizes on the fact that malignant breast tissue conducts electricity much better than normal breast tissue, and therefore appears as bright white spots on the computer screen. This test is currently used as an adjunct for mammography to help sort out what needs to be biopsied.

The electrical impedance scanning device, which does not emit any radiation, consists of a handheld scanning probe and a computer screen that displays two-dimensional images of the breast. An electrode patch similar to the one used for an electrocardiogram is placed on the patient's arm. A very small amount of electric current (about the same amount used by a small penlight battery) is transmitted through the patch and into the body. The current travels through the breast, where it is measured by the scanning probe placed over the breast, generating an image from the measurements of electrical impedance.

The scanner sends the image directly to a computer, allowing the radiologist to move the probe around the breast to get the best view of the area being examined.

The device may reduce the number of biopsies needed to determine whether a mass is cancerous and may help doctors figure out who should have a BIOPSY. It is not available at many centers and studies need to be done before it is widely used. It is not yet clear if it is sufficiently sensitive or specific.

It is not approved as a screening device for BREAST CANCER. However, if techniques like this can be developed as a screening tool, it would be useful: it is portable, inexpensive and can be used in dense breasts of younger women. Although this device has not been studied in patients with implanted electronic devices such as pacemakers, it is not recommended for use on such patients.

electromagnetic fields and breast cancer Overhead power lines do not increase breast cancer risk, according to an extremely thorough 2003 New York study of nearly 600 cancer patients and 600 healthy volunteers. All study participants were longtime residents of New York's Long Island, specifically Nassau or Suffolk County, areas whose populations have unusually high rates of breast cancer.

The disparity between the rates of breast cancer in industrialized and less-industrialized regions has led to many hypotheses, including the theory that exposure to electromagnetic fields may suppress melatonin level and therefore may increase the risk of breast cancer.

In this current study Stony Brook University researchers investigated whether strong electric fields might be the breast cancer culprit and found no association between electromagnetic field levels and breast cancer risk on Long Island.

Scientists in the study did not just map overhead power lines; they also took electromagnetic field readings from various spots in all the residents' houses, including 24-hour measurements. They took readings from electric lines in the ground and also interviewed each resident.

An earlier study of electric fields and cancer, in Seattle, reached similar conclusions. A third study of the issue is ongoing in California.

electromagnetic radiation   See ELECTROMAGNETIC FIELDS.

Ellence (epirubicin hydrochloride)   CHEMOTHERAPY drug approved in 1999 for use as part of ADJUVANT TREATMENT in patients whose BREAST CANCER has spread to the lymph nodes under the arm after surgery. Ellence has been used to treat nearly 1 million women with breast cancer worldwide. It is the first and only chemotherapy agent approved by the Food and Drug Administration for the adjuvant treatment of node-positive early breast cancer.

Ellence approval was based on data from a trial demonstrating that in combination with CYCLOPHOSPHAMIDE and fluorouracil, it offers patients with early breast cancer greater relapse-free and overall survival rate benefits than a current standard adjuvant therapy, cyclophosphamide, methotrexate, fluorouracil (CMF). CMF and another common adjuvant chemotherapy, ADRIAMYCIN and CYTOXAN (AC), have been shown to have similar survival rates.

With roughly 75,000 women eligible for adjuvant therapy each year, a treatment regimen based on Ellence holds the potential for saving thousands of women who have early breast cancer when used as an alternative to a CMF regimen.

Side Effects
Side effects may include NAUSEA and vomiting, DIARRHEA, mouth sores, dehydration, fever, infection, pain, and burning or stinging at the injection site. Other side effects include HAIR LOSS, ANEMIA, loss of menstrual cycle, FATIGUE, HOT FLASHES, and rash or itch. Side effects involving the heart are a known risk of treatment with this class of drugs.

Long-term treatment with Ellence can cause leukemia, which may not be seen for up to three years after treatment. Ellence may cause premature menopause in women.

ENCOREplus   A community-based program, sponsored by the YWCA, that helps women who need early-detection education, breast and cervical cancer screening, and support services. The program also provides women under treatment for and recovering from BREAST CANCER with a combined peer group/support and exercise program.

The ENCOREplus program is designed to decrease inequalities in health care by removing barriers to access and promoting effective community-based outreach, education, and referral to clinical services and support systems.

The program components include the following:

- Community outreach and breast health education
- Referral to low- or no-cost breast and cervical screening
- Resources, information, and advocacy
- Peer group support and exercise for women who are being treated for or recovering from breast cancer

For contact information, see Appendix I.

endocrine therapy   Treatment for BREAST CANCER in which the hormonal balance of the body is changed to prevent HORMONE-dependent cancer cells from multiplying. This can include the use of TAMOXIFEN and (in premenopausal women) shutting off the ovaries either with medication or by surgical removal. In postmenopausal women the AROMATASE INHIBITORS may be used.

endostatin A drug known as an ANGIOGENESIS INHIBITOR that was heralded in 1998 for its ability in animal research to starve a malignant tumor by drying up its source of blood. Human tests of endostatin were launched in 1999 at the M. D. Anderson Cancer Center, the University of Wisconsin, and the Dana-Farber Cancer Center.

Studies proved that endostatin may have some modest activity against BREAST CANCER. Endostatin can decrease blood flow to some tumors in patients and promote death in cancer and blood vessel cells. Researchers concluded that the drug, even at different dosages, was both safe for and well tolerated by the 25 patients who received it. Patients used the drug for a median period of 69 days. In two patients, there was evidence of minor antitumor activity—several tumors were observed to shrink—but no long-term responses were seen. All patients, who suffered from a variety of advanced cancers and had no other treatments available to them, eventually died.

Scientists believe that the science behind the angiogenesis inhibitions is very exciting, but the saga of endostatin shows again how difficult it is to predict what will work well in the treatment of patients and their breast cancers. Cancer is unpredictable and experts predict that many types of treatments will be necessary to control this disease.

Angiogenesis inhibitors such as endostatin have helped scientists understand cancer better, and may be used in the future treatment of breast malignancies.

epidermal growth factor receptor (ErbB1) See HER-2.

epirubicin See ELLENCE.

erb B-2 See ONCOGENE.

erythropoietin (EPO, Epogen, Procrit) Produced in the adult kidney, this substance triggers the production of red blood cells. It can be used as a drug to reverse anemia in patients with breast cancer who are receiving CHEMOTHERAPY.

esophagitis Inflammation of the esophagus. It occurs occasionally as a direct result of taking CHEMOTHERAPY drugs for BREAST CANCER. Esophagitis can lead to bleeding, painful ulcers, and infection. However, sores in the esophagus are usually temporary and develop generally between five and 14 days after chemotherapy. They heal completely once chemotherapy is finished.

estrogen A female HORMONE secreted by the ovaries that is essential for menstruation, reproduction, and development of secondary sex characteristics, such as breasts. Estrogen stimulates the normal growth of breast tissue both during adolescence and during pregnancy, when breast cells differentiate (specialize) so they can produce milk.

Evidence suggests that the longer a woman is exposed to estrogen (whether made by her body or taken as a drug), the more likely she is to develop BREAST CANCER. For example, breast cancer risk is somewhat increased among women who begin menstruation at an early age (before age 12), experience menopause late (after age 55), never have children or have the first child after age 30, or take hormone replacement therapy for long periods. Each of these factors increases the amount of time a woman's body is exposed to estrogen.

In between the growth of the breast and the first pregnancy, breast cells are exposed to estrogen. If a woman does not become pregnant until after she turns 30, there is a long period when her breast cells are exposed to estrogen and have not differentiated. If she never becomes pregnant, the cells never differentiate. In both cases, the breast cells become vulnerable over time to cancerous changes as a result of their long exposure to estrogen while being undifferentiated.

A woman's chances of breast cancer development drops with each successive pregnancy.

HRT and Breast Cancer

When hormone replacement was first developed, doctors simply administered estrogen alone (ESTROGEN REPLACEMENT THERAPY, or ERT). ERT helped relieve the symptoms of menopause and appeared to provide protection against heart disease and bone fractures, problems that often occur in older women. But doctors discovered that it also increased the risk of endometrial cancer—cancer of the uterine lining. They later found that adding the hormone progesterone to estrogen (the treatment was now called HORMONE REPLACEMENT THERAPY or HRT) protection against endometrial cancer.

The link between estrogen and cancer is the reason why women who have had breast cancer, or who were at high risk, were always discouraged from taking HRT.

Despite improvements in HRT for postmenopausal women, further risks have been discovered. The largest randomized study ever to look at combined HRT in healthy postmenopausal women was stopped early, in July 2002, when researchers found an increased risk of breast cancer among participants. The study was stopped because of ethical concerns due to the clear risk for study subjects.

The researchers looked at more than 16,000 healthy postmenopausal women who were part of the Women's Health Initiative (WHI), a trial funded by the National Institutes of Health. Each woman was between the ages of 50 and 79 and still had an intact uterus. The women began taking either a combination estrogen–progesterone pill or a placebo each day, starting in the mid-1990s. The women were supposed to be followed for an average of eight and a half years, and the researchers were to check the results twice each year. The last scheduled review (May 2002) showed the results were significant enough to stop the trial after just over five years. At the time of the study, 38 percent of postmenopausal American women were on HRT.

According to the study, the rate of breast cancers was 26 percent higher among those who had HRT as opposed to those who had placebo. The rate for heart disease was 29 percent higher, stroke rate was 41 percent higher, and blood clot rates were more than twice as high in those who had HRT.

HRT did have some benefits, however. The rate of colorectal cancer was 37 percent lower in the HRT group, and the rate of bone fractures was 24 percent lower. Endometrial cancer rates were about the same in both groups. The WHI study report, along with an editorial recommending against the long-term use of HRT by healthy post-

menopausal women, was published in the July 17, 2002, issue of the *Journal of the American Medical Association.*

Given these results, researchers recommend that clinicians stop prescribing HRT for long-term use. Nonetheless, although the increased risk of breast cancer and other conditions may make HRT unsuitable for prevention in healthy people, the overall risk for each woman is still rather small. For example, the 36 percent increased risk of breast cancer is based on the finding that during 10 years, among 10,000 women receiving combination HRT there will be 38 cases of breast cancer while among 10,000 women taking a placebo, there will be 30 cases. The same holds true for heart disease (37 cases per 10,000 women per year with HRT, versus 30 cases per 10,000 women per year with placebo) and blood clots (34 cases per 10,000 women per year with HRT, versus 16 cases per 10,000 women per year with placebo). Still, there is a risk, and it would probably increase as the length of time taking combination HRT increased.

The AMERICAN CANCER SOCIETY acknowledged that deciding whether to take HRT, particularly estrogen plus progestin, will be more difficult now and recommended that women who are taking HRT discuss this recent finding with their doctors. The effects of ERT on women who no longer have an intact uterus are being studied in a separate WHI clinical trial, with results expected in 2005.

estrogen receptor assay (ERA) A test that is done on breast cancer tissue to determine whether tumor is nourished by estrogen (estrogen receptor positive, ER+) or not (estrogen receptor negative, ER-). Tumors that are hormone dependent may respond to treatment with hormonal therapy. These ER+ tumors tend to be less aggressive and respond better to treatment than ER- tumors.

estrogen-receptor-positive (ER+) tumor BREAST CANCER tumor that contains receptors for the hormones estrogen and progesterone. These receptors are located on the cell surface and regulate breast tissue growth in response to changing hormone levels. About two-thirds of all breast cancer tumors are ER+; two-thirds of these ER+ tumors also contain receptors to progesterone and are also considered PR+. (PR+ tumors require an intact estrogen receptor.) Younger women tend to have fewer ER+ breast tumors. Tumors that have many estrogen receptors tend to be less aggressive, respond well to hormone therapy, and have a better prognosis than tumors that do not have them.

estrogen replacement therapy (ERT)   The use of ESTROGEN to replace estrogen a woman no longer produces herself because of natural or induced menopause. Once recommended for women without a uterus as a way of easing menopause symptoms, research released in 2004 found that women who took estrogen alone after menopause had a significantly increased risk of stroke and a possible higher risk of dementia, according to the National Institutes of Health (NIH). The NIH decided to stop the estrogen-only study a year before its planned completion because enough data had been collected to assess overall risks and benefits.

The government ended the last major study of estrogen early because of the health risks, noting that estrogen alone is not as bad as when it is combined it with the hormone progestin—but officials advise that estrogen still is too risky for long-term use.

Surprisingly, estrogen alone did not increase the risk of breast cancer, a surprise to researchers, since the estrogen-progestin combination had increased that risk by 26 percent.

For a long time, doctors had thought that using estrogen (alone or together with progestin) would keep women healthier after menopause by reducing heart attacks and keeping the brain sharp. However, millions of women abandoned the estrogen-progestin combination in 2002, when a major federal study concluded that those pills raised the risk of breast cancer, strokes, and heart attacks. At that time, the scientists were not sure whether estrogen alone was as risky. (Only women who have undergone a hysterectomy can even consider taking estrogen alone; in other women, progestin use with estrogen is crucial to protect against uterine cancer.)

Then, in March 2004, the NIH shut down its study of estrogen-only use as well, telling the 11,000 women enrolled to quit their pills, essentially ending hope that estrogen alone would have

some usefulness that the hormone combination did not. The women in the study were healthy 50- to 79-year-olds, who took either estrogen or a dummy pill for nearly seven years. The study's primary purpose was to see if estrogen could prevent heart disease after menopause.

In stopping the study, the government revealed that estrogen alone increased the risk of a stroke as much as combination estrogen-progestin does. For every 10,000 women, those taking hormones suffer eight more strokes per year than nonhormone users. At the same time, estrogen alone had no effect on heart disease. (In contrast, the estrogen-progestin combination increases heart attack risk by 29 percent.)

Neither type of hormone therapy seems good for women's brains. Preliminary data from a related study of women 65 and older suggest those taking estrogen alone were more likely to suffer some degree of dementia than those taking a placebo. Likewise, scientists announced in 2003 that the estrogen-progestin combination doubled the risk of Alzheimer's and other forms of dementia.

Benefits

Estrogen (and estrogen-progestin) decrease the risk of a hip fracture from bone-thinning osteoporosis, although only women who cannot take one of the nation's many other osteoporosis treatments should consider estrogen for that use, according to the government.

European Organisation for Research and Treatment of Cancer (EORTC)   An international nonprofit group that conducts, coordinates, and stimulates laboratory and clinical research in Europe to improve the management of cancer. Because comprehensive research in this field is often beyond the means of individual European laboratories and hospitals, the organization creates the opportunity for multidisciplinary, multinational collaborations of basic research scientists and clinicians from the European continent.

The ultimate goals of the EORTC are to improve the standard of cancer treatment in Europe through the development of new drugs and innovative approaches and to test more effective treatments with drugs, surgery, and RADIATION THERAPY.

The international organization was founded under Belgian law in 1962 by eminent oncologists working in the main cancer research institutes of Switzerland and the European Union (EU) countries. Named Groupe Européen de Chimiothérapie Anticancéreuse, it became the European Organisation for Research and Treatment of Cancer in 1968. For contact information, see Appendix I.

Evista   A SELECTIVE ESTROGEN RECEPTOR MODULATOR (SERM) that acts as an estrogen and an antiestrogen simultaneously. It is in the same class of drugs as TAMOXIFEN, and is very closely related to tamoxifen both in benefits and side effects.

Doctors have used Evista (raloxifene) since December of 1997, when it was approved by the U.S. Food and Drug Administration (FDA) for the prevention of osteoporosis in postmenopausal women. Subsequently, large studies testing its effectiveness against osteoporosis have shown that women who take the drug have fewer BREAST CANCERS than women who take a placebo.

One of these studies was the Multiple Outcomes of Raloxifene Evaluation trial, designed to study the effects of raloxifene on osteoporosis in postmenopausal women. In this study, researchers also tracked rates of breast cancer and observed a 54 percent reduction in the risk of breast cancer among women who took raloxifene. The results of this study were reported in the June 16, 1999, issue of the *Journal of the American Medical Association.*

However, women in that study were not assigned to Evista or placebo based on breast cancer risk, so the finding may be partly due to chance. This is currently under study.

In one recent study, researchers compared the effects of Evista and of placebo in women who had high and low levels of estrogen in their blood. The study found that women who had high levels of estrogen who took Evista had about one-fifth the rate of breast cancer compared to women on placebo. But among women with low estradiol levels, who were already at low risk of getting breast cancer, taking Evista did not decrease risk further.

STAR Study

Raloxifene is currently being compared with tamoxifen in the Study of Tamoxifen and Ralox-

ifene (STAR), one of the largest breast cancer prevention trials ever undertaken. STAR is also the first trial to compare a drug proved to reduce the probability of breast cancer development with another drug that has the potential to reduce breast cancer risk. All participants—22,000 postmenopausal women—will receive one or the other drug for five years at more than 400 sites in the United States, Puerto Rico, and Canada.

Tamoxifen (Nolvadex) proved in the BREAST CANCER PREVENTION TRIAL to reduce breast cancer incidence by 49 percent in women who were at increased risk of the disease. The FDA approved the use of tamoxifen to reduce the incidence of breast cancer in women at increased risk of the disease in October 1998. It has been approved by the FDA to treat breast cancer for more than 20 years and has been in clinical trials for about 30 years.

The trial is limited to postmenopausal women because raloxifene has not been adequately tested for safety in premenopausal women.

Side Effects

Serious side effects are known to occur in women who take tamoxifen, including endometrial cancer, blood clots in the leg or lung, and possibly stroke. Raloxifene is not believed to cause endometrial cancer, but it shares the other side effects.

Information about the side effects of raloxifene is limited because it has been studied for only about five years, and fewer women have been studied during that time for this drug than for tamoxifen. Studies of raloxifene have generally involved women who received the drug to determine its effect on osteoporosis, and the durations of both therapy and follow-up have been short.

Other side effects include hot flashes (which may often be controlled with herbal supplements or additional medication) and/or leg cramps (which may be reduced by drinking tonic water, which contains quinine).

See also NATIONAL SURGICAL ADJUVANT BREAST AND BOWEL PROJECT; STAR.

excisional biopsy   A surgical procedure in which an entire lump or suspicious area in the breast is removed and then examined under a microscope for diagnosis.

See also BIOPSY.

exemestane   See AROMASIN.

exercise   Studies suggest that exercise may reduce the risk of BREAST CANCER, perhaps by influencing age at first menstruation, lowering ESTROGEN level, decreasing weight gain and overall weight, and enhancing the immune system. Regular exercise may decrease the risk of breast cancer in younger women and lower the chance of cancer recurrence in women who already have had breast cancer.

Exercise helps the body use food and fiber optimally, build lean muscle, and burn calories. A sedentary lifestyle contributes to obesity, and obesity is a risk factor for heart disease, diabetes, and many cancers, including cancer of the breast.

The amount of exercise needed to provide protection against breast cancer, however, is controversial. Some studies say that only 30 minutes of moderate exercise a day—not necessarily at one time—is enough; others indicate the benefit may result exclusively from vigorous exercise.

In one 2001 study, women who were active on the job or doing housework had a lower risk of breast cancer. Moderate activity was related to the greatest risk reduction. The study found women benefited from activity from housework and on the job, but that work carried a slightly greater benefit.

Some studies have reported that athletes who exercised vigorously and participated in competitive sports had a lower risk of breast cancer than nonathletes. Others have reported that women who did not participate in competitive sports but who exercised three hours a week throughout their reproductive years had a lower risk of breast cancer than did women who never exercised.

Among 11 studies looked at together, eight reported a decrease in the risk of breast cancer in premenopausal, postmenopausal, or all women with high levels of physical activity compared to women with low levels of activity. In the three studies in which exercise was not found to influence breast cancer risk, most of the women were younger and premenopausal. These results suggest that exercise may have a different influence on premenopausal versus postmenopausal breast cancer risk.

The inconsistency of the results in these studies may also be due to differences in study design and the ways women reported their level of physical activity. Researchers are continuing to design studies to determine more specifically the relationship between exercise and breast cancer and to give women suggestions for incorporating appropriate levels of exercise in their daily routine.

The relationship between exercise and breast cancer is complicated and difficult to study. Researchers must consider established risk factors for breast cancer, such as family history or age at time of first menstrual cycle, first pregnancy, and at menopause. In addition, women who exercise may be different in other ways from women who do not exercise. For example, women who exercise may be less likely to smoke, may be leaner, and may eat differently than women who do not exercise. Researchers must consider all of these factors when trying to assess the influence of exercise on the risk of breast cancer.

In animal studies of exercise and breast cancer risk, results depended on the kind of exercise program used. Animals that exercised by using an exercise wheel placed in their cage had fewer breast tumors than animals that did not have an exercise wheel. In other studies, a motorized treadmill was used to control the animal's level and frequency of exercise. Some researchers reported that this type of exercise (called involuntary exercise) reduced the incidence of breast tumors; others reported that it either had no effect or increased the incidence of tumors. The stress of involuntary exercise may influence the growth of breast tumors and account for the mixed results in these studies.

Usually, researchers measure work-related and leisure time activities separately to try to determine their effects on breast cancer risk independently.

Activity on the Job

According to several large studies of work-related activity, women who reported a high level of physical activity at work had an 18 to 52 percent reduction in their risk of breast cancer development when compared to women with low levels of activity at work. In some of these studies, level of work-related activity was determined by classifying women according to their job. Farmers, nurses, and nurses' aides were classified as having a high level of physical activity; teachers, salespeople, and waitresses were classified as having a moderate level; and most office professionals were classified as having little activity. In other studies, the level of work-related activity was determined by asking women to rate how physically active they are at work. The differences in the ways researchers determined level of work-related activity may be one reason why these studies reported such differences in risk reduction.

Recreation and Breast Cancer

In studies of recreational activity, women who exercised during their leisure time were reported to have between 12 and 60 percent reductions in their risk of breast cancer. This range in risk reduction may be due to differences in study design, such as the ways the researchers measured or defined different levels of physical activity and questioned women about their level of activity. Some of the researchers focused their attention on athletes; others asked women to describe their own level of activity.

Exercise for Patients with Breast Cancer

Several studies have reported that exercise benefits women diagnosed with breast cancer both during and after surgery, chemotherapy, and/or radiation. Getting modest amounts of exercise, even just an easy half-hour walk a day, appears to substantially improve women's chances of surviving breast cancer.

In fact, a 2004 study found that women who exercised after breast cancer reduced their chance of dying from the disease by one-quarter to one-half, depending on how active they were. Just how exercise might do this is still unclear, though experts have several theories. Exercise might also reduce breast cancer by burning up stored fat that produces estrogen, which in turn can fuel breast cancer growth. In addition, women who get exercise are less likely to develop many common health problems, including heart disease, high blood pressure, osteoporosis and diabetes.

The results were based on the NURSES' HEALTH STUDY, which has followed the health of almost 122,000 female nurses since 1976. The researchers looked at physical activity in 2,167 women who were diagnosed with breast cancer after the study began. During up to 16 years of follow-up, those who got lots of exercise were most likely to survive their disease, although even a little bit of exercise helped. Most of the women walked for exercise. Those who walked one to three hours a week at a leisurely 3 mph lowered their risk of dying from breast cancer by one-quarter, compared with the most sedentary women. Those who walked between three and eight hours a week cut their risk in half.

Typically, doctors recommend at least 45 minutes of moderate to vigorous exercise five times a week. Even modest exercise can have major benefits, researchers note. Women with breast cancer who exercised also report having higher self-esteem, improved body image, less nausea during chemotherapy, and less fatigue, depression, and insomnia. Women who exercise also had better physical performance and a better quality of life.

Weight gain is also a troublesome and potentially serious problem for patients with breast cancer who are undergoing chemotherapy. In one study, patients who gained more weight during treatment were more likely to relapse and more likely to die of breast cancer than patients who gained less weight. Patients with breast cancer who exercise while having treatment may gain less weight than patients who do not exercise.

Exercise Recommendations

Women need to consider their age, health, and overall fitness level and consult a doctor before starting any exercise program. Government experts recommend that Americans aim for light to moderate physical activity for at least 30 minutes five or more times per week. If this schedule is not possible, women should try to participate in physical activity at least three times per week.

There is no clear recommendation as to whether exercise is more helpful during adolescence, during adulthood, or throughout life. It may be important to exercise during the teenage years because this may be a critical period for the development of breast cancer. One study demonstrated that women younger than age 40 who averaged 3.8 hours of exercise per week during their reproductive years had about a 60 percent decrease in their risk of breast cancer. Another study reported that women who were athletes in college remained more physically active than nonathletes later in life, and their risk of breast cancer was reduced by about 50 percent. Other researchers have not found that exercise during adolescence is more helpful than current exercise habits.

The AMERICAN CANCER SOCIETY (ACS) is putting a new emphasis on exercise as a way to reduce cancer. The organization recommends that for cancer prevention adults have at least 30 minutes of moderate activity, such as a brisk walk, five days a week. In addition, the ACS believes that 45 minutes or more of moderate to vigorous activity five or more days a week may further reduce breast cancer risk. "Vigorous activity" can range from jogging to martial arts, basketball, or masonry work. This level of exercise can reduce the risk of breast cancer by a third.

The society also recommends that children and adolescents do moderate to vigorous physical activity at least 60 minutes a day, five days a week. The goal is to create lifetime habits that will prevent youngsters from becoming overweight or obese.

familial breast cancer   BREAST CANCER that occurs in families more often than would be expected by chance.

family history   Having a family member with BREAST CANCER increases a woman's risk of developing the disease. This risk is minimal if only one distant relative has the disease but higher if a close relative (such as mother, sister, or daughter) has breast cancer. If there are multiple relatives with breast cancer, the risk may be extremely high.

In some cases, the increased risk is caused by sharing genetic traits that are known to contribute to breast cancer, such as the *BRCA1* or *BRCA2* genes or the *P-TEN* GENE (see BREAST CANCER SUSCEPTIBILITY GENES).

Women in families with a strong history of breast cancer should consider talking to a genetic counselor about getting tested to see if they have inherited a mutation in the *BRCA1* or *2* gene.

If the genetic blood test is positive and reveals that the woman has inherited an abnormal, cancer-causing gene, screening tests may be administered more often to check for breast cancer (MAMMOGRAMS and MRI scans). Screening tests also may be considered for ovarian cancer (ultrasound tests and CA125 blood tests), because women who have inherited a *BRCA1* or *2* malformation are at higher risk for developing ovarian cancer as well.

Women with the *BRCA1* or *2* gene also may consider preventive surgery—either removing the ovaries or removing the breasts before cancer develops.

For women who lack the gene but have a positive family history, screening guidelines should be carefully followed, and the women should consider taking other risks and strategies, such as taking TAMOXIFEN, to prevent the development of breast cancer.

Fareston (toremifene citrate)   An antihormone type of CHEMOTHERAPY tablet approved in 1997 for the treatment of metastatic BREAST CANCER in postmenopausal women who have estrogen-receptor-positive or receptor-unknown tumors. It works by blocking ESTROGEN so that the cancer cells that depend on estrogen to divide stop growing and die.

Side effects include HOT FLASHES, vaginal discharge and bleeding, and "flare" reactions (temporary increase in tumor or bone pain that ends within a week or two) when the drug is started.

Both TAMOXIFEN and Fareston may be administered after breast cancer surgery to prevent cancer recurrence. Tamoxifen has been proved to decrease the recurrence of breast cancer and prolong life, but there are risks in taking tamoxifen, including an increase in risk of endometrial cancer. Since Fareston and tamoxifen are very similar in their chemical makeup, experts hope that Fareston will work as well as tamoxifen, but with fewer side effects. Fareston has been shown to be as effective against metastatic breast cancer as tamoxifen, and the U.S. Food and Drug Administration's advisory committee determined that the two drugs were therapeutically equivalent in terms of response rate.

The North American Fareston vs. Tamoxifen Adjuvant Trial for Breast Cancer is comparing Fareston with tamoxifen to see which is a better treatment for breast cancer.

Faslodex   See FULVESTRANT.

fatigue The most common side effect experienced by cancer patients, occurring as a result of the cancer or treatment. Although it occurs most frequently in those who are having treatment, overwhelming fatigue may continue after treatment ends.

Scientists are not sure of its exact cause; some researchers believe fatigue may be caused by the waste products produced as a tumor shrinks, or may be related to the energy the body needs to fight cancer. Others believe fatigue may be related to interruptions in the signals sent through the nervous system. A low blood count (ANEMIA) as a result of chemotherapy, sleep disturbances, stress, depression, poor diet, infection, or other medication side effects can all contribute to this exhaustion.

Symptoms

The symptoms of cancer-related fatigue are different from normal feelings of being tired. Fatigue can begin suddenly and be all-consuming; naps may not help. Fatigue can be physically and emotionally draining on the patient as well as the family. General weakness may be accompanied by limb heaviness, decreased ability to concentrate, sleeplessness, and/or irritability.

Diagnosis

Patients with this type of extreme tiredness should consult a health-care provider, who will conduct simple tests, including a blood count to check for anemia or infection and a physical examination.

Treatment

If symptoms are fatigue related, there are several things patients can do to help manage those symptoms. It is important to eat healthy, appetite-stimulating foods. The complex carbohydrates found in pasta, fresh fruits, and whole grain breads provide long-term energy. Studies have shown that a moderate amount of exercise may actually help improve energy level.

Sleep is also important. Patients should go to bed at a regular time each day and follow a regular routine.

It is also important to make sure that treatable causes of fatigue (anemia, depression, low thyroid) are ruled out.

fat necrosis A hard, noncancerous lump caused by destruction of fat cells in the breast due to trauma or injury. Fat necrosis occurs as the body tries to repair damaged breast tissue. The affected area may sometimes be replaced with firm scar tissue that may then swell or become tender. Symptoms of fat necrosis usually subside within a month. Although fat necrosis is harmless, the lump may feel like a breast tumor; it also may be mistaken for cancer on a mammogram. A BIOPSY can confirm fat necrosis.

Femara (letrozole) A type of HORMONE used to treat advanced BREAST CANCER in postmenopausal women. It works by blocking ESTROGEN, thus stopping the growth of estrogen-hungry cancer cells. Approved in 1997 for the treatment of advanced breast cancer in postmenopausal women, it received additional approval in 2001 for first-line treatment of postmenopausal women whose tumor was either hormone-receptor positive or hormone-receptor unknown and whose cancer had spread locally or throughout the body. Given in pill form, it can cause bone or muscle pain and (less often) headaches, fatigue, nausea, or hot flashes. A 2003 study found Femara effective in continuing to reduce risk of recurrence in women who had completed five years of tamoxifen therapy.

fibroadenoma The most common solid tumor of the breast. Fibroadenomas are benign rubbery growths that move easily within the breast but do not contain fluid. They are not related to the development of breast cancer. Fibroadenomas range in size from tiny lumps that cannot be felt but may show up on a mammogram to large growths that can be easily felt. On a mammogram, a fibroadenoma appears as a smooth area with distinct edges.

Most fibroadenomas grow smaller over time, but some may grow larger and cause discomfort. Because most masses in very young women are benign, doctors may simply watch the growth carefully. Ultrasound may help confirm the diagnosis.

Typically fibroadenomas are not cancerous, but if the lump contains certain types of cells, a woman may have a three times higher risk of developing breast cancer. A rare type of cancer occurs in about 1 percent of fibroadenomas. This is why doctors

˙usually recommend a biopsy in older women. A fibroadenoma may be removed surgically if required but can usually be left alone.

fibrocystic breast changes A noncancerous breast condition in which multiple CYSTS or lumpy areas develop in one or both breasts. It can be accompanied by discomfort or pain that fluctuates with the menstrual cycle. Cysts are fluid-filled sacs that feel like soft lumps or tender spots in the breast. They are found most often in women ages 30 to 50 and in postmenopausal women who are taking hormones. Typically, a cyst is not cancerous and does not increase a woman's risk of future breast cancer, although a rare type of cancer does occur in about 1 percent of cysts. Large cysts can be treated by aspiration of the fluid they contain.

A breast lump that should be checked is one that does not change with a woman's menstrual cycle. Any persistent lump or thickening should be evaluated by a trained medical professional.

financial issues Treating BREAST CANCER can be very expensive, but health insurance plans usually cover much of the cost. Patients who belong to a health maintenance organization (HMO) or preferred provider organization (PPO) should become familiar with their provider choices and their financial responsibility if they receive care "out of network" from a doctor not covered by the health plan.

Patients with breast cancer who do not have insurance should contact their local Social Security Office to determine whether they qualify for Supplemental Security Income (SSI) or Social Security Disability Insurance (SSDI). The medical requirements and disability determination process are the same in both programs. However, whereas eligibility for SSDI is based on employment history, SSI is based on financial need.

Free Hospital Care

Patients with breast cancer who do not have insurance can also receive care from hospitals who receive federal grants from Hill-Burton Funds that allow hospitals and nursing homes to provide low-cost or no-cost medical care. To receive a listing of hospitals or nursing homes participating in the Hill-Burton program, patients can call (800) 638-0742.

Prescription Drugs

Most major pharmaceutical companies have patient-assistance programs that offer a free three-month supply of medication to those who cannot afford their prescriptions. To obtain guidelines and a listing of participating companies, patients can call the Pharmaceutical Manufacturers' Association at (800) 762-4636. The medication request must be completed by a physician.

Free Air Transportation

Many nonprofit agencies offer free air transportation for patients who travel treatment centers, relying on private pilots who donate their time and use their own planes. Patients can obtain a list of these services at http://www.aircareall.org. In addition, major airlines sometimes offer reduced or no-cost travel through an assistance program.

Local Transportation

For local travel assistance to and from treatments, a hospital social worker may be able to provide van service or cab/bus vouchers. Some local AMERICAN CANCER SOCIETY offices run volunteer transportation programs or provide funds to reimburse travel expenses. Some communities offer MediVans for those who qualify as a result of illness or disability. Local nursing homes, park districts, or YMCAs also may offer van transportation to local hospitals. In addition, many communities offer seniors reduced-fare taxi service within the community.

Temporary Housing

Temporary housing is sometimes required by patients with breast cancer who must travel for consultation or treatment or for families who visit hospitalized patients. The American Cancer Society may be able to arrange a low-cost hotel room for those receiving treatment. In addition, many hospitals negotiate discount rates at local hotels or provide dormitory-style housing.

The NATIONAL ASSOCIATION OF HOSPITALITY HOUSES (800-542-9730) also provides referral information to anyone in need of lodging while undergoing treatment away from home.

Utilities

Assistance programs are offered by many gas, electric, water, and phone companies for patients with breast cancer who may have trouble paying monthly bills. Many states have regulations that prohibit companies from turning off utilities; a doctor or social worker may need to write a letter describing why the services are medically necessary. The regulations do not lessen a patient's responsibility for paying bills but may allow families more time or lower monthly payments. In an emergency, local help lines and social service agencies may be able to provide one-time emergency help with utility bills.

Home Care/Respite

Some insurance plans offer coverage for home care ranging from skilled nursing to companions. If companion care is not a covered benefit, patients can contact various agencies for assistance.

Respite care allows the caregiver a few hours each week to take a break while someone watches over the patient. Many caregivers use this time to run errands, take care of personal health needs, or just unwind.

Local respite caregivers can be located by calling the National Respite Locator at (800) 773-5433. The locator service can also provide a listing of qualifying conditions.

In addition, the National Federation of Interfaith Volunteer Caregivers, a not-for-profit group that oversees 400 regional offices, sends volunteers into the homes of people who need care, company, and supervision. They can be reached at (800) 350-7438.

Medical Supplies

The Cancer Fund of America (800-578-5284) can provide necessary nonprescription medical items such as nutritional supplements. Items available vary, as the group receives donated products from companies. Patients or family members can call and be placed in their database for specific needs.

Food Programs

Meals on Wheels coordinates thousands of programs throughout the United States dedicated to delivering meals to those who are homebound. Some programs require a small donation; eligibility is determined by each program. For a local referral to Meals on Wheels, patients can contact the national office at (616) 530-0929.

Viatical Settlement Companies

Viatical companies purchase a patient's life insurance policy at a discounted rate, providing money for patients to use however they want. The seller, in turn, signs over the policy to the viatical company.

In general, any life insurance policy (group or individual) can be sold, but the rate of return and eligibility criteria vary with each company. However, patients should consider tax implications and the effect of a viatical settlement on their eligibility for assistance programs.

A free brochure, "Viatical Settlements: A Guide for People with Terminal Illnesses," is available from the Federal Trade Commission at (202) 326-2222. The National Viatical Association (202) 347-7361) offers a listing of viatical companies.

Life Insurance Loans

LifeWise Family Financial Security, Inc., allows patients to take out a loan against their existing life insurance policy if their life expectancy is five years or less. There is no obligation to repay the loan, but the option is available, thereby creating a different option from selling an insurance policy to a viatical company. If a patient chooses not to repay the loan, the life insurance policy proceeds are the sole source of repayment. All surplus funds are remitted to the patient's family. LifeWise has counselors available to answer any questions and publishes *The Financial Resource Guide: A Comprehensive, Step-by-Step Reference for Individuals Facing Life-Threatening or Terminal Illnesses.* Advice from counselors and a copy of the guide are available by calling (800) 219-7385.

fine needle aspiration   Procedure to remove cells or fluid from tissues by using a needle with an empty syringe. Cells or breast fluid is extracted by pulling back on the plunger and then is analyzed by a physician for cancer cells.

See also BIOPSY.

fish and breast cancer   Eating fish has no association with BREAST CANCER risk, according to 10 of 13 studies. Of the three that did see a connection between eating fish and breast cancer risk, two reported an increase in risk and one reported a decrease in risk. There is evidence that fish oils slow the development of mammary cancer in animals, but the research in humans is less clear. The studies described examined fish in general rather than fish oil.

Fish living in contaminated waters can accumulate environmental contaminants, and studies of breast cancer in women who eat sport fish caught in contaminated waters have not been conducted. These concerns would not include fish bought in grocery stores, which are tested by the U.S. Food and Drug Administration.

five-year survival rate   The percentage of people who survive five years or longer with a disease. Although the rates are based on the most recent information available, they may include data from patients treated several years earlier. Although still statistically valid, five-year survival rates may not reflect advances in cancer treatment, which often occur very quickly. These numbers are statistics and may guide decision-making but do not help lessen individual risk.

flap surgery   See BREAST RECONSTRUCTION.

flavonoids   A large family of plant substances formerly designated as vitamin F. However, flavonoids are neither vitamins nor essential nutrients. They occur often in pigments and in fruits (especially citrus fruits, purple berries, apples, and grapes), as well as in vegetables, tea, and whole grains. Flavonoids include flavones (such as quercetin), ISOFLAVONES (from soybeans), flavonones (such as rutin in citrus), anthocyanins (blue, purple, and red plant pigments), and flavonoids (including tannins).

Flavonoids found in fruit, vegetables, chocolate, tea, wine, and grape juice reduce cellular oxidative stress and may be associated with a reduced risk of cancer. They can act as antioxidants to prevent FREE RADICAL damage and oxidation that triggers inflammation. (Free radicals are harmful, highly reactive molecules that tear electrons away from nearby molecules to replace missing electrons.) Concord grape juice is one example of a potent, long-lasting antioxidant.

The amounts of key flavonoids in foods and beverages have been determined, but the quantity of a certain flavonoids that should be consumed to help prevent breast cancer is uncertain. How flavonoids are processed in the intestine, how they are absorbed, and how they are assimilated by the body remain unknown.

flow cytometry   A test done on cancerous tissues that shows the aggressiveness of a breast tumor. The test shows how many cells are in the dividing stage at one time, commonly referred to as the S phase, and the (DNA) content of the cancer, referred to as the ploidy. This information reveals how rapidly the tumor is growing. However, it is not clear how much flow cytometry adds to other known prognostic functions such as node positivity, ER+, grade and size of breast cancer.

foam breast prosthesis   A type of inexpensive breast prosthesis, primarily used for its shape, that replaces a breast that has been removed during mastectomy. Although some foam prostheses are weighted, most do not match the weight or movement of a natural breast.

folic acid (folate)   A B-complex vitamin being studied as a cancer prevention agent. Some experts believe that folic acid may help prevent breast cells from mutating and may help strengthen the immune system. It also may help lower cardiovascular risk.

free radicals   Highly charged destructive forms of oxygen generated by each cell in the body that destroy cellular membranes through the oxidation process. Free radicals can damage important cellular molecules such as DNA or lipids in other parts of the cell.

Because free radicals are essential to many reactions in the body (they are generated by the immune system to fend off microbes and help the digestive system break down food), they should not be entirely destroyed. It is only when their levels become too high that damage can occur.

Free radical damage can be offset by molecules called ANTIOXIDANTS, which neutralize free radicals before they can damage cells. Antioxidants include BETA-CAROTENE, selenium, and vitamins E and C. It is still not clear exactly what role these vitamins have in the prevention of disease, nor is it clear whether it is better to have a diet high in these antioxidants or if supplements should be added.

free transverse rectus abdominis muscle flap
See TRANSVERSE RECTUS ABDOMINIS MYOCUTANEOUS FLAP.

frozen section A technique in which a part of the BIOPSY tissue is frozen immediately after removal, and a thin slice is then mounted on a microscope slide, enabling a pathologist to analyze it in just a few minutes for a diagnosis. While this is almost always able to distinguish benign from malignant lesions, permanent sections give much more information and enable the pathologists to do special stains for estrogen and progesterone.

frozen shoulder A rare complication of axial LYMPH NODE removal in which the patient's shoulder is painful and severely restricted in range of motion. The common name for arthrofibrosis or adhesive capsulitis, it can occur in anyone, but is more common in diabetics and after injury, immobility, or surgery.

Cause

Frozen shoulder occurs when inflammation in a joint triggers the formation of a protein called fibrin, which causes clotting, forming a sticky substance in the joint. Fibrin causes the folds in the tissue surrounding the joint to stick to each other and prevents full motion of the joint.

Prevention

Because this complication is rare, techniques to prevent it are not known. Doctors recommend gentle range-of-motion arm exercises after MASTECTOMY to maintain mobility.

Treatment

Treatment for frozen shoulder usually includes physical therapy and sometimes medication. Heat should not be applied directly after breast surgery (even though it may feel good) or during radiation therapy.

An active exercise program, using weights or rubber tubing to strengthen the affected muscles,

helps improve the range of motion. Activities such as swimming, using overhead pulleys, and performing dance movements in which the arms are taken up over the head can be enjoyable ways to get through painful restoration of lost motion.

fruits and vegetables There is some evidence that eating five daily servings of fruits and vegetables decreases a woman's risk of developing cancer.

Most studies report that eating vegetables is more strongly linked to cancer risk reduction than consuming fruits is. Especially beneficial are carrots, other yellow-orange vegetables such as squash and sweet potatoes, and dark-green vegetables, such as broccoli and spinach. All of these foods are good sources of nutrients such as vitamin C and CAROTENOIDS. Several studies have reported that consuming foods that contain high levels of vitamin C or carotenoids, some of which can serve as sources of vitamin A, may reduce a woman's risk of BREAST CANCER.

There is also some evidence that raw vegetables may be more helpful in protecting against breast cancer than cooked vegetables. This effect may occur because some of the natural chemicals found in vegetables are damaged by heat.

There are several different ways that the natural chemicals found in fruits and vegetables may help reduce the risk of breast cancer and other cancers. They may stimulate cell differentiation and stop cell division. A compound in fruits and vegetables, such as carotenoid-derived vitamin A, that encourages a cell to differentiate interferes with the process of uncontrolled abnormal division typical of cancer cells.

These substances also may act as antioxidants. Free molecules of oxygen within cells (called FREE RADICALS) can damage cells. They are produced by the cell as natural by-products of normal cell activities, or in response to contact with something harmful in its environment. Antioxidants such as vitamin E absorb free radicals.

Natural chemicals may increase the activity of detoxifying enzymes that make cancer-causing compounds harmless. Some chemicals in fruits and vegetables, such as dithiolthiones in broccoli, have been shown to increase the activity of detoxifying enzymes in the body.

Finally, eating fruits and vegetables may strengthen the immune system, which is the body's defense against cancer. They also may alter ESTROGEN levels. Estrogen is normally broken down into different forms in the body. Some compounds in fruits and vegetables, such as glucosinolates in broccoli, break down estrogen into weaker forms of the hormone. Women who do not have breast cancer seem to have higher levels of the weaker forms of estrogen than do women with breast cancer.

Helpful Amounts

In the NURSES' HEALTH STUDY, researchers reported a 17 percent lower rate of breast cancer among women who consumed at least two servings a day of fruits and vegetables compared to those who ate less than one serving a day.

The health benefits of eating fruits and vegetables have prompted the NATIONAL CANCER INSTITUTE and the Produce for Better Health Foundation to cosponsor the national "5 a Day for Better Health" program, which is designed to encourage people to consume at least five servings of fruits and vegetables each day. A serving is

- One piece of fresh fruit
- Six ounces (three-quarter cup) 100-percent fruit juice
- One-half cup of cooked vegetables or canned fruit
- One cup of leafy vegetables or salad
- One handful (one-quarter cup) of dried fruit
- One-half cup of dried peas or beans

Best Fruits and Vegetables

Researchers have identified and isolated many natural substances in fruits and vegetables that may prevent or help combat breast cancer, including CAROTENOIDS, vitamins C and E, FOLIC ACID, selenium, dietary fiber, dithiolthiones and glucosinolates, and phytoestrogens.

Carotenoids   These chemicals are found in yellow and orange vegetables and fruits, and in dark-green leafy vegetables. Some fruits and vegetables contain particularly high amounts of specific carotenoids: sweet potatoes and carrots are high in BETA-CAROTENE; kale, spinach, parsley, and mustard greens have high levels of LUTEIN; tomatoes have a high level of LYCOPENE. Some carotenoids can be converted to vitamin A in the body; foods that are particularly high in these carotenoids include cantaloupe, carrots, and sweet potatoes.

Vitamin C   This vitamin is found in citrus fruits (and juices) such as grapefruits and oranges. Other good sources of vitamin C include green peppers, cauliflower, broccoli, tomatoes, strawberries, melons, cabbage, and leafy green vegetables.

Vitamin E   Foods high in vitamin E include broccoli, kohlrabi, cilantro, turnip greens, spinach, avocados, blueberries, mangos, ripe olives, and especially nuts. Other plant sources of vitamin E include vegetable oils and whole grains.

Folic acid   This vitamin is found in relatively high concentrations in green leafy vegetables, asparagus, lima beans, broccoli, beets, and several types of beans. It is present in moderate amounts in oranges and orange juice.

Selenium   Selenium is a mineral that plants obtain from the soil; the more selenium in the soil, the higher the concentration in plants. Many animal studies have demonstrated anticancer effects of selenium in the form of supplements or in selenium-enriched foods such as garlic grown in selenium-rich soil.

Dietary fiber   Most fruits and vegetables contain fiber; those that have the most include apples, blackberries, grapefruits, oranges, raspberries, and broccoli.

Dithiolthiones and glucosinolates   These natural chemicals are found exclusively in cruciferous vegetables such as brussels sprouts, cauliflower, cabbage, broccoli, rutabaga, and turnips.

Phytoestrogens   These plant estrogens may decrease the level of estrogen circulating in the body, but there is controversy about whether they are helpful or harmful in the prevention and treatment of breast cancer. Studies are inconclusive. Foods high in phytoestrogens include soybeans, dried beans and peas, and bean sprouts.

Other natural substances in fruits and vegetables currently being studied include isothiocyanates and thiocyanates in brussels sprouts; FLAVONOIDS in berries; coumarins in citrus fruits; phenols in almost all fruits and vegetables; protease inhibitors in legumes; plant sterols in vegetables; ISOFLAVONES, saponins, and inositol hexaphosphate in soybeans; allium compounds in garlic; limonene in citrus fruit oils; and resveratrol in grapes.

Vegetarian Diet and Breast Cancer

Two studies were unable to show an association between a vegetarian diet and a lower risk of breast cancer. Although a few studies report lower levels of estrogen in vegetarian women, experts say there is not enough information to determine whether a vegetarian diet reduces the risk of breast cancer.

Patients with Breast Cancer

One study reported that women who ate fruits and vegetables high in nutrients such as beta-carotene before they were diagnosed with breast cancer had better survival rates after development of the disease. Two others found no association between diet and breast cancer mortality rate. However, since the natural chemicals found in fruits and vegetables have been shown to influence cancer cells in many different ways, experts say it is possible that continuing to eat fruits and vegetables after receiving a diagnosis of breast cancer may help to fight the progression of the disease and help women stay healthy.

Recommendations

There are many easy and convenient ways for women to add more nutritious fruits and vegetables to their diet. Women should snack on carrots or peppers or fruit, eat a sweet potato instead of a white potato or substitute spinach or another dark-green leafy vegetable for iceberg lettuce in a salad, and so on.

full-field digital tomosynthesis (TOMO)   A new breast imaging technique that not only can increase the visibility of breast lesions but dramatically reduce the number of patients called back for a second mammogram because the first screening mammogram was ambiguous.

TOMO allows doctors to take multiple projections of the breast at different angles, which are then reconstructed into a three-dimensional data set. Each slice can be looked at individually and assessed without confusing overlap from surrounding structures. The ability to look at individual slices of the breast is a real asset.

TOMO is also more comfortable for the patient, since her breasts need to be compressed only once (compared to twice for the standard two-view mammogram). Moreover, the patient sits during the procedure, and the overall radiation dosage is lower.

fulvestrant (Faslodex)   A type of hormonal therapy approved for use in postmenopausal women with hormone-receptor-positive metastatic breast cancer that has progressed after therapy with a hormonal treatment such as TAMOXIFEN. After a BREAST CANCER BIOPSY, hormone receptor tests on the tumor tissue can determine whether the cancer is responsive to estrogen (estrogen-receptor positive). Estrogen-receptor positive breast cancers may respond to treatment with an anti-estrogen therapy, such as tamoxifen, which blocks the estrogen receptor.

Faslodex may be an effective alternative for patients who are not successfully treated with tamoxifen because of the way it works; instead of blocking the estrogen receptor, Faslodex targets and degrades the estrogen receptors present in breast cancer cells.

The effectiveness of Faslodex was demonstrated in clinical trials comparing the drug to the AROMATASE INHIBITOR Arimidex (anastrozole), which works by reducing the amount of estrogen in the body.

Ongoing studies are looking at both Aromasin and Faslodex in the treatment of early breast cancer.

Side Effects

Women should not take Faslodex during pregnancy. Faslodex is given as a monthly injection, not as a daily pill. Because it is administered intramuscularly, it should not be used in patients with certain blood disorders or in patients receiving blood thinners.

The most common side effects are nausea, vomiting, constipation, diarrhea, abdominal pain, headache, back pain, hot flashes, sore throat, and injection site reactions with mild, transient pain and inflammation.

galactoceles Benign milk-filled CYSTS that can occur in women who are pregnant or BREAST-FEEDING. These cysts usually appear as smooth, movable lumps. As with cysts, galactoceles do not usually need to be treated. If the diagnosis is uncertain or the galactocele is causing discomfort, it can be drained with a thin needle.

garlic A bulb that has been used as a health tonic by civilizations for thousands of years. More recently, some studies have found that garlic can inhibit the growth of BREAST CANCER. Researchers have shown that if a compound called diallyldisulfide (formed when raw garlic is cut or crushed) is injected into tumors, they can be reduced by half. Another compound (S-allylcysteine) can stop cancer-causing agents from binding to human breast cells.

Research on laboratory mice has indicated that garlic may help boost the immune system, thereby reducing the growth of cancerous cells. In one study, white blood cells from garlic eaters were able to kill 139 percent more tumor cells than white blood cells from non–garlic eaters.

Because garlic is nontoxic and relatively cheap, experts do not hesitate to recommend its use. Cooks should remember to peel garlic and let it sit for 15 minutes before cooking for more effective cancer-fighting benefits. According to nutrition experts, peeling garlic releases an enzyme called allinase, starting a series of chemical reactions that help protect against cancer. But the protective substances require 15 minutes to form. Peeling garlic and immediately starting to cook with it inactivate the allinase and destroy garlic's cancer-fighting properties.

See also DIET.

gene profiles Profiles of a woman's genetic expression may someday help determine whether or not a woman who has BREAST CANCER would respond to certain CHEMOTHERAPY treatments. Yet patients react differently to chemotherapy drugs, and some women do not respond to treatment at all. However, since there is currently no way to distinguish between women who might respond and those who probably will not, all eligible patients are treated the same way.

In one Texas study, researchers took biopsy samples from primary breast tumors of 24 patients before treatment and then measured tumor response to DOCETAXEL. Different gene expression profiles were associated with different responses to the drug. Tumors that were sensitive to treatment had higher expression of genes involved in the cell cycle, protein transport, and protein modification, whereas resistant tumors showed enhanced expression of some transcriptional and signal transduction genes. This study helps to define the molecular portrait of cancers that respond to docetaxel, one of the most active agents in breast cancer treatment. This type of molecular profiling could have important implications for defining the best treatment for individual patients and could reduce unproductive treatment, unnecessary toxicity, and overall cost.

genes and breast cancer Virtually every cancer is caused by mutations of DNA, the genetic material that controls cell behavior. In some cases of breast cancer, a person's DNA may be altered by the activation of ONCOGENES (mutated genes that cause cells to grow out of control) or by the disabling of SUPPRESSOR GENES (normal genes that control cell growth and prevent cells from dividing too rapidly).

Experts believe that most genetic damage is caused by environmental factors, such as exposure to chemicals, radiation, smoke and pollution; saturated fat in the diet; or viruses. In addition, cell mutations may occur by mistake as cells divide. These mistakes can also be inherited; that is why some cancers run in families.

Within the past few years, researchers have identified two inherited genes linked to an increased risk for the development of breast cancer: BRCA1 and BRCA2. A person who inherits one of these genes has a 50 to 80 percent chance of development of breast cancer in her lifetime.

See also BREAST CANCER SUSCEPTIBILITY GENES; FAMILY HISTORY; GENETIC MARKERS; GENETIC TESTING; HEREDITY AND CANCER.

genetic markers   Alterations in DNA that may indicate an increased risk of development of a specific disease or disorder.

See also BREAST CANCER SUSCEPTIBILITY GENES; FAMILY HISTORY; GENES AND BREAST CANCER; HEREDITY AND CANCER.

genetic testing   A blood test that determines genetic alterations that may be linked to BREAST CANCER. People may choose genetic testing to determine more clearly why they contracted cancer, to clarify risk to their children, to define the appropriateness of particular surveillance approaches, or to aid in decision making about risk-reducing prophylactic mastectomy.

However, the majority of cancers are not caused by genetic mutations, so testing is not indicated except in very specific circumstances. A genetic counselor can help make recommendations about the usefulness of testing in those with a strong family history or very early onset of breast cancer.

See also FAMILY HISTORY; GENES AND BREAST CANCER; GENETIC MARKERS; HEREDITY AND CANCER.

genistein   A PHYTOESTROGEN (plant estrogen) produced by SOY PRODUCTS.

Gilda Radner Familial Ovarian Cancer Registry
An international registry of families with two or more relatives who have ovarian cancer. In addi-

tion to ovarian cancer research, the registry offers a helpline, education, information, and peer support for women who have a high risk of ovarian cancer.

The registry is pursuing research into causes of familial ovarian cancer, hoping to identify new genes associated with familial ovarian cancer, and improving genetic and psychosocial counseling for individuals and families. Researchers also hope to identify lifestyle choices, such as use of oral contraceptives or hormone replacement therapy, that reduce ovarian cancer risk in women who may be more susceptible to the disease. With that aim, the registry is collecting family histories, medical records, and tissue samples from women who have ovarian cancer. For contact information, see Appendix I.

Gilda's Clubs   Nonprofit places where all who have any type of cancer, and their families and friends, build social and emotional support as a supplement to medical care. Free of charge, Gilda's Clubs offer support and networking groups, lectures, workshops, and social events in a nonresidential homelike setting. Funding is solicited from private individuals, corporations, and foundations.

The Gilda's Club program is composed of the following elements, which are offered in every clubhouse:

- *Support and Networking Groups:* These include weekly wellness groups for those living with cancer, family groups for family members and friends, and monthly networking groups on a particular kind of cancer or topic of common interest (prostate cancer, young adulthood cancer, living solo with cancer, and so on).
- *Lectures and Workshops:* Typical lecture topics, which are selected on the basis of members' interests, include stress reduction, nutrition, talking to your children about cancer, and managing pain. Major workshop areas include art and other forms of self-expression, meditation, exercise and yoga, and cooking.
- *Social Activities:* A range of gatherings, including potluck suppers with music, karaoke nights, joke fests, comedy nights, and major celebrations around special holidays.

- *Team Convene:* Two-hour sessions requested by a person who has cancer or a family member to create a network to provide support at the time of diagnosis and during any challenging situations that may follow. Sessions include all significant friends and family in a member's life, who join to provide support for transportation, food preparation, child care, or other necessities.
- *Family Focus:* A meeting facilitated by a staff member designed to enlist all family members as a resource and help them learn together how to live with cancer. It seeks to identify and discuss family beliefs about cancer, critical family issues, and immediate practical problems as well as solutions.
- *Noogieland:* In a special area of every clubhouse, activities are conducted for children affected by cancer. Most Gilda's Clubs also have several kinds of activities for teens, who frequently volunteer in many parts of the clubhouse.

Gilda's Club is named in memory of the comedian Gilda Radner, who died of ovarian cancer in 1989. Radner is best known for her work on NBC's *Saturday Night Live;* her book, *It's Always Something,* describes her life with cancer. Gilda's Club was founded by Joanna Bull, Gilda's cancer psychotherapist, with the help of Gilda's husband, Gene Wilder; Joel Siegel; and other friends.

All Gilda's Clubs have a warm and welcoming homelike atmosphere, with a living room for reading and relaxing; support group rooms for weekly sessions led by licensed professionals; a workshop area for meditation, nutrition, stress reduction, and art projects; Noogieland, a playroom for kids and teens; an It's Always Something room, a quiet place for personal time; and a large Community Meeting Room for potluck suppers, jokefests, and lectures.

ginseng (*Panax ginseng*) An herb whose root some people believe may have anticancer effects. Most cancer experts in the United States have said there is insufficient evidence demonstrating that Siberian ginseng is an effective treatment for cancer. Likewise, most experts believe there is no scientific evidence that ginseng is effective in reducing the side effects of chemotherapy or radiation therapy, and there have been no human studies of its safety or long-term effects. Although some practitioners claim that the herb enables chemotherapy drugs to penetrate cancer cells more easily, there has been no scientific evidence to support the claim.

Siberian ginseng is an herb that grows in Siberia, China, Korea, and Japan. *Siberian ginseng* should not be confused with *Asian ginseng* or *American ginseng,* which belong to a different family of herbs.

Herbalists have long prescribed Siberian ginseng to relieve menopausal symptoms, to treat cancer, and to reduce the toxic effects of chemotherapy and radiation therapy. After the Chernobyl nuclear reactor disaster, Russian and Ukrainian citizens reportedly received the herb to counter the effects of radiation poisoning. But few animal studies of Siberian ginseng have been published in peer-reviewed medical journals. In addition, lack of standardization of extracts, study methods, and doses makes it difficult to draw conclusions regarding effectiveness.

Controversy

Proponents point to the results collected from a number of animal and human studies, which show that *Panax ginseng* may indeed reduce the risk of several types of cancer, according to a report in *Cancer Causes and Control,* a medical journal published in the Netherlands. In one 1980 study in Korea, red ginseng extract inhibited the formation of lung tumors in rats. In another study in 1983 using mice, a 75 percent reduction in LIVER CANCER was reported.

But even proponents caution that although *Panax ginseng* has shown cancer-preventive effects, the evidence is not conclusive.

There have been only a few studies of ginseng use on humans. One study, conducted by the Korean researcher Taik Koo Yun, found that among more than 4,600 people above the age of 40, ginseng users were approximately 70 percent less likely to have cancer, when compared to those who did not take the herb. They also found that the more frequently ginseng was consumed, the lower the risk of cancer.

The AMERICAN CANCER SOCIETY (ACS) has offered no official position on ginseng as a cancer treatment or prevention agent and cautions that ginseng has not yet been adequately tested. Noting that the studies that were conducted produced contradictory results, the ACS also points out the lack of standardization among ginseng products.

Safety/Dosage

Siberian ginseng is on the approval list of Commission E (Germany's herbal regulatory agency), and ginseng supplements are available in tablets and liquid extracts. However, there is no standardization for the purity and strength of ginseng, as several different plants have the same common name. Consumers who buy ginseng should consider the source and the product. No federal agency enforces quality control over these ingredients, and studies of 54 ginseng products found that 25 percent contained no ginseng at all; 60 percent contained only trace amounts.

The powdered or cut root can be brewed as a tea; an average dose is two to three grams per day. Typically, Siberian ginseng is consumed regularly for six to eight weeks, followed by a one- or two-week break before resuming.

Health risks associated with Siberian ginseng have not been established, although side effects seem to be rare. A few cases of diarrhea and insomnia have been reported, and people who have high blood pressure should avoid the supplements. There have been no studies of Siberian ginseng's long-term effects.

Constituent Ingredients

Most botanists recognize three medicinal species, *Panax ginseng* (Chinese, Siberian, or Korean ginseng), *P. pseudo-ginseng* (Japanese ginseng), and *P. quinquefolium* (American ginseng), although the term *ginseng* has referred to any of 22 different plants, usually of the genus *Panax*, used as a tonic and restorative.

P. ginseng—both red and white versions, which proponents say fight cancer growth—gets its pharmaceutical properties from 34 compounds, collectively called ginsenosides or panaxosides, that share a common steroidlike chemical structure.

Ginsenosides are PHYTOESTROGENS that may be expected to have effects similar to those of soy. Although ginsenosides are structurally similar, studies have demonstrated markedly different biochemical effects among different ones.

goserelin acetate   See ZOLADEX.

grade   A measure of how abnormal the BREAST CANCER cells appear under a microscope. Grades of breast cancer tumors are measured by three or four degrees of severity.

Grade 1 tumors are unaggressive under the microscope. The cells appear closely related to normal and structural units are present. In higher grade cancers the cells are undifferentiated; the cells are dividing; and the cells make a solid sheet. Higher grade tumors are more likely to recur and so treatment decisions may be made based partly on grade, together with size, node status, and estrogen receptor status.

granisetron   See KYTRIL.

granular cell tumor   A rare benign tumor that is usually found in the mouth or skin but extremely rarely may be detected in the breast. Most granular cell tumors of the breast are identified as hard, firm lumps that may be fixed to the skin. It appears much like a cancer. Doctors typically diagnose granular cell tumors by a fine needle or needle core BIOPSY and then surgically remove the tumors along with a surrounding margin of breast tissue. Granular cell tumors do not indicate higher risk of development of BREAST CANCER.

granulocyte colony-stimulating factor   A COLONY-STIMULATING FACTOR that triggers the production of a type of white blood cell called a neutrophil. Granulocyte colony-stimulating factor is a CYTOKINE that belongs to the family of drugs called hematopoietic (blood-forming) agents.

These drugs are given to prevent infections in those likely to have low blood counts as a result of CHEMOTHERAPY. They are given as subcutaneous injections either daily or once each chemotherapy cycle.

Side Effects

Granulocyte colony-stimulating factors may cause bone pain, but otherwise tend to be well tolerated, although they are expensive.

grapes   Fruits that contain FLAVONOIDS, substances found in pigments and in some fruits (especially citrus fruits, purple berries, and apples), as well as in vegetables, tea, and whole grains. Flavonoids in grape juice—especially Concord grape juice—have been found to reduce cellular oxidative stress and therefore may be associated with a reduced risk of cancer. They can act as antioxidants to prevent FREE RADICAL damage and the oxidation that trigger inflammation. (Free radicals are harmful, highly reactive molecules that tear electrons away from nearby molecules to make up for their deficiency.)

Flavonoids include flavones (such as quercetin), ISOFLAVONES (from soybeans), flavonones (such as rutin in citrus), anthocyanins (blue, purple, and red plant pigments), and flavononols (including tannins).

The amounts of key flavonoids in foods and beverages have been determined, but the quantity of a certain flavonoid that should be consumed to help prevent breast cancer is uncertain. How flavonoids are processed in the intestine, how they are absorbed, and how they are assimilated by the body remain unknown.

group therapy A combination of individual and group treatment for patients with BREAST CANCER can provide an opportunity to give and receive emotional support and learn from the experiences of others. To be most effective, groups should be made up of women at similar stages of the disease and led by psychologists or other mental health professionals who have experience in breast cancer treatment.

Whether aimed at individuals or groups, psychological interventions strive to help women adjust to their diagnosis, cope with treatment, and come to terms with the disease's impact on their life. Psychologists typically ask open-ended questions about patients' assumptions, ideas for living more fully, and other matters. Although negative thoughts and feelings are addressed, most psychological interventions focus on problem solving as women meet each new challenge.

Researchers know that stress suppresses the body's ability to protect itself. Whether group therapy or emotional support can prolong life after diagnosis is unclear. One study, for example, found that patients who had advanced breast cancer who had group therapy lived longer than those who did not. Other studies found no such benefit.

hair loss   Known medically as alopecia, this is one of the most well-known side effects of the CHEMOTHERAPY treatments often prescribed for patients with BREAST CANCER. The fast-growing hair follicle cells are affected by chemotherapy, causing brittle hair that breaks off at the scalp or is spontaneously released from the follicle. Although a few drugs used to treat breast cancer do not cause hair loss (or cause slight hair loss), most do cause partial or complete hair loss for a time.

The amount of hair lost depends on the type of drug or combination of drugs used, the dosage given, and the person's individual reaction to the drug. If hair loss is going to happen, it usually begins within a few weeks of the start of treatment, although rarely it can start within a few days. Body hair may be lost as well, and some drugs even trigger loss of the eyelashes and eyebrows; however, this loss is usually less severe, since growth is less active in these hair follicles than on the scalp.

Hair loss can profoundly affect a patient's quality of life and psychological well-being. In fact, alopecia can cause loss of self-confidence, depression, and grief reactions.

If patients do lose their hair as a result of chemotherapy, it grows back once treatment is over. However, the color or texture may be different, and hair often grows back curly, no matter how straight it was originally. Hair starts to regrow shortly after chemotherapy is completed.

Halsted's mastectomy   See MASTECTOMY.

hand and foot syndrome   A condition marked by redness, tenderness, and peeling of the hands and feet that may occur as a side effect of certain chemotherapy drugs—especially Doxil and Xeloda.

Occasionally, the skin reactions can be severe, causing blistering. The syndrome is known medically as palmar-plantar erythrodysthesia.

Prevention/Treatment

It can be prevented or lessened by regular and intensive use of creams on the hands and feet, but at times, chemotherapy doses need to be reduced.

health insurance   The cost of treating BREAST CANCER can be high, but health insurance plans usually cover much of the cost. Patients who belong to a health maintenance organization (HMO) or preferred provider organization (PPO) should become familiar with their provider choices and their financial responsibility if they receive care "out of network" from a doctor not covered by the health plan.

SSI and SSDI

Patients with breast cancer who do not have insurance should contact their local Social Security Office to determine whether they qualify for Supplemental Security Income (SSI) or SOCIAL SECURITY DISABILITY INSURANCE (SSDI). The medical requirements and disability determination process are the same under both programs. However, whereas eligibility for SSDI is based on employment history, SSI is based on financial need.

Medicare/Medicaid

Since 1998, Medicare has covered mammography screening for the early detection of breast cancer, for all women with Medicare over 40. Medicare will also cover a baseline MAMMOGRAM for women beneficiaries between 35 and 39.

Under Medicaid, diagnostic mammograms are a mandated service and states must cover them. Screening mammograms, however, are provided by states as an optional service; most states cover screening mammograms in fee-for-service Medicaid. In addition, virtually all Medicaid managed care plans offer preventive services, including mammography, to their enrollees.

The Health Care Financing Administration (HCFA) has urged states to provide annual mammography screening to Medicaid beneficiaries at age 40; HCFA will continue to provide federal matching payments for annual mammography screening services.

Hill-Burton Coverage

Patients with breast cancer who are without insurance also can receive care from hospitals that receive federal grants from Hill-Burton Funds that allow hospitals and nursing homes to provide low-cost or no-cost medical care. To receive a listing of hospitals or nursing homes participating in the Hill-Burton program, patients can call (800) 638-0742.

Other Coverage

The Centers for Disease Control (CDC) sponsors the NATIONAL BREAST AND CERVICAL CANCER EARLY DETECTION PROGRAM, which offers free or low-cost mammography screening to uninsured, low-income, elderly, minority, and Native American women nationwide. In October 1996 the program went nationwide, with funding for all 50 states. In 2001, the program served 371,865 women. The Native American Breast and Cervical Cancer Treatment Technical Amendment Act of 2001, signed by President Bush in January 2002, amends title XIX of the Social Security Act to expand Medicaid coverage for Native American breast or cervical cancer patients.

See also FINANCIAL ISSUES.

hematopoietic growth factors See COLONY-STIMULATING FACTORS.

hematopoietic stem cell transplantation A combination term now used to include both BONE MARROW TRANSPLANTATION and PERIPHERAL BLOOD STEM CELL TRANSPLANTATION. Both of these treatments allow the use of particularly high dosages of CHEMOTHERAPY and/or TOTAL BODY IRRADIATION to kill breast cancer cells. This treatment kills both cancer cells and the blood-forming (hematopoietic) stem cells in the patient's bone marrow. They are replaced by stem cells that are removed from the patient before chemotherapy or by stem cells donated by someone else.

While these techniques appeared to be very exciting in the early 1990s, randomized trials proved transplants were no more effective than chemotherapy in the ADJUVANT TREATMENT of women with very high risk breast cancer.

HER-2 (human epidermal growth factor receptor-2) A receptor that goes awry in 20 percent to 30 percent of breast cancers and that can be affected by a drug called trastuzumab (HERCEPTIN), which kills cancer cells that carry excess HER-2. Although Herceptin was approved as a breast cancer treatment by the U.S. Food and Drug Administration in September 1998, until recently scientists did not know precisely how it interacts with the HER-2 receptor.

The HER-2 receptor behaves differently than its relatives HER-1, HER-3, and HER-4 do: although all four proteins are similar in the sequence of their building blocks, only excess HER-2 level leads to uncontrolled cell growth in the lab and breast cancer in people. Like its relatives, the HER-2 receptor is embedded in the cell membrane, partially outside the cell and partially inside. The extracellular part is the receptor's "on" switch. Through this region, HER receptors join into pairs to become fully active and trigger events that eventually result in cell division. Comparisons of HER family structures reveal that a few key changes in the sequence make all the difference for HER-2.

Specifically, HER-2 does not need to be "opened" in order to pair with another HER; that is why extra HER-2 can cause cancer, and why no one has found any small molecules that bind to it. It is unlikely that any natural small molecules for HER-2 exists—it just does not need one to work.

The extracellular regions of all the HER proteins are made up of four structurally distinct *domains,* I, II, III, and IV. In HER-1 and -3, a fingerlike projection in domain II keeps it connected to domain IV, forming a bracelet like loop. In HER-2, however, a tight interaction between domains I and III prevents the bracelet formation. Thus, domain IV is available for binding to Herceptin, and domain II for pairing with other HER proteins.

Herceptin (trastuzumab) A MONOCLONAL ANTIBODY protein that belongs to a class of synthetic substances called BIOLOGIC RESPONSE MODIFIERS. Herceptin is a protein that fits like a lock and key into a protein on certain BREAST CANCER cells. The protein (antigen) on the breast cancer cell is called human epidermal growth factor receptor-2 (HER-2). Once Herceptin attaches to the cell, it draws other immune cells to help kill the cancer cell.

This injectable CHEMOTHERAPY drug was approved in 1998 for use alone in certain patients who have tried chemotherapy with little success. It is also approved as a first-line treatment for breast cancer that has spread, when used in combination with paclitaxel (TAXOL).

Side Effects

Herceptin can cause ventricular dysfunction and congestive heart failure. The incidence and severity of heart problems are particularly high in patients who receive Herceptin together with anthracyclines and cyclophosphamide (CYTOXAN).

A study released in March 2002 shows that Herceptin not only blocks a factor that spurs tumor growth but also slows the flow of blood the tumors need to grow. If so, that could make the drug a competitor to several cancer treatments under development for reducing blood flow to tumors.

Tumors secrete various growth factors that cause the body to produce blood vessels that feed tumors the oxygen and nutrients they need. Many companies are developing drugs that block one or more of the growth factors, hoping to stop the vessels from forming and thereby starving the tumors. But according to some scientists, there is mounting evidence that blocking only one growth factor is not effective because tumors can rely on others instead.

Herceptin seems to make the blood vessels that supply the tumors less abnormal. That means that more chemotherapy drugs may be able to reach the tumors and may explain why combining Herceptin with chemotherapy, produces better results than either treatment does separately.

Scientists from the Salk Institute have identified the probable link between Herceptin and cardiac failure. The results may also explain why a common combination drug regimen that includes Herceptin is particularly toxic.

Herceptin targets the protein HER-2 (for a protein related to human epidermal growth factor receptor), which is produced in excess in some breast cancer cells. The recent study shows that the version of HER-2 used in mice, called erb B-2, is needed for proper heart cell function. It was considered possible that Herceptin triggered heart problems in a number of ways, but now it appears that the drug's direct action on erb B-2 is the culprit. It should be possible to engineer new generations of drugs that would sidestep Herceptin's harmful effects on heart function.

It appears that the loss of erb B-2 function caused by Herceptin makes cardiac muscle more susceptible to anthracycline toxicity. Therefore, it may be appropriate to examine different combinations of chemotherapy drugs with Herceptin in order to eliminate the increased risk of heart disease associated with combined Herceptin–anthracycline therapy.

heredity and breast cancer Having a mother or other first-degree relative who had BREAST CANCER does not mean it is likely or certain that a woman will get breast cancer. Even if a woman has the breast cancer gene alteration (*BRCA1* or *2*), she may not develop breast cancer. Experts do not know why some women get breast cancer and others do not. However, making healthy lifestyle choices about DIET, EXERCISE, and ALCOHOL will certainly pay off by lower cardiovascular disease and may help lower breast cancer risk.

Indicators that a woman is at risk for inherited breast cancer include the following:

- A family member who has breast cancer that develops at a young age
- A family member who has breast cancer that strikes in both breasts or at two different locations in one breast
- Two or more members of one generation who have breast cancer
- Particular tumor site combinations seen within one family, especially breast and ovary

See also BREAST CANCER SUSCEPTIBILITY GENES; FAMILY HISTORY; GENES AND CANCER.

HER-2/neu A gene that controls human epidermal growth factor receptor-2 (HER-2), a specific protein that controls cell growth. In 1981, laboratory biologists identified the *neu* gene in a rat tumor, which when mutated, worked as a switch that turned normal cells into cancerous ones. Four years later, scientists found a similar human gene that they called *HER-2/neu.*

Since then, evidence has mounted that the *HER-2/neu* gene may be altered in at least 25 percent of all breast cancer tumors, and patients who have the altered form of the gene tend to have the most aggressive disease. Scientists have also noted the importance of *HER-2/neu* as a marker of tumor aggressiveness in cancers of the ovary, endometrium, and salivary glands.

HER-2/neu is an example of an ONCOGENE (cancer gene) that speeds up the growth of malignant cells. Like many oncogenes, the normal version of the *HER-2/neu* gene is harmless and plays a key role in early development and cell growth. But many tumors contain too many copies of the *HER-2/neu* gene, which may also carry genetic changes that cause the gene to be turned on constantly. Combined with other potent alterations in a cell's genes, this mechanism leads to the uncontrolled growth of cancer.

If a woman's cancer is a *HER-2/neu* positive and involves lymph nodes it may be more aggressive. Studies are testing whether herceptin given after chemotherapy decreases the chance of cancer returning. For a woman with metastatic cancer that is H2N+, herceptin should be given alone or with chemotherapy. Some studies suggest different responses to specific chemotherapy or hormone treatments in patients who are H2N+ or H2N–.

Hispanics/Latinas and breast cancer Hispanic/Latina women have lower breast cancer rates than non-Hispanic white women. However, studies also show that despite their lower breast cancer rates, if they get breast cancer, Hispanic/Latina women are more likely to die of the disease. This is most likely due to the fact that Hispanic/Latina women are less likely to have screening MAMMOGRAMS and are therefore more likely to be diagnosed at later stages of breast cancer. They also tend to obtain health-care services less often than other ethnic groups.

Studies consistently show that lower rates of diagnosis among Hispanic and Latina women are linked to low income, low levels of education, lack of health insurance, inability to speak English, lack of awareness of breast cancer risks and screening methods, and lack of physician referrals.

See also RACE AND BREAST CANCER.

history of breast cancer Incidents of breast cancer were first recorded by early Egyptians, whose popular treatment was burning off of the diseased tissue. Surgery was also used in Egyptian times as a treatment for breast cancer, but it was an extremely radical treatment, as there was no way to anesthetize patients or treat infection.

According to the doctrines of the Greek physician Caudius Galen (C.E. 130–200), whose works on physiology and anatomy dominated medical thought through the Middle Ages, the primary cause of breast cancer is "melancholia." Galen recommended special diets together with treatments such as exorcism and the use of topical applications.

During the Renaissance, the Flemish anatomist Andreas Vesalius questioned the medical doctrines of Aristotle and Galen. He recommended MASTECTOMY, as well as sutures instead of cautery to control the bleeding during surgery.

The fact that breast cancer could and did spread to the regional lymph nodes under the armpit, and that this indicated a poor prognosis, was not understood until the early 18th century. This observation was a major breakthrough and is the current basis on which physicians today make recommendations about chemotherapy or hormonal treatments after surgery.

Though early treatments for breast cancer were primitive, some women actually survived and lived a normal life after therapy. According to historians, in 1700 a nurse at L'Hotel Dieu Hospital in Quebec City who had breast cancer had a mastectomy. She recovered and lived for another 30 years.

During the mid-1800s, surgeons first began to keep detailed records of breast cancer, which indicated that even those treated by mastectomy had a high rate of recurrence within eight years—especially when the glands or lymph nodes were affected. Nevertheless, doctors still generally removed the breast and the surrounding glands in an effort to prevent further tumor development.

By the late 1800s, radical mastectomies, as well as the removal of axillary nodes, were commonly carried out in an effort to stop the spread or recurrence of breast cancer. Because surgery was so dangerous, procedures were performed on locally advanced cancers. Patients who survived for three years were considered "cured." Statistics kept at the time by Johns Hopkins Hospital indicate that only 12 percent of patients survived for 10 years.

Between the 1930s and the 1950s doctors gradually began to improve the treatment of breast cancer, focusing on clinical methods of classifying the stage and progression of the disease. STAGING systems that divided breast cancer into two distinct patient groups with outlooks predicted on the basis of clearly defined clinical signs were developed. Stages I and II represented operable or curable groups of cases; stage III indicated locally advanced disease in which surgery was not a viable option; and stage IV described distant metastases.

Survival rates improved dramatically during the 20th century. Ten-year survival rates after mastectomies improved from about 10 percent in the 1920s to about 50 percent in the 1950s. The hormonal basis for many breast cancers was understood by the early 1900s.

TAMOXIFEN was developed in the 1960s and has made an enormous difference for tens of thousands of women. Chemotherapy, developed in the 1950s but not widely used in breast cancer until the 1980s, has led to decreased mortality.

Survival rates continue to improve as breast cancer is diagnosed earlier because of mammograms and patient awareness. Although more women are diagnosed, fewer are dying.

The life expectancy of a woman until the 1920s was only about 40 years because of infection and childbirth. Because breast cancer occurs in older women, as women live longer, breast cancer is becoming more common.

HLA See HUMAN LEUKOCYTE ANTIGEN.

1H-nuclear magnetic resonance spectroscopic imaging A noninvasive imaging method of detecting and measuring activity at the cellular level, this type of imaging is also called proton magnetic resonance spectroscopic imaging. It is used in conjunction with MAGNETIC RESONANCE IMAGING to provide spatial information about BREAST TISSUE.

See also DIAGNOSIS OF BREAST CANCER.

hormonal therapy A type of treatment that keeps BREAST CANCER cells from getting the HORMONES they need to grow. Hormones are chemicals that circulate in the bloodstream and are produced by glands in the body. ESTROGEN and PROGESTERONE are types of hormones that affect the way some breast cancer grows.

If tests show that breast cancer cells have estrogen and progesterone receptors (proteins found on some cancer cells to which estrogen and progesterone will attach), then changing the body's hormone levels or altering the cancer cells' estrogen receptors can treat the cancer.

This can be done in premenopausal women by surgically removing the ovaries or blocking them with medications and in postmenopausal women by preventing transformation of adrenal steroids and estrogen by aromatase inhibitors. In both pre- and postmenopausal women, TAMOXIFEN can be used to alter the patient's estrogen receptors.

Hormonal therapy is not CHEMOTHERAPY, but like chemotherapy it may be used after surgery as ADJUVANT TREATMENT, preventing risk of recurrence, or as treatment for metastatic disease. The type of hormonal therapy used is determined by menstrual status as well as by any other medical problems the woman may have.

If a woman is premenopausal, in the United States removal of her ovaries or suppressing them medically is rarely used as adjuvant treatment, although there is currently a large study under way testing whether it should be used. Ovary removal or suppression is commonly practiced in Europe, however, and may be as effective as chemotherapy. In the United States, tamoxifen is usually used instead. If the cancer has spread, removal of the ovaries is often considered.

In postmenopausal women, tamoxifen or ARO-MATASE INHIBITORS are used both as adjuvant treatment and for metastatic disease. Choice of method is based on other factors: Tamoxifen increases blood clots of uterine cancer; FULVESTRANT (which destroys the estrogen receptors) and aromatase inhibitors may worsen osteoporosis.

Other hormonal treatments include Megace (a progesterone that may cause significant weight gain) and estrogen (which has a very high risk of blood clots).

hormone   A substance secreted by various organs in the body that helps regulate growth, metabolism, and reproduction. Some hormones are used in postsurgical treatment for breast and other cancers.

Exposure to hormones (especially ESTROGEN) is suspected to increase a woman's risk of development of breast cancer. Estrogen stimulates normal breast cells from a girl's first menstrual cycle, through the birth of a child and breast-feeding until the onset of menopause. It is this lifetime exposure to estrogen that is believed to put a woman at risk for breast cancer.

This does not mean experts know for sure that estrogen or other hormones cause BREAST CANCER. What they do know is that a woman who begins her menstrual cycle before age 12, has her first child after age 30, or goes through menopause after age 55—in other words, who has been exposed longer to estrogen—has an increased risk of breast cancer.

hormone receptors   Certain proteins on the surface of some BREAST CANCER cells that indicate the cancer may rely on ESTROGEN to grow. If these estrogen and PROGESTERONE receptors are present on the cell surface, as determined at the time of biopsy, then hormone treatments that alter estrogen levels or the estrogen receptor can be used as adjuvant therapy or as treatment of metastatic disease. Tumors in younger women are sometimes hormone-receptor positive; in older women they are usually positive. The outcome of women with hormone-receptor-positive breast cancer is often better than that of estrogen-negative women.

hormone replacement therapy (HRT)   Treatment used in postmenopausal women to restore ESTROGEN levels. PROGESTERONE is added to estrogen because estrogen alone causes uterine cancer. HRT is used to prevent hot flashes and other menopausal symptoms and to decrease the risk of osteoporosis, and for many years it was used because doctors thought it might prevent heart disease. However, a large trial was stopped in 2003 when researchers not only found that HRT did not prevent heart disease but confirmed that HRT increased the risk of breast cancer and heart disease.

When hormone replacement was first developed in the 1960s, doctors simply administered estrogen alone, calling the treatment ESTROGEN REPLACEMENT THERAPY (ERT). ERT helped to ease the symptoms of menopause, and appeared to protect against heart disease and bone fractures—problems that often occur in older women. But doctors discovered that ERT also increased the risk of cancer of the uterine lining. By adding progesterone to estrogen (and renaming the treatment "hormone replacement therapy"), the uterus was protected against endometrial cancer. Initially, the regimen seemed to have all the benefits attributed to ERT. Thousands of women were given HRT to "stay young" and prevent heart disease.

However, although experts thought they knew the benefits and risks of HRT, a large randomized controlled trial was undertaken to prove HRT was safe. Instead, this trial proved that HRT did not prevent heart disease, and increased the risk of breast cancer. As a result, the study—the Women's Health Initiative (WHI)—was stopped in July 2002 (three years early) when researchers identified an increased risk of breast cancer among participants. At the time, 38 percent of postmenopausal women were taking HRT. Experts found that a woman's risk of developing breast cancer is increased by about 26 percent if she uses HRT. This increased risk declines over time once a woman stops taking hormones. The WHI study report of the 16,000 postmenopausal women participants was published in the July 17, 2002 *Journal of the American Medical Association,* along with an editorial warning against the long-term use of HRT.

Study participants receiving HRT were also found to be at higher risk for coronary heart disease and blood clots, although HRT did seem to lower the risk of colorectal cancer and bone fractures. Overall, however, the risks outweighed the benefits, researchers concluded.

The 2002 study did not assess short-term use of HRT to prevent menopausal symptoms, such as hot flashes, so it is difficult to draw conclusions about this, researchers note. However, other studies have suggested no increased risk of breast cancer with short-term use to prevent menopausal symptoms.

In the WHI study, the rate of breast cancers was 26 percent higher among those receiving HRT as opposed to those getting placebo. The rate for heart disease was 29 percent higher, stroke rates were 41 percent higher, and blood clot rates were more than twice as high in those women who were having HRT.

HRT did have some benefits, however. The rate of colorectal cancer was 37 percent lower in the HRT group, and the rate of bone fractures was 24 percent lower. Endometrial cancer rates were about the same in both groups.

Although the increased risk of breast cancer and other conditions may make HRT unsuitable for prevention in healthy people, the overall risk for each woman is still very small. For example, the 26 percent increased risk of breast cancer is based on the finding that during one year, among 10,000 women receiving combination HRT there are 38 cases of breast cancer, while among 10,000 women taking a placebo, there are 30 cases. The same holds true for heart disease (37 cases per 10,000 women per year with HRT, versus 30 cases per 10,000 women per year with placebo) and blood clots (34 cases per 10,000 women per year with HRT, versus 16 cases per 10,000 women per year with placebo). Still, there is a risk, and it would probably increase as the time taking combination HRT increased.

The American Cancer Society acknowledged that decisions to use hormone replacement therapy (particularly estrogen plus progestin) will be more difficult now and recommended that women who are taking hormone replacement therapy discuss this recent finding with their doctors.

Short-term hormone use may still be considered. It is also important to note that the risk of breast cancer is seen in current users, and that eventually after stopping HRT a woman's risk returns to normal.

hormones in food   While a variety of HORMONES are produced by the human body that are essential for normal development of healthy tissues, steroid hormones used as medications (such as HORMONE REPLACEMENT THERAPY) have been found to influence cancer risk. There is no such clear link between human health and the use of hormones in animals that provide meat or dairy products. The amount of steroid hormone that is eaten in meat from a treated animal is negligible compared to what the human body produces each day. However, the BREAST CANCER risk for women who eat meat from hormone-treated animals has not been compared with the risk for women who eat meat from untreated animals, and any definitive conclusions need to be made from a large study.

Hormones are produced naturally in the body. They control important functions, such as growth, development, and reproduction. Certain hormones can make young animals gain weight faster. They help reduce the waiting time and the amount of feed eaten by an animal before slaughter in meat industries. In dairy cows, hormones can be used to increase milk production. Thus, hormones can increase the profitability of the meat and dairy industries. As early as the 1930s, farmers realized that cows injected with bovine growth hormone (bGH) from the pituitary glands produced more milk. In the 1980s, it became possible to produce large quantities of pure bGH. In 1993, the U.S. Food and Drug Administration (FDA) approved recombinant bovine growth hormone (rbGH), also known as bovine somatotropin (rbST), for use in dairy cattle. Recent estimates by the manufacturer of this hormone indicate that 30 percent of the cows in the United States may be treated with rbGH. Breast cancer can take many years to develop, so it is too early to study the breast cancer risk of women who drink milk and eat milk products from hormone-treated animals. However, there are no data as of now that suggest that breast cancer risk is higher in women who drink milk from these cows.

Hormones Approved for Use in Animals

There are six different kinds of steroid hormones that are currently approved by the FDA for use in food production in the United States: estradiol, progesterone, testosterone, zeranol, trenbolone acetate, and melengestrol acetate. Estradiol and progesterone are natural female sex hormones; testosterone is the natural male sex hormone; zeranol, trenbolone acetate, and melengestrol acetate are synthetic growth promoters. Currently, federal regulations allow these hormones to be used on growing cattle and sheep, but not on chickens, turkeys, ducks, or pigs. The FDA also allows the use of rbGH to increase milk production in dairy cattle; it is not allowed in beef cattle.

Steroid hormones are usually released into the animal from a pellet placed under the skin of the ear; the ears are thrown away at slaughter. Federal regulations prohibit the use of pellet implants in other parts of the animal, which can cause higher levels of hormone residues in the edible meat. Melengestrol acetate is available in a form that can be added to animal feed. Dairy cattle may be injected under the skin with rbGH.

Because estradiol, progesterone, and testosterone are made naturally by animals, the government cannot monitor agricultural use of these hormones. It is not possible to distinguish between the hormones used for treatment and those made by the animal's own body.

However, it is possible to detect residues of DES, zeranol, and trenbolone acetate in meat. The Food Safety Inspection Service of the U.S. Department of Agriculture monitors meat from cattle for zerano,l trenbolone, and DES residues, although DES is banned in food products.

Because the levels of naturally produced hormones vary from animal to animal and it is not possible to differentiate between the hormones produced naturally by animals and those used to treat them, determining exactly how much of the hormone used for treatment remains in the meat or the milk is difficult. Studies indicate that if correct treatment and slaughter procedures are followed, the levels of these hormones may be slightly higher in the treated animal's meat or milk but still within the normal range of natural variation known to occur in untreated animals. Scientists are currently trying to develop better methods to measure steroid hormone residues in edible meat from a treated animal.

Puberty and Hormones

Early puberty in girls is associated with a higher risk for breast cancer; height, weight, diet, exercise, and family history all influence onset of puberty. Although some experts suspect that steroid hormones in food cause early puberty in girls, exposure to higher-than-natural levels of steroid hormones through hormone-treated meat or poultry has never been documented. The trend toward earlier puberty is primarily tied to better health and nutrition.

Hormones in Milk

FDA scientists have concluded that eating foods that have slightly higher levels of rbGH would not affect human health because the amount of rbGH that is in milk or milk products as a result of treatment of the animals is insignificant compared to the amount of growth hormone naturally produced by a woman's body. Also, rbGH is a protein hormone that is broken down during digestion. The rbGH hormone used on dairy cattle is effective in promoting growth in cows but not in humans. Scientists know that rbGH is not recognized as a hormone by human cells.

Although the wholesomeness of milk is not affected by rbGH treatment, some subtle changes do take place in the treated animal. The growth hormone typically acts by triggering the cells to make other chemicals, called growth factors. These growth factors actually cause the increase in growth rate and milk production. Milk from rbGH-treated cattle has been found to have slightly higher levels of the naturally produced protein called insulin-like growth factor-1 (IGF-1).

Scientists have considered the evidence from studies of cancer risk in people who have naturally high body levels of IGF-1. Higher levels of IGF-1 in blood were found in women with breast cancer when compared to women without breast cancer in the Harvard-based NURSES' HEALTH STUDY. Scientists are investigating whether IGF-1 is just present at higher levels in patients with breast cancer or has a role in increasing the risk for the disease. In the laboratory, breast cancer cells in the test tube grow at a faster rate when bathed in a solution containing IGF-1. However, IGF-1 also plays an important role in helping normal cells grow. From the few studies done, experts cannot conclude whether or not IGF-1 increases breast cancer risk.

FDA scientists have concluded that IGF-1 in milk is unlikely to present any human food safety concern for a variety of reasons. First, in milk from untreated cows, IGF-1 levels vary, depending on the number of calves a cow has and the lactation stage. IGF-1 is also present in human breast milk, at levels higher than in hormone-treated cow's milk. Moreover, IGF-1 in milk is not expected to act as a growth factor in people who drink it because it is digested in the stomach, which breaks down its chemical structure. Furthermore, IGF-1 needs to be injected into the blood to have a growth-promoting effect, and increased IGF-1 levels in food are not expected to result in higher blood levels of IGF-1 in humans who eat the food.

The debate on whether growth hormones should or should not be used for food production has become a political issue. In 1989, the European Union banned all meat from animals treated with steroid growth hormones. The use of steroid hormones for beef cattle is permitted in Canada. Countries within the European Union do not allow the use of the protein hormone rbGH for dairy cattle. In 1999, the Canadian government refused approval for the sale of rbGH for dairy cattle, on the basis of concerns about the health effects, including mastitis, in treated animals.

hormone therapy   See HORMONAL THERAPY.

hospice   A concept, rather than a place, that focuses on a holistic model of services designed neither to hasten nor to postpone death, but rather to make a patient's final days weeks or months as positive and symptom-free as possible. The concept of hospice is based on a philosophy of caring that respects and values the dignity and worth of each person. Although hospices care for people approaching death, they cherish and emphasize life by helping patients and their families live each day to the fullest. There are almost 3,000 hospice and palliative care organizations in the United States. Most emphasize keeping patients at home, although a few hospices offer care in a hospice facility.

Typically, a family member serves as the primary caregiver and, when appropriate, helps make decisions for the terminally ill individual. Hospice is a medical benefit covered by most insurance plans, enabling patients to live at home at the end of their life and receive care from an integrated hospice team of nurses, medical social workers, physical and occupational therapists, nutritionists, home aid workers, pastoral counselors, and trained volunteers. Patients can continue to be treated by their own physician or by the hospice physician. Members of the hospice staff make regular visits to assess the patient and provide additional care or other services and are on call 24 hours a day, seven days a week.

The hospice team develops a care plan that meets each patient's individual needs for pain management and symptom control and outlines the medical and support services required, such as nursing care, personal care (dressing, bathing), social services, physician visits, counseling, and homemaker services. It also identifies the medical equipment, tests, procedures, medication, and treatments necessary to provide high-quality comfort care.

While patients are at home, all necessary symptom-relieving medications are provided by hospice workers, along with any necessary special medical equipment. In emergencies, hospice workers take patients to a hospital or hospice inpatient unit designed to be as homelike as possible. Inpatient respite care is also available to provide a break for families.

Besides medical aid, hospice workers help patients with practical support (such as shopping) and emotional support, including life-closure, grief, and spiritual counseling. Depending on the hospice's resources, it may also provide other services such as art, touch, and music therapy.

Hospice care is available as a benefit under Medicare Part A, which is designed to provide patients with a terminal illness, and their families, with special support and services not otherwise covered by Medicare. Under the Medicare hospice benefit, beneficiaries choose to receive noncurative treatment and services for their terminal illness by waiving the standard Medicare benefits for treatment of a terminal illness. However, the beneficiary may continue to access standard Medicare benefits for treatment of conditions unrelated to the terminal illness. Medicare law states that to qualify for hospice care, a patient must have "a medical prognosis that life expectancy is six months or less if the illness runs its normal course." However, it is difficult to predict how much time is left to a cancer patient, and beneficiaries are not restricted to six months of coverage by hospice rules.

See also HOSPICE FOUNDATION OF AMERICA; NATIONAL HOSPICE AND PALLIATIVE CARE ORGANIZATION.

Hospice Education Institute   An independent nonprofit organization, founded in 1985, that serves a wide range of individuals and organizations interested in improving and expanding HOSPICE and palliative care throughout the United States and around the world. The institute works to inform, educate, and support people seeking or providing care for the dying and the bereaved, or those coping with loss or advanced illness.

The institute offers seminars, books, and pamphlets, and a range of programs. These programs include HOSPICELINK, which maintains a directory of hospice programs and a program offering small gifts to patients and their families. For contact information, see Appendix I.

Hospice Foundation of America   A nonprofit organization that promotes HOSPICE care and educates professionals and those they serve about caregiving, terminal illness, loss, and bereavement. The foundation provides leadership in the development and application of hospice and its philosophy of care. Hospice Foundation, Inc., was chartered in 1982 as a way to help raise money for hospices operating in South Florida, before passage of the Medicare hospice benefit. In 1990, the foundation expanded its scope to a national level in order to provide leadership in the entire spectrum of end-of-life issues.

To reflect its national scope more accurately, in 1992 the foundation opened a Washington, D.C., office, and in 1994 it changed the name of Hospice Foundation, Inc., to Hospice Foundation of America. For contact information, see Appendix I.

HospiceLink   A service offered by the HOSPICE EDUCATION INSTITUTE that maintains a computerized directory of all hospice and palliative care programs in the United States. The toll-free telephone number (800-331-1620) provides referrals to hospice and palliative care programs, as well as general information about the principles and practices of good hospice and palliative care. For contact information, see Appendix I.

hot flashes   A sensation of heat and flushing that occurs suddenly and may be associated with menopause or some medications.

human epidermal growth factor receptor-2   See HER-2/NEU.

hydrazine   A compound found in tobacco plants, tobacco smoke, and some types of mushrooms that has been used as an unconventional therapy to treat the severe weight loss and loss of appetite that may accompany advanced stages of cancer. Although it is widely available in Europe, it is available in the United States only to those patients who are participating in research studies. The ability of hydrazine sulfate to improve quality of life among cancer patients—especially in terms of nutritional status—remains controversial, as does its effect on tumor growth.

6-hydroxymethylacylfulvene   See IROFULVEN.

hyperplasia   An abnormal excessive growth of cells in the lining of a gland.

I Can Cope program A patient education program supported by the AMERICAN CANCER SOCIETY that is designed to help patients, families, and friends cope with the day-to-day issues of living with BREAST CANCER. For contact information, see Appendix I.

immune system Complex system by which the body protects itself from outside invaders that are harmful to it.

immunosuppression The condition of having a lowered resistance to disease. In the treatment of cancer, immunosuppression is often a temporary result of lowering of white blood cell count by CHEMOTHERAPY administration.

immunotherapy A treatment that stimulates the body's own defense mechanisms to combat diseases such as cancer. These therapies have been successful in treating some types of kidney cancer, melanoma and some blood malignancies. As basic research teaches doctors more about the immune system, experts will be able to refine these therapies and use them more effectively.

implant radiation See BRACHYTHERAPY.

incidence of breast cancer The incidence of BREAST CANCER has been rising for the past two decades. Much of the increase is associated with increased screening by physical examination and mammography. However, screening alone does not seem to explain this entirely; other factors include aging of the population, later childbirth, and use of HORMONE REPLACEMENT THERAPY.

Breast cancer is the most common form of cancer among women in the United States, and in the past 50 years, a woman's lifetime risk of breast cancer has nearly tripled. In the 1940s, a woman's lifetime risk of breast cancer was one in 22. In the year 2002, the risk was one in eight.

In 2002, an estimated 203,500 women in the United States were diagnosed with invasive breast cancer, and 54,300 were diagnosed with ductal carcinoma in situ, a noninvasive cancer contained in the milk ducts.

Despite the rising incidence, the death rate from breast cancer is dropping. More women die of lung cancer; the death rate in women with lung cancer has increased 150 percent in the past 20 years.

incisional biopsy A surgical incision made through the skin to remove a portion of a suspected breast lump or breast tissue.

See also BIOPSY.

indoles A group of plant chemicals that bind to cancer-causing chemicals, activating enzymes that destroy the chemicals and prevent damage to cells. Indoles fall within a much larger group called organosulfur compounds, which are found in CRUCIFEROUS VEGETABLES such as broccoli, bok choy, cabbage, kale, brussels sprouts, and turnips.

induction therapy Treatment designed to be used as a first step toward shrinking a BREAST CANCER tumor. This can be done either with chemotherapy or hormone therapy. It is often used if a cancer is too large to be treated with a LUMPECTOMY. Induction treatment shrinks the cancer and then surgery can be done.

infection   Patients with BREAST CANCER who are undergoing CHEMOTHERAPY are at greater risk for development of life-threatening infections because the drugs affect the bone marrow, inhibiting production of infection-fighting white blood cells. The blood cells are usually at their lowest level from seven to 14 days after the chemotherapy treatment, although the level varies with the type of chemotherapy.

Most infections are caused by bacteria normally found on the skin and in the mouth, intestines, and genital tract. However, if counts are expected to be low, then patients should be careful to avoid exposure to those with illness. Sometimes the cause of an infection may not be known.

Symptoms include the following:

- Fever above 100°F or 38°C
- Shaking, chills
- Sweating
- Diarrhea
- Urgency to urinate or burning urination
- Severe cough or sore throat
- Unusual vaginal discharge or itching
- Redness, swelling, or tenderness, especially around a wound, sore, ostomy, pimple, rectal area, or catheter site
- Sinus pain or pressure
- Earaches, headaches, or stiff neck
- Blisters on the lips or skin, or mouth sores

Treatment

If patients contract an infection when their white blood cell level is very low, they often need evaluation with blood cultures and exams. Sometimes X-rays or samples of urine and stool are taken. Antibiotics are often given, either by mouth or, sometimes, through the veins. If a chemotherapy is known to cause very low counts or carry very high infection risks, growth factors (such as Neupogen) are sometimes given to stimulate the bone marrow and prevent low white blood counts.

Prevention

Chemotherapy patients can prevent a great many infections by being careful not to injure themselves or eat potentially tainted food. Patients should wash their hands often during the day, especially before meals and after using the toilet or touching animals. The rectal area should be cleaned gently but thoroughly after each bowel movement.

Patients should avoid crowds during those periods when their white counts are lowest and should stay away from people who have contagious diseases such as colds, flu, measles, or chickenpox. Patients should also avoid contact with children who have recently received live virus vaccines such as chickenpox and oral polio vaccines, since they may be contagious to people who have a low blood cell count.

Patients should be careful to prevent breaking of the skin when using scissors or nail scissors, knives, or razors and should not squeeze or scratch pimples or insect bites. Cuts and scrapes that do occur should be cleaned daily with warm water, soap, and an antiseptic, until healed. Good oral hygiene and daily baths can help prevent infections, and lotion or oil can soften and heal skin that has become dry and cracked. Protective gloves should be worn when gardening or cleaning up after others.

Patients should avoid contact with animal litter boxes and waste, bird cages, and fish tanks and prevent standing water in bird baths, flower vases, or humidifiers. They should not have any immunizations, such as flu or pneumonia shots, without checking with a doctor first and should avoid raw animal products such as sushi, raw beef, or uncooked eggs.

infiltrating breast cancer   See INVASIVE BREAST CANCER.

infiltrating ductal cell carcinoma (IDC)   See INVASIVE DUCTAL CARCINOMA.

infiltrating lobular carcinoma   See INVASIVE LOBULAR CARCINOMA.

inflammatory breast cancer   An uncommon type of locally advanced BREAST CANCER in which the breast feels warm and looks red and swollen because cancer cells have blocked the lymph vessels in the skin of the breast. The skin of the breast may also show a pitted appearance called *peau d'orange* (French for "the skin of an orange"). Inflammatory breast cancer accounts for about 1 percent of invasive breast cancers. This type of cancer is quite likely to spread to lymph nodes under the arm, and often has spread to other organs by the time of diagnosis.

The name for this type of breast cancer was chosen many years ago because doctors thought the breast tissue was inflamed. In fact, the skin changes typical of this type of cancer are not due to inflammation but rather to spread of cancer cells within the lymphatic channels of the skin. Often this diagnosis is detected as women are treated for mastitis.

Inflammatory breast cancer has a higher chance of spreading and a worse prognosis than typical invasive ductal or lobular cancers. Inflammatory breast cancer is automatically classified as stage IIIB unless it has already spread to other organs at the time of diagnosis. Such spread, common with inflammatory breast cancer, advances classification to stage IV.

Diagnosis

A biopsy can confirm the diagnosis of inflammatory breast cancer.

Treatment

Because this type of cancer is very aggressive, surgical removal (even MASTECTOMY) does not control it locally. Therefore, aggressive CHEMOTHERAPY is usually given as a first step to dramatically reduce the skin changes. After chemotherapy, mastectomy and RADIATION THERAPY to destroy any cancer left in the breast and chest wall.

Potential New Treatments

Researchers are studying the effectiveness of high-dose chemotherapy combined with bone marrow or peripheral blood STEM CELL transplantation (replacing blood-forming cells destroyed by treatment) in an attempt to improve the outcome of this type of breast cancer. They are also studying BIOLOGICAL THERAPY (stimulating the immune system to fight the cancer), new chemotherapy and hormonal drugs, and new combinations of chemotherapy and hormonal drugs.

inflammatory carcinoma of the breast See INFLAMMATORY BREAST CANCER.

informed consent A process in which a person learns key facts about a treatment, including potential risks and benefits, before deciding whether or not to proceed. Informed consent is given before surgery, radiation, chemotherapy, or any other treatments that could cause harm. Most informed consent forms are signed by the patient or a legal representative. Clinical trials also require informed consent.

in situ Medical term that means "in place." It is used to describe cancer that is localized and confined to one area. BREAST CANCER in situ is considered to be a very early stage of cancer.

insurance coverage See HEALTH INSURANCE.

intraductal carcinoma Cancer that occurs within the duct of the breast, known more commonly as DUCTAL CARCINOMA IN SITU.

intraductal papilloma A noncancerous wartlike growth that grows inside the breast, often in the large milk ducts near the nipple, causing NIPPLE DISCHARGE that may be bloody. Multiple papillomas may sometimes be found farther from the nipple.

Papillomas are usually diagnosed by imaging the breast duct with a DUCTOGRAM or by removing a portion of the affected duct. Typically, surgeons remove the papilloma and a segment of the duct where the papilloma is found, usually through an incision at the edge of the areola.

Of the benign conditions that cause suspicious nipple discharge, about half are caused by papillomas, and the other half are a mixture of fibrocystic conditions or DUCT ECTASIA.

invasive breast cancer Breast cancer that has spread outside its site of origin (the duct or lobule) and is growing into the surrounding breast tissue. See BREAST CANCER for full description.

invasive (infiltrating) ductal carcinoma (IDC) See DUCTAL CARCINOMA.

invasive lobular cancer A type of cancer that starts in cells that make up the lobules at the end of the ducts where milk is made and stored. Invasive lobular BREAST CANCER starts when a single cell in the lobule of the breast begins to divide and grow in an abnormal way.

Invasive lobular breast cancer is uncommon, affecting about 10 to 15 percent of all women who have breast cancer. It can occur at any age but more commonly affects women 45 to 55 years old. Men can also have invasive lobular breast cancer, but very rarely.

Symptoms

Unlike other forms of breast cancer, invasive lobular cancer is more likely to show up as a thickening of the breast rather than a definite hard lump. Because the symptoms can be vague, these cancers may sometimes grow to a larger size than other breast cancers before they are diagnosed.

Diagnosis

A number of tests can diagnose invasive lobular breast cancer, including a MAMMOGRAM, ultrasound, FINE NEEDLE ASPIRATION, and NEEDLE BIOPSY. However, invasive lobular breast cancer can sometimes be hard to diagnose because there is no lump that is easily detected by touch. It is also more difficult to see on a mammogram because the white MICROCALCIFICATIONS that appear on a mammogram with other types of breast cancer are not usually formed by invasive lobular cancers.

Treatment

There are a number of possible treatments for invasive lobular breast cancer, including surgery, chemotherapy, and radiation therapy.

Surgery   As is typical for most types of breast cancer, surgery is usually the first treatment. This may be a MASTECTOMY (removal of the whole breast) or a LUMPECTOMY (wide local excision, or removal of the cancer and an area of normal tissue around it). If a lumpectomy is possible, there is a chance that a second operation may be necessary to make sure that a clear enough area of tissue around the lump (clear margin) is taken. In some cases, to get a clear area of tissue it may be necessary that the whole breast be removed.

Invasive lobular cancer can sometimes affect more than one area within the breast. If this is the case, the surgeon may recommend a mastectomy.

The surgeon may remove some or all of the lymph nodes in the axilla (glands in the armpit) to find out whether any further treatment is needed.

Chemotherapy   After surgery, the doctor may recommend a course of chemotherapy to reduce the risk of cancer recurrence elsewhere in the body.

Radiation therapy   Women who have had a lumpectomy are always given radiation therapy to reduce the risk of cancer recurrence in the same breast. Women who have had a mastectomy may not need radiation therapy.

Hormonal treatment   Women whose tumor is estrogen-receptor positive (the tumor depends on estrogen to grow) are offered the hormone therapy drug tamoxifen or an AROMATASE INHIBITOR after all other treatment is completed. Most invasive lobular cancers are estrogen-receptor positive.

inverted nipple   The turning inward of the nipple. This is usually a congenital condition, but if it occurs where it had not previously existed, it can be a sign of BREAST CANCER.

4'-iodo-4'-deoxydoxorubicin   An ANTINEOPLASTIC ANTIBIOTIC used as a CHEMOTHERAPY drug.

isoflavones   Plant compounds found in SOY PRODUCTS that may help prevent cancer. Isoflavones are very similar to the human ESTROGEN HORMONE in chemical shape and properties but are much weaker and their biological action is still not fully understood. Studies show that at certain levels in the body, isoflavones may mimic human ESTROGEN—but they also may block estrogen in the body. Moreover, isoflavones work differently in different parts of the human body. The effect of isoflavones also depends on other factors, such as the number of estrogen receptors and the level of human estrogen in the body.

Isoflavones are believed to work differently in premenopausal women than they do in postmenopausal women. Research suggests that eating soy products may decrease the risk of breast cancer in premenopausal women. Dietary isoflavones can affect menstrual cycle length, which is one of the risk factors for breast cancer. Some experts believe that Asian women have a lower risk for breast cancer because they have longer menstrual cycles and lower estrogen concentrations in the body. On the other hand, there is little proof that soy intake decreases the risk of breast cancer in post-menopausal women.

One recent study did confirm that a diet rich in plant estrogens might protect against breast cancer. It showed that the lower the risk of breast cancer, the higher the level of such estrogens in the urine.

Contraindications

Consumers also should understand that soy foods and isoflavone extracts (pills or tablets) are not the same. Although there is little danger of overdose of soy foods, experts do not know the safe maximal dosage for isoflavone supplements.

Women who have been diagnosed with estrogen-receptor-positive breast cancer should be cautious about eating soy, because plant estrogens in soybeans may act as estrogen in the body. Eat-ing large amounts of soy products could therefore be harmful for women who have this specific type of breast cancer. Other researchers believe that the weaker plant estrogens such as those in soy may block the estrogen receptors and thus be helpful.

Women who are taking TAMOXIFEN should also talk to their physician about soy intake, because tamoxifen works by attaching to estrogen-receptor sites. To get the most benefit from tamoxifen, experts recommend women restrict their intake of weak plant estrogens. Women who are not taking tamoxifen or who do not have a history of estrogen-positive breast cancer may find that weak plant estrogens help protect against breast cancer.

2IT-BAD monoclonal antibody 170   A type of MONOCLONAL ANTIBODY used in cancer detection or therapy. Monoclonal antibodies are laboratory-produced substances that can locate and bind to cancer cells.

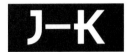

Japanese populations and cancer See ASIAN-AMERICAN WOMEN AND BREAST CANCER.

Karnofsky Performance Status (KPS) A standard way of measuring the ability of cancer patients to perform ordinary tasks. The scores range from 0 to 100; a higher score indicates a better ability to carry out daily activities. KPS may be used to determine a patient's prognosis to direct treatment, to measure changes in functioning, or to decide whether a patient should be included in a clinical trial.

Kytril (granisetron) A drug, given either intravenously (IV) or as a pill, that can help control the acute episodes of NAUSEA and vomiting that occur within 24 to 48 hours after CHEMOTHERAPY. It is not effective in controlling delayed nausea and vomiting.

Kytril belongs to a general class of drugs called serotonin antagonists, which act by blocking two pathways of serotonin release, preventing nausea and vomiting. Kytril binds to the serotonin receptors in the stomach lining, preventing the stimulation of the vomiting center and the chemoreceptor trigger zone in the brain.

Typically, Kytril is administered immediately before IV chemotherapy; pills can then be taken for a day or two to help ward off nausea and vomiting afterward.

lactation Breast-feeding for a long period of time is linked to a decrease in the risk of BREAST CANCER, probably because of the suppression of ESTROGEN and other HORMONES during this time. In fact, the longer mothers breast-feed their infants and the more children they give birth to, the lower their risk for breast cancer, according to an Oxford University study.

After analyzing data involving 150,000 women in 30 countries, Canadian scientists found that the relative risk of development of breast cancer dropped by 4.3 percent for every year of breast-feeding, in addition to a 7 percent decrease for every child born.

Other studies have found that women who first breast-feed at an early age have an even lower risk. Researchers found that if women who do not breast-feed or who breast-feed for less than three months were to do so for four to 12 months, breast cancer among premenopausal women could be reduced by 11 percent. If all women with children breast-fed for 24 months or longer, however, the incidence might be reduced by nearly 25 percent. This reduction would be even greater among women who first breast-fed at an early age.

However, the patterns of breast-feeding in industrialized nations is different than in other parts of the world. It is not clear that breast-feeding in the United States is as protective as constant breast-feeding.

Laetrile A purified form of the chemical amygdalin, a substance found in the pits of many fruits and in numerous plants, which some people have used as a cancer treatment. However, Laetrile has exhibited little anticancer activity in animal studies and no anticancer activity in human clinical trials and is not approved for use in the United States.

Used as a poison in ancient Egypt, laetrile was first used as a cancer treatment in Russia in 1845 and in the United States in the 1920s. Some people thought that the cyanide contained in laetrile might fight cancer. In the 1970s, laetrile gained popularity as an anticancer agent, and by 1978 more than 70,000 individuals in the United States were reported to have been treated with it.

Laetrile is a combination of the words *levorotatory* and *mandelonitrile*, which are used to describe amygdalin, a plant compound that contains sugar and produces cyanide. Laetrile has been used for cancer treatment both as a single agent and in combination with a metabolic therapy program that consists of specialized diet, high-dose vitamin supplements, and pancreatic enzymes.

In the United States, researchers must file an Investigational New Drug (IND) application with the U.S. Food and Drug Administration (FDA) to conduct clinical drug research in human subjects. In 1970, an application for an IND to study laetrile was filed by the McNaughton Foundation in San Ysidro, California. Although the request was approved at first, it was later rejected because animal research suggested that laetrile was probably not effective and because there were questions about how the proposed study was to be conducted. Laetrile supporters viewed this reversal as an attempt by the U.S. government to block access to new and promising cancer therapies, and they increased pressure to legalize the drug. Court cases in Oklahoma, Massachusetts, New Jersey, and California challenged the FDA's role in determining which drugs should be available to cancer patients. Consequently, laetrile was legalized in more than 20 states during the 1970s. In 1980, the U.S. Supreme Court overturned decisions by the lower courts, reaffirming the FDA's position that drugs must be proved to be both safe and effective before they can be sold. As a result, the use of laetrile as a cancer therapy is not approved in the United States, although in Mexico laetrile continues to be manufactured and widely administered as an anti-cancer treatment.

Although the names *laetrile, Laetrile,* and *amygdalin* are often used interchangeably, they are not the same product. The chemical composition of U.S.-patented Laetrile (mandelonitrile-beta-glucuronide), a semisynthetic derivative of amygdalin, is different from the laetrile/amygdalin produced in Mexico (mandelonitrile beta-D-gentiobioside), which is made from crushed apricot pits. Mandelonitrile, which contains cyanide, is a structural component of both products.

Laetrile can be taken as a pill or injection. Outside the United States, it is commonly given intravenously at first, followed by dosages in pill form. The incidence of cyanide poisoning is much higher when laetrile is taken by mouth because intestinal bacteria and some commonly eaten plants contain enzymes that activate the release of cyanide after laetrile has been ingested.

Side Effects

The side effects associated with laetrile treatment are much the same as the symptoms of cyanide poisoning, including NAUSEA and vomiting, headache, dizziness, bluish skin discoloration, liver damage, low blood pressure, droopy upper eyelid, difficulty walking due to damaged nerves, fever, mental confusion, coma, and death. These side effects are increased if the patient takes laetrile and then immediately eats raw almonds or crushed fruit pits, high doses of vitamin C, or fruits and vegetables that contain beta-glucosidase (such as celery, peaches, bean sprouts, and carrots).

laser lumpectomy This new therapy combines high-tech imaging and lasers and may enable doctors to destroy cancerous breast tumors without surgery. MAGNETIC RESONANCE IMAGING (MRI) allows doctors to see the tumor as they treat the patient, placing a needle into the tumor and then advancing a fiber-optic wire through the needle to apply laser heat for about 10 minutes. This technique, called ablation, destroys the tumor.

In a 1999 study at the University of Arkansas a total of 26 treatments were performed on 15 patients, and a pathological study of the laser lumpectomy zones confirmed that all of the tissue identified by MRI and targeted by laser was destroyed.

The MRI allows the doctor to see clearly the edges of the tumor; in traditional lumpectomies, surgeons often cannot determine where the tumor ends and have to go back and surgically remove more tissue to get clear margins.

Interactive MRI-guided laser LUMPECTOMY may provide results with less pain. The procedure can be performed on an outpatient basis, and the patient is given only a local anesthetic. After the procedure, the patient typically requires only a mild pain reliever. The needle puncture heals within a few days, and the tumor mass should be resorbed within weeks, leaving little or no cosmetic defect. The patient then receives radiation treatment. A sentinel node procedure also is performed.

The interactive MRI used in the study is called rotating delivery of excitation off-resonance (RODEO MRI). RODEO uses computer software to accentuate the contrast of the breast tissue so it is plainly visible. Currently, it is available for clinical trials only at six institutions, so this treatment is far from standard.

latissimus dorsi flaps A surgical procedure after a MASTECTOMY in which the broad fan-shaped back muscle (latissimus dorsi) and the overlying skin are used to create a breast during BREAST RECONSTRUCTION. A SALINE IMPLANT is usually inserted as well.

Because the latissimus dorsi flap is usually thinner and smaller than the TRANSVERSE RECTUS ABDOMINIS MYOCUTANEOUS (TRAM) FLAP, this procedure may be more appropriate for reconstructing a smaller breast. The latissimus dorsi flap procedure typically takes two to four hours of surgery with general anesthesia and usually requires a two- to three-day hospital stay. Women can usually resume daily activities after two to three weeks. There may be some temporary or permanent muscle weakness, difficulty with movement in the back and shoulder, and a scar on the back, which can usually be hidden in the bra line. There also may be more scars on the reconstructed breast.

lavage See DUCTAL LAVAGE.

LCIS   See LOBULAR CARCINOMA IN SITU.

leptomeningeal carcinoma   A type of secondary cancer that involves the meninges, the tissue lining the brain and spinal cord. This rare complication of BREAST CANCER occurs when the cancer spreads by way of the bloodstream to the meninges.

Symptoms
Signs of this cancer include headache, mental changes, uncoordinated movements, facial distortions, seizures, nausea, and vomiting.

Diagnosis
This type of cancer is diagnosed by MAGNETIC RESONANCE IMAGING (MRI) and lumbar puncture (spinal tap).

Treatment
This type of cancer is very difficult to treat and carries a grave prognosis. Treatment may include any combination of steroids, CHEMOTHERAPY, and RADIATION THERAPY. Because the prognosis is so grim, some decide not to pursue therapy. However, if therapy is undertaken, chemotherapy is given directly into the spinal fluid by means of a reservoir. This line or IV port is implanted by neurosurgeons in the skull, and then chemotherapy is administered directly into the brain lining.

lesbians and breast cancer   Lesbians appear to have a greater risk for BREAST CANCER than other women, not because of their sexual orientation, but because they are less likely to have children (not having children is a risk factor for breast cancer).

In addition, for many women, reproductive health issues are their main link to the health-care system. Although a woman may see her doctor primarily about reproductive health, the visit often leads to other health-care procedures such as clinical breast exams or MAMMOGRAMS. But because fewer lesbians have children and therefore may not seek routine health care, they may have less encouragement to have these important tests for early detection of breast cancer.

When cancer is detected at an early stage, it can often be treated successfully. Steps lesbians can take are to find a doctor who is sensitive to their health issues and to see that doctor on a regular basis—especially for clinical breast exams and mammograms.

leukopenia   A condition in which there are too few white cells in a patient's blood. This may occur as a side effect of CHEMOTHERAPY treatment.

lifestyle and breast cancer   Scientists have identified many factors that contribute to the development of BREAST CANCER, including a number of preventable lifestyle factors. Avoiding these risk factors whenever possible could have a significant effect on a person's probability of having cancer. The main risk factors fall under the following categories.

Alcohol
ALCOHOL consumption has been linked with an increased risk of breast cancer. People who enjoy alcohol should drink moderately—for men, this means no more than two drinks a day. For women, just one drink a day is considered moderate. Folic acid may prevent the increase in breast cancer associated with alcohol.

Diet
Researchers are sure that DIET makes a difference to health. In some cases, eating too little of certain foods can increase the risk of some types of cancer. Eating a diet rich in fruits, vegetables, whole grains, and other plant-based foods is associated with a reduced chance of cancer development. Diet also has a major influence on cholesterol, which affects the risk of cardiovascular disease.

Sedentary Lifestyle
Studies have shown that people who get regular EXERCISE are less likely to have breast cancer. One theory suggests that exercise decreases a woman's amount of ESTROGEN. An excess of estrogen is linked to the development of breast cancer. Again, as with diet, the most important reason to exercise is to prevent heart disease.

Obesity
Although study results related to cancer have been conflicting, with some showing an increased risk and others not showing such a link, obesity does appear to be linked to some types of breast cancer.

This link may be due to the fact that body fat produces estrogen, which is linked to the development of breast cancer, is produced by body fat. This link is seen only in menopausal women.

Hormones

Some types of malignant tumors need HORMONES to grow, and so increasing the amount of hormones in the body could increase the risk of breast cancers.

Birth control pills Current or former use of oral contraceptives among women ages 35 to 64 did not significantly increase the risk of breast cancer, according to the Women's Contraceptive and Reproductive Experience study.

Hormone replacement The estrogen and progestin component of the Women's Health Initiative concluded in 2002 that postmenopausal women who take combined estrogen and progestin therapy have an increased risk of invasive breast cancer. After an average of five years of follow-up for each of more than 16,000 women in the study, the study found a 26 percent increase in breast cancer risk as compared to that in women taking placebo. The biggest risk is in women who have used HRT for more than 10 years. Still, most women who develop breast cancer on HRT would otherwise have developed it even without HRT. It is not as significant a risk factor as age of puberty or time of first pregnancy.

lifetime risk The overall lifetime risk that a woman will have BREAST CANCER is one in eight. However, this does not mean she has a one in eight chance at any moment of breast cancer development. In fact, this risk changes over time, depending on her age.

Age	Risk
30	1 in 2,525
35	1 in 622
40	1 in 217
45	1 in 93
50	1 in 50
55	1 in 33
60	1 in 24
65	1 in 17
70	1 in 14
75	1 in 11
80	1 in 10
85	1 in 9
Lifetime	1 in 8

Li-Fraumeni syndrome (LFS) A very rare condition in which there is an altered gene in a family that dramatically increases risk of BREAST CANCER (among other cancers, including soft tissue or bone sarcoma, brain tumors, osteosarcoma, leukemia, or adrenocortical cancer) before age 45. Although most types of hereditary cancer syndromes involve only one or two specific types of tumors, families who have LFS are at risk for a wide range of malignancies.

Cause An inherited inborn or spontaneous defect in the *p53* gene causes this syndrome. The *p53* mutations were reported first in 1990; subsequent studies have shown that more than two-thirds of families who have LFS have inherited mutations of one of the two copies of the *p53* tumor suppressor gene; the second copy is normal. Mutations in certain areas of the gene produce more aggressive cancers than others.

limited field radiation therapy A type of RADIATION THERAPY for BREAST CANCER in which the radiation is directed only at the tumor site instead of the entire breast. Whole breast radiation therapy is part of standard treatment for women who have early-stage breast cancer who have had breast-conserving surgery. However, it has never been clear how much tissue surrounding the tumor area needs to be irradiated, and whole-breast radiation therapy has been associated with both acute and chronic toxicity.

Data from a five-year study suggest that limited field radiation therapy may be as effective as whole-breast radiation therapy in preventing breast cancer recurrence in women treated with breast-conserving surgery. In the study, conducted by researchers at William Beaumont Hospital in Royal Oak, Michigan, scientists compared the results in 199 women treated with limited field radiation therapy with those in 199 women treated with whole-breast radiation therapy. All of the women had early-stage breast cancer and were treated with breast-conserving surgery. Women in the two groups were matched by age, tumor size, lymph-node status, margins of excision, estrogen receptor status, and use of adjuvant tamoxifen therapy.

After five years, there was no difference in the median time to recurrence or the rate of local recurrence between women in the two treatment groups; nor was there any difference in the rates of spread of the disease, disease-free survival, overall survival, or cause-specific survival.

The results suggest that, in appropriately selected early-stage patients with breast cancer, limited field radiation therapy may be able to control disease after breast-conserving therapy. The results raise the question of whether whole-breast radiation therapy is necessary for certain low-risk patients.

Several European Phase III trials are comparing standard whole-breast radiation therapy with limited field radiation therapy using different techniques and radiation schedules. Data from these studies may provide more information on how much breast tissue needs to be treated and the range of patients appropriately managed with limited field radiation therapy.

However, scientists caution that these studies are small and brief. Extended follow-up will be needed to determine any late recurrences or late toxicity, which may not appear for 10 or more years.

liver metastases   See SECONDARY LIVER CANCER.

lobular carcinoma in situ (LCIS)   See BREAST CANCER.

localized breast cancer   Cancer of the breast that is confined to the site where it originated, with no sign that it has spread into the lymph nodes or beyond.

Look Good . . . Feel Better (LGFB) Program   A free, nonmedical national public service program founded in 1989 supported by corporate donors to help women deal with appearance-related changes caused by cancer treatment. The Look Good . . . Feel Better program was developed by the Cosmetic, Toiletry, and Fragrance Association, the AMERICAN CANCER SOCIETY (ACS), and the National Cosmetology Association. Today, LGFB group programs are held in every state and Puerto Rico. Teen and Spanish programs, self-help mailer kits, online programs, and a 24-hour hotline are also offered, and numerous independent international LGFB programs are available. International LGFB programs are also offered by sister organizations.

The Luzca Bien . . . Siéntase Mejor is the Spanish version that offers bilingual group programs

(English and Spanish) for Hispanic women in 14 locations: Albuquerque, Brownsville (Texas), Chicago, Dallas, Denver, Houston, Los Angeles, Miami, New York City, Phoenix, San Antonio, San Diego, San Francisco, and Washington, D.C. Spanish-language materials are available nationwide upon request.

The Look Good . . . Feel Better for Teens group offers programs for teen girls and boys in 13 cities—Boston, Columbus (Ohio), Denver, Durham (North Carolina), Houston, Memphis, New Haven, New York City, Palo Alto, Philadelphia, Rochester (Minnesota), Tampa, and Washington, D.C.—plus the 2bMe website with online demos.

Each two-hour, hands-on workshop includes a 12-step skin care/makeup application lesson, demonstration of options for dealing with hair loss, and discussion of nail-care techniques. Held at comprehensive care clinics, hospitals, ACS offices, and community centers, local group programs are organized by the ACS, facilitated by LGFB-certified cosmetologists, and aided by general volunteers. Patients in various stages of treatment receive makeover tips and personal attention from professionals trained to meet their needs. They also use and take home complimentary cosmetic kits in their appropriate skin tones (light, medium, dark, extra dark) with helpful instruction booklets. Professional advice is provided on wigs, scarves, and accessories. (Teen sessions also include social and health tips.)

"Just for You" self-help kits in English or Spanish with 30-minute video and makeover tips booklet are offered free to patients who cannot locally access LGFB. Call (800) 395-LOOK to request a kit. For contact information, see Appendix I.

lumpectomy   A surgical procedure in which only the cancerous tumor in the breast is removed. Any form of surgery that removes only part of the breast is considered breast-conserving or breast preservation surgery; it may be called quadrantectomy or wedge resection.

Technically, a lumpectomy is a partial MASTECTOMY, because part of the breast is removed—although exactly how much can vary a great deal from one woman to another. In a lumpectomy, the surgeon removes not just the tumor but also an area of healthy tissue surrounding the tumor; if cancer cells are found in the margins of the breast tissue that was removed, the surgeon performs a second surgery (called a reexcision) to try to remove the remaining cancer and obtain CLEAR MARGINS. Some women need several such surgeries before clear margins are obtained.

After a successful lumpectomy, most women receive five to seven weeks of radiation therapy to eliminate any cancer cells that may be left in the remaining breast tissue. Evidence shows that lumpectomy followed by radiation is as effective as mastectomy for women who have cancer in only one area of the breast and whose tumor is smaller than four centimeters and removed with clear margins.

Although the combination of lumpectomy and radiation is an excellent option for many women with breast cancer, it is not the best treatment for everyone. A woman may choose not to have a lumpectomy if she already has had radiation to the same breast for an earlier breast cancer, has extensive cancer in the breast or two or more separate areas of cancer in the same breast, or has a small breast and a large tumor, so that removing the tumor would be extremely disfiguring. Women also may choose mastectomy if multiple attempts to obtain clear margins have been unsuccessful, she has a connective tissue disease, or she is pregnant. Sometimes a woman may choose a mastectomy if she learns she carries the *BRCA* gene after discovering the lump. Other women cannot commit themselves to the daily schedule of radiation therapy or simply believe they would feel more comfortable with a mastectomy.

The risk of recurrence in the breast after lumpectomy (with clear margins) and radiation ranges between 5 percent and 15 percent; the average is about 10 percent. The larger the cancer, the closer the margins; the younger the patient, the more aggressive the cancer; the greater the number of lymph nodes involved, the higher the risk of recurrence.

lung metastasis The spread of cancer to the lungs. The lungs are a common site to which BREAST CANCER cells spread, since all the blood from the heart flows through the lungs.

Treatment

Treatment depends on a number of factors, including the type of lung cancer; the size, location, and extent of the tumor; and the patient's health. Many different treatments and combinations of treatments may be used to control lung cancer and to improve quality of life by reducing symptoms.

Surgery The type of surgery a doctor performs depends on the location of the tumor in the lung. An operation to remove only a small part of the lung is called a segmental or wedge resection. When the surgeon removes an entire lobe of the lung, the procedure is called a lobectomy; pneumonectomy is the removal of an entire lung. Some tumors are inoperable because of the size or location, and some patients cannot have surgery for other medical reasons.

Chemotherapy Even after cancer has been removed from the lung, cancer cells may still be present in nearby tissue or elsewhere in the body. CHEMOTHERAPY may be used to control cancer growth or to relieve symptoms. Chemotherapy drugs typically used for all types of lung cancer include DOXORUBICIN, cisplatin, and CYCLOPHOSPHAMIDE.

Radiation RADIATION THERAPY may also be used to relieve shortness of breath. Lung cancer is usually treated with external radiation, but this malignancy can also be treated with an implant containing radioactive material placed directly into or near the tumor.

Laser treatment Photodynamic therapy (PDT) is a type of laser treatment in which a specific chemical is injected into the bloodstream and absorbed by cells all over the body. The chemical rapidly leaves normal cells but remains in cancer cells for a longer time. A laser light aimed at the cancer activates the chemical, which then kills the cancer cells that have absorbed it. PDT may be used to reduce symptoms of lung cancer—for example, to control bleeding or to relieve breathing problems due to blocked airways—when the cancer cannot be removed through surgery. It also may be used to treat very small tumors in patients for whom the usual treatments for lung cancer are not appropriate.

lycopene One of more than 600 PHYTOCHEMICALS called CAROTENOIDS that have very powerful disease-fighting capabilities. Lycopene is associated with the red color in tomatoes; tomato-based products such as tomato sauce, tomato soup, and tomato juice are the most concentrated source of lycopene.

Cooked tomato sauces are associated with greater health benefits than uncooked tomatoes, because the heating process makes lycopene more easily absorbed by the body. Also, lycopene is fat-soluble, meaning that in order for the body to absorb it, it has to be eaten with at least a small amount of fat. Lycopene has been associated with a reduced risk for many cancers.

lymphadenectomy   Removal of LYMPH NODES to check for the extent of the spread of BREAST CANCER. When breast cancer is being staged to determine whether it has spread, the surgeon will remove some of the lymph nodes to see whether any malignant cells have spread there. Presence of cancer cells in the lymph nodes suggests that the cancer has spread from the primary site and is likely to spread to other parts of the body.

See also SENTINEL-NODE BIOPSY.

lymphatic system   A network of capillaries, vessels, ducts, nodes, and organs that produce, filter, and carry lymph, a colorless liquid that bathes the body's tissues and contains cells to help the body fight infection. As lymph is slowly moved through larger and larger lymphatic vessels, it passes through LYMPH NODES that filter out substances harmful to the body; these nodes also contain lymphocytes and other cells that activate the immune system to fight disease. Eventually, lymph flows into one of two large ducts in the neck. The right lymphatic duct collects lymph from the right arm and the right side of the head and chest and empties into the large vein under the right collarbone. The left lymphatic duct collects lymph from both legs, the left arm, and the left side of the head and chest and empties into the large vein under the left collarbone.

The lymphatic system collects excess fluid and proteins from the tissues and carries them back to the bloodstream. Swelling (LYMPHEDEMA) may occur if there is an increase in the amount of fluid, proteins, and other substances in the body tissues caused by problems in the blood capillaries and veins or due to a blockage in the lymphatic system.

lymphatic vessels   Thin, tubular structures that make up the LYMPHATIC SYSTEM, which removes cellular waste from the body by filtering it through the LYMPH NODES.

See also LYMPH NODE STATUS.

lymphedema   A fluid buildup that may collect in the arms or legs when LYMPHATIC VESSELS or LYMPH NODES are blocked or removed. Left untreated, this stagnant fluid interferes with wound healing and provides a culture medium for bacteria that can result in infection.

If lymph nodes are removed, there is always a risk of development of lymphedema, either immediately after surgery, or weeks, months, or even years later. The risk is increased by any infection of the arm on the side of the axillary lymph node. Air travel occasionally has also been linked to the onset of lymphedema in people who have had cancer surgery, probably as a result of the decreased cabin pressure. This is why cancer patients prone to lymphedema might consider a compression garment (a special sleeve or stocking) when flying.

Risk Factors

There are a number of risk factors for the development of lymphedema:

- Untreated or recurrent breast cancer if it involves nodes under the arm
- Axillary radiation alone
- Infections in the arm or hand
- Removal of the axillary lymph nodes, especially combined with radiation

Symptoms

Lymphedema can cause symptoms such as a feeling of fullness in the limb; tightened skin; decreased flexibility in the hand or wrist; problems fitting into clothing; or tightness of a ring, wristwatch, or bracelet. A patient in the early stages of lymphedema has swelling that indents with pressure but remains soft. The swelling may easily improve by supporting the arm or leg in a raised position, gently exercising, and wearing elastic support garments.

However, continued problems with the lymphatic system cause the lymphatic vessels to expand; as lymph flows back into the body tissues, the condition worsens. This causes pain, heat, redness, and swelling as the body tries to get rid of the extra fluid. The skin becomes hard and stiff, and the condition no longer improves with raised support of the arm or leg, gentle exercise, or elastic support garments.

Stages

Lymphedema develops in a number of stages, from mild to severe (referred to as stages 1, 2, and 3).

Stage 1 (spontaneously reversible): In the initial stage of lymphedema, tissue appears "pitted" when pressed by fingertips. Typically, on waking in the morning the affected area looks normal.

Stage 2 (spontaneously irreversible): In this intermediate stage, the tissue now has a spongy consistency and bounces back when pressed by fingertips, with no pitting. The area begins to harden and get larger.

Stage 3 (lymphostatic elephantiasis): In this advanced stage, the swelling is irreversible and the affected area has usually grown quite large. The tissue is hard and unresponsive. This condition rarely occurs but can be debilitating.

Acute Lymphedema

There are four types of acute lymphedema, which may be treated with different aspects of decongestive therapy such as manual lymphatic drainage, bandaging, proper skin care and diet, compression garments (sleeves or stockings), or remedial exercises.

The first type of acute lymphedema is mild and lasts only a short time, appearing immediately after surgery to remove the lymph nodes. The affected limb may be warm and slightly red but is usually not painful. The limb generally improves within a week if it is supported in a raised position and if the patient periodically contracts the muscles in the affected arm or leg (such as by making a fist and releasing it).

The second type of acute lymphedema occurs six to eight weeks after surgery or during radiation therapy. This type may be caused by inflammation of either lymphatic vessels or veins, producing a limb that is tender, warm, and red. It is treated by keeping the limb supported in a raised position and taking anti-inflammatory drugs. Antibiotics also are given to treat an underlying infection.

The third type of acute lymphedema occurs after an insect bite, minor injury, or burn that causes an infection of the skin. The affected area is red, very tender, and hot and is treated by supporting the affected arm or leg in a raised position and taking antibiotics. Using a compression pump or wrapping the affected area with elastic bandages should not be done during the early stages of infection. Mild redness may continue after the infection.

The fourth and most common type of acute lymphedema develops very slowly and may become noticeable only two years or more after surgery—or not until many years after cancer treatment. The patient may experience discomfort of the skin or aching in the neck and shoulders or spine and hips caused by stretching of the soft tissues, overuse of muscles, or posture changes caused by increased weight of the arm or leg.

Temporary versus Chronic Lymphedema

Temporary lymphedema lasts less than six months and does not involve hardening of the skin. A patient may be more likely to have lymphedema if there is

- A surgical drain that leaks protein into the surgical site
- Inflammation
- Inability to move the limb
- Temporary loss of lymphatic function
- Blockage of a vein by a blood clot or inflammation of a vein

Chronic (long-term) lymphedema is the most difficult of all types of swelling to treat; it occurs when the damaged lymphatic system of the affected area is not able to handle the increased need for fluid drainage from the body tissues. This may happen

- After a tumor recurs or spreads to the lymph nodes
- After an infection of the lymphatic vessels

- After periods of inability to move the limbs
- After radiation therapy or surgery
- When early signs of lymphedema have not been controlled
- When a vein is blocked by a blood clot

Those who have chronic lymphedema are at increased risk of infection. No effective treatment is yet available for patients who have advanced chronic lymphedema. Once the body tissues have been repeatedly stretched, lymphedema may recur more readily.

Prevention

Poor drainage of the lymphatic system due to surgery to remove the lymph nodes or radiation therapy may make the affected arm or leg more susceptible to serious infection. Even a minor infection may lead to severe lymphedema.

It is important that patients take precautions to prevent injury and infection, since lymphedema can occur 30 years or more after surgery. The skin must be protected to avoid cracks, infections, scratches, or burns. Any infection of the skin must be treated promptly. Gloves should be worn while cleaning and gardening.

Because lymphatic drainage is improved during exercise, exercise can help prevent lymphedema. Patients with breast cancer should do hand and arm exercises after mastectomy, but should only increase activity and weights slowly.

lymph node dissection   The removal of the LYMPH NODES from a specific area.

lymph nodes   Small oval structures, ranging in size from a pinhead to a bean, that filter germs and foreign substances from LYMPH (the clear fluid that bathes many of the body's organs). When lymph nodes trap germs, they swell; that is why a swollen lymph gland is often a sign of infection or disease. A valuable part of the immune system, lymph nodes are linked via LYMPHATIC VESSELS throughout the body. Lymph nodes can be found under the arms, behind the knee and ears, in the groin, and in the abdominal cavity.

See also LYMPHEDEMA; SENTINEL-NODE BIOPSY.

lymph node status   The determination of whether a LYMPH NODE contains malignant cells (positive) or does not (negative). Negative lymph nodes are associated with less aggressive types of breast cancer and a better ultimate prognosis. During surgery, a number of lymph nodes are removed so the lab can check for malignant cells. More recently, SENTINEL-NODE BIOPSY allows a surgeon to determine which node would likely be the first one that cancer cells would reach; if this node is clear, it is likely that the rest are clear also.

macrobiotic diet A mostly vegetarian diet that advocates believe can prevent disease by adjusting food, lifestyle, relationships, and environment. Macrobiotic diet proponents believe that everything in the world (including cancer) has two opposite forces: yin and yang. The diet is planned to correct any imbalances of yin and yang that could lead to ill health or cancer.

The modern macrobiotic diet is comprised of 50 percent whole cereal and grains, 20 percent to 30 percent vegetables, 5 percent to 10 percent soups, and 5 percent to 10 percent beans and sea vegetables. Foods that may occasionally be eaten include fish, seafood, seasonal fruits, nuts, seeds, and other natural snacks. Sugar and meat are not allowed in a macrobiotic diet.

The NATIONAL CANCER INSTITUTE (NCI) and the AMERICAN CANCER SOCIETY believe that adhering to a strict macrobiotic diet is not effective in treating or preventing cancer.

Diet critics warn that the modern macrobiotic diet may not provide enough of certain nutrients, including protein, vitamins D and B_{12}, and the minerals zinc, calcium, and iron. An earlier version of the macrobiotic diet that included only grains has been associated with severe malnutrition and even death. According to the NCI, no clinical trials that show health benefits of macrobiotic diet have been conducted. However, it is low in fat, high in vegetables and fiber, so it may be a heart-healthy diet.

macrocalcifications Coarse calcium deposits in the breast that can be seen on a MAMMOGRAM, usually caused by changes in the breast as a result of old injuries, inflammation, or aging. They are usually benign and do not usually require biopsy.

About half of all American women older than age 50 have some macrocalcifications; they also appear in about 10 percent of women younger than age 50.

macrocyst A CYST in the breast that is large enough to be felt with the fingers.

magnetic resonance elastography (MRE) A new imaging technique that can detect breast tumors by using a combination of sound waves and MAGNETIC RESONANCE IMAGING (MRI) to evaluate the mechanical properties of tissues within the breast, according to Mayo Clinic researchers. In the future, this could mean earlier and more reliable diagnosis of BREAST CANCER.

Malignant breast tumors tend to be much harder than normal tissues and most benign tumors. This explains why breast cancer is often detected by physical examination simply on the basis of a very hard lump in the breast. The MRE technique was tested on six healthy women and six women with known breast cancer. The images of women with breast cancer demonstrated areas of high tissue stiffness corresponding to the known tumors. On average, the stiffness of the breast cancer tissue was more than four times higher than that of the surrounding tissue.

Standard imaging techniques such as computed tomography, ultrasonography, and MRI do not provide information about the mechanical properties of tissue. This new imaging technology allows scientists to look at tissues in a way that has never before been possible, combining the sensitivity of MRI with evaluation of tissue hardness. This could reduce false positives and unneeded biopsies.

magnetic resonance imaging (MRI) An imaging method that uses magnets and not radiation to take pictures. Very detailed pictures of the breast interior can be taken when the contrast agent gadolinium is applied. These can be used to sort out whether a lump is cancerous or benign. Studies are now under way to determine if MRI can be used as a screening tool in women without lumps or radiologic abnormalities. However, MRI has many false positives, resulting in unnecessary biopsies, and also may not be as effective in picking up precancerous conditions.

Although many experts believe that most women are well served by MAMMOGRAPHY and do not need MRI (this costly test is not always covered by health insurance), women at high risk for BREAST CANCER may benefit from this high-tech test. In one 2002 study, comparing mammograms and MRIs in 179 women younger than age 50 at high risk for early-onset breast cancer, 13 breast cancers were found. MRI detected all of them, whereas mammogram detected only six. Researchers point out that younger women in particular have dense breast tissue that is more difficult to evaluate with a mammogram than with MRI. Women with a genetic predisposition to breast cancer also may benefit from screening with both MRI and mammograms.

More testing is needed to confirm the value of MRI in breast cancer screenings. In the meantime, it will continue to be an important complementary tool in the detection of breast cancer.

mammaglobin (MG) A novel gene that has been detected in BREAST CANCERS at rates many times higher than in normal breast tissue. In 1998, researchers discovered a new gene with a sequence similar to that of *MG*. Accordingly, this gene was named *mammaglobin B (MGB)*, and the original mammaglobin gene was renamed *MGA*. *MGA*, *MGB*, and several related genes, such as lipophilin B (*LPB*), are localized in a dense cluster on chromosome 11q12.2, and all have been associated with human breast cancer.

In one study *MGA* was found more frequently in estrogen-receptor-positive cancers. Among the 97 cancers studied, nearly half (41 percent) were positive for *MGA* and *MGB*, and 78 percent of cancers expressed at least one of these genes. *MGB* was found in four of 15 nonmalignant breast tissues.

Experts believe that these findings could have important consequences for breast cancer screening. Because *MGA* is primarily confined to breast tissue, this gene may be one of the first relatively mammary-specific markers. It could be used to detect tiny breast cancer cells in lymph nodes, peripheral blood, and bone marrow; identify metastases of unknown origin; and help with early detection of breast cancer.

mammary duct ectasia See DUCT ECTASIA.

mammary glands The breast tissue that includes the glands that produce milk and the ducts that carry milk to the nipples.

mammogram An X-ray of the breast to identify potential breast malignancies. Experts recommend that women have regularly scheduled screening mammograms and CLINICAL BREAST EXAMS. A screening mammogram, which looks for breast changes in women who have no signs of breast cancer, is the best tool available for finding breast cancer early. Mammograms can often detect a breast lump before it can be felt, and a mammogram can show small deposits of calcium (called MICROCALCIFICATIONS) that may be an early sign of cancer.

The NATIONAL CANCER INSTITUTE recommends that women in their forties or older have screening mammograms every one to two years. Women who are at increased risk for breast cancer should seek medical advice about when to begin having mammograms and how often to be screened. For example, a doctor may recommend that a woman at increased risk begin screening before age 40 or change her screening intervals.

The following strong risk factors may be used to justify yearly screening in women between 40 and 50 years old and perhaps even regular mammography at an earlier age (30 to 35):

- Previous breast cancer
- *BRCA1* or *BRCA2* mutations

- Mother, sister, or daughter who has a history of breast cancer
- ATYPICAL HYPERPLASIA found on any previous breast BIOPSY
- At least 75 percent of breast classified as dense tissue on mammogram at age 45 to 49
- Two or more previous breast biopsies, even if the results were benign

If an area of the breast looks suspicious on the screening mammogram, additional mammograms may be needed. Depending on the results, the doctor may advise the woman to have a biopsy.

Although mammograms are the best way to find breast abnormalities early, they are not perfect. A mammogram may miss some cancers that are present (false negative result) or may find things that turn out not to be cancer (false positive result). In addition, detecting a tumor early does not guarantee that a woman's life will be saved, because some fast-growing breast cancers may have spread to other parts of the body before being detected. Nevertheless, studies show that having mammograms reduces the risk of dying of breast cancer.

To ensure that she has a good-quality mammogram, a woman should

- Ask to see the U.S. Food and Drug Administration (FDA) certificate that is issued to all facilities that meet high professional standards of safety and quality.
- Use a facility that either specializes in mammograms or performs many mammograms each day.
- Continue to go to the same facility on a regular basis so that the mammograms can be compared from year to year.
- Keep a list of the dates of previous mammograms, biopsies, or other breast treatments as well as the places they were carried out.

If a woman has had mammograms at another facility, she should obtain the X-rays to make sure they are available to the radiologist at the current examination. On the day of the examination, a woman should not wear deodorant, since this can interfere with the mammogram by appearing on the X-ray film as tiny spots. If a woman's breasts are usually tender the week before her period, she should avoid mammograms during this time. Ideally, the best time for a woman to have a mammogram is one week after her period.

A woman should describe any breast symptoms or problems to the technologist performing the examination. She also should be prepared to discuss any pertinent history such as prior surgeries, hormone use, and family or personal history of breast cancer. Any new findings or problems in the breasts should also be discussed with a doctor or nurse before having a mammogram.

During the procedure, a technologist (usually a woman) positions the breasts for the mammogram. Women may feel some discomfort when the breasts are compressed, but there should not be pain.

All mammogram facilities are now required to send results of the mammogram to the patient within 30 days. A woman should be contacted within five business days if there is a problem with the mammogram result. If a woman does not hear from her doctor within 10 days, she should not assume that the mammogram finding was normal—she should call the doctor or the facility.

Paying for a Mammogram

Mammogram costs, or a portion of them, are covered by MEDICARE, MEDICAID, and most private health plans. Low-cost mammograms are available in most communities. The AMERICAN CANCER SOCIETY (800-ACS-2345) can provide information about local facilities.

mammogram, baseline   Usually a patient's first screening MAMMOGRAM, the baseline mammogram provides a basis for comparison when later mammograms are conducted. Women should always try to keep track of when and where they have had each mammogram because doctors need to compare earlier films to help interpret current or future mammograms. Women who do not have a baseline mammogram are more likely to need extra views, follow-up exams, and biopsies.

See also MAMMOGRAM, SCREENING; MAMMOGRAM, DIAGNOSTIC; MAMMOGRAM, DIGITAL.

mammogram, contrast digital   See CONTRAST DIGITAL MAMMOGRAPHY.

mammogram, diagnostic A MAMMOGRAM taken when a suspicious finding is present on the screening mammogram. A screening mammogram is just two views of the breast; a diagnostic mammogram may include extra views, magnified views, or extra compression of the breast.

mammogram, digital See DIGITAL MAMMOGRAPHY.

mammogram, screening The annual MAMMOGRAM a physician prescribes for a woman to check for BREAST CANCER, which usually involves two X-ray views of each breast. The best time to schedule a screening mammogram is about seven days after a woman's period, as breasts are less tender then.

mammogram facility A hospital or clinic where MAMMOGRAMS are performed. Many facilities can offer mammogram services, and some institutions are better than others. Many experts suggest that to get a good mammogram, a woman go to a place where people specialize in mammography.

Comparison shopping for a good mammogram facility is not easy, since the government does not gather much of the information that experts say women need. Women in rural areas may have to travel long distances to find doctors who meet the experts' standards. Even high-technology radiology clinics in upscale neighborhoods may be staffed with doctors who do not have the training, experience, or knack to read mammograms well.

The MAMMOGRAPHY QUALITY STANDARDS ACT (MQSA) requires mammography facilities to adhere to strict quality standards. For example, mammography facilities must give women written results of their mammogram in easy-to-understand language within 30 days of the mammogram. Patients may also obtain their original mammogram (not a copy) from the facility so they may compare the results with those of previous mammograms.

Women do not need to be referred by a physician to have a mammogram at most facilities. Women who do not have a primary physician or do not wish to be referred by their physician may "self-refer" at most facilities. Self-referred patients who have no doctor receive both the simplified report and the report designated for the physician.

If an abnormality is found on the patient's mammogram, the facility is required to notify the patient and her physician (if appropriate) and recommend a suitable course of action. Women who do not receive their mammogram results within 30 days should contact the mammography facility and ask for the results. Women should not assume their mammogram result is normal if they do not receive the results. Facility certification can now be extended to include U.S. Food and Drug Administration (FDA)–approved DIGITAL MAMMOGRAPHY units.

A woman can locate a nearby certified mammogram facility by visiting the Web site of the Center for Devices and Radiological Health of the FDA. This Web site (http://www.accessdata.fda.gov/scripts/cdrh/cfdocs/cfmqsa/search.cfm) includes an extensive Mammography Site Database; women may search for a nearby mammography clinic by entering their state and zip code.

The following regulations govern every mammography facility in the United States:

- Physicians who interpret mammograms, radiological technologists who perform mammography, and medical physicists who survey mammography equipment must have adequate training and experience.
- Each mammography facility must have an effective quality control program and maintain thorough records.
- Each facility must submit typical mammography images (X-rays) to the FDA for review. The FDA evaluates the quality and amount of radiation used to obtain the images (radiation levels are required to be low).
- Each mammography facility must develop systems for following up on mammograms that reveal abnormalities and for obtaining biopsy results.
- Each mammography facility must undergo yearly inspections by FDA- or state-certified inspectors.

As of April 1, 2004, there were 9,079 MQSA-certified mammography facilities in the United States and its territories.

To get a good mammogram, a woman should

- Find a clinic where doctors read large numbers of mammograms, far beyond the 480 a year required by the FDA.
- Look for doctors who completed fellowships in mammography or who spend at least half their time reading mammograms.
- Look for clinics where two doctors independently interpret every film.
- Ask about medical audits, which show whether a doctor sends too many women for biopsies.
- Use open-records laws to obtain a clinic's inspection reports, which list violations. A woman should be wary of citations for equipment failures or missing quality control records.

A woman should *not*

- Press for an instant interpretation of her film. A day's delay through "batch" reading can maximize a doctor's power of concentration.
- Put too much faith in a doctor who is board certified in radiology. Many doctors passed the board before the late 1980s, before mammography was added to the exam. In any case, the number of practice mammograms it now includes does not reflect the rigors of real-world screening.
- Judge doctors by the lawsuits they have lost for misreading mammograms. Even the best doctors miss some cancers.
- Put too much faith in promising but still-unproven technologies such as digital X-ray machinery and computer programs that look for cancers doctors might miss.
- Have a mammogram done on Mother's Day, when many clinics offer free or discounted exams. These programs can swamp the doctors and rush the reading.

mammography A special series of X-rays that show images of the soft tissues of the breast, designed to help find BREAST CANCER early, when it can still be cured. Yearly MAMMOGRAMS are recommended for women older than 40 even if they have no signs of breast cancer, and for younger women who have symptoms of breast cancer or who have a high risk of breast cancer. The entire procedure for a screening mammogram takes about 20 minutes.

About 10 percent of women have a suspicious mammogram that requires further testing. Of women with these suspicious mammograms, only 8 percent to 10 percent need a biopsy—and most of those biopsies do not detect cancer. In other words, only one or two mammograms of every 1,000 precede a diagnosis of cancer.

The modern mammography machine is used only for breast X-rays to produce high-quality pictures with a low radiation dose (usually about 0.1 to 0.2 rad per picture). In the past there were concerns about radiation risks, but today's machines pose a minimum risk, if any. For example, a woman who receives radiation as a treatment for breast cancer receives several thousand rads, whereas a woman who has had a mammogram every year for 50 years will have received only between 20 to 40 rads. Moreover, the type of X-ray used for the breasts does not penetrate tissue as easily as the X-ray used for routine films of chest, arms, or legs.

During a mammogram, the breast is squeezed between two plates to spread the tissue apart and to allow a lower dose of radiation. This procedure produces a black-and-white image of the breast tissue on a large sheet of film, which is interpreted by a radiologist. Reading mammograms is difficult because there is a wide range in what is considered normal, and the appearance of the breast on a mammogram varies a great deal from woman to woman. This is why it is extremely helpful for a radiologist to have previous X-ray films from the same woman for comparison.

Abnormal Findings

A mammogram may reveal tiny white spots on the film, which are tiny mineral deposits within the breast tissue called calcifications, or may highlight a suspicious mass.

Calcifications MACROCALCIFICATIONS are large calcium deposits that appear in the breast as a result of aging, old injuries, or inflammation. These deposits are related to noncancerous conditions and do not require a biopsy. Macrocalcifications occur in about half of all women older than age 50 and in one of 10 women younger than age 50.

MICROCALCIFICATIONS are tiny specks of calcium in the breast that may appear alone or in clusters. The shape and location of microcalcifications can help a radiologist determine how likely it is that the areas are malignant. In some cases, microcalcifications do not require a biopsy, but only a follow-up mammogram within three to six months. In other cases, the microcalcifications are suspicious and a BIOPSY is recommended.

Mass A mass may occur with or without calcifications and can be caused by benign breast conditions or by breast cancer. Some masses can be monitored with periodic mammography; others may need a biopsy. The size, shape, and margins of the mass help the radiologist to determine the likelihood of cancer. Many masses turn out to be CYSTS (benign collections of fluid); to confirm that a mass is really a cyst, a doctor must either order a breast ultrasound or remove some fluid with a needle.

If a mass is not a cyst, then the patient may need more imaging tests. Prior mammograms may help show that a mass has remained unchanged for many years, indicating a benign condition.

If a mass raises a significant suspicion of cancer, tissue must be removed for examination under the microscope to determine whether it is cancer. This can be done with needle biopsy or open surgical biopsy.

Screening Mammograms

A screening mammogram is an X-ray of the breast of a woman who has no breast complaints. Screening mammography is designed to find cancer when it is still too small to be felt by a doctor or patient. Finding small breast cancers early by a screening mammogram greatly improves a woman's chance for successful treatment. A screening mammogram usually involves two X-rays of each breast.

Results from a recent compilation of many studies found 17 percent fewer deaths from breast cancer among women in their 40s who had mammograms. The AMERICAN CANCER SOCIETY (ACS) believes that the benefits of a yearly mammogram for women 40 and older outweigh the effects of minimal exposure to radiation and of occasional false positive results that require a biopsy of benign conditions.

Because mammograms cannot find all breast cancers, the ACS recommends women that are older than 40 who do not have symptoms get regular mammograms, have yearly CLINICAL BREAST EXAMS by a health-care professional, and perform monthly BREAST SELF-EXAMINATIONS. These guidelines apply only to women at usual risk for breast cancer who have no symptoms of breast cancer. For women 20 to 39 who have no symptoms of breast cancer, the society recommends a physical examination of the breast every three years, performed by a health-care professional.

Women at high risk for breast cancer should discuss their situation with their doctor. In some cases, mammograms should be started before age 40 and a more frequent schedule of early detection tests may be appropriate. For example, doctors recommend that a baseline mammogram be done at age 25 for women whose genetic testing results show changes in breast cancer susceptibility genes (*BRCA1* and/or *BRCA2*).

Diagnostic Mammograms

A woman who has either a breast symptom (such as a breast mass) or a screening mammogram result that shows an abnormality is scheduled for a diagnostic mammogram. A diagnostic mammogram involves more pictures to allow the RADIOLOGIST to study the breast's condition carefully. Specific images known as cone views with magnification are used to make a small area of altered breast tissue easier to evaluate.

As a result of the diagnostic mammogram, the doctor may suggest that a biopsy is needed to tell whether or not the lesion is cancer. If a biopsy is recommended, the woman should discuss the different types of biopsy with her doctor to determine which method is best for her.

Breast Image Reporting and Data System

The American College of Radiology has developed a standard way of describing mammogram findings by giving the results a code numbered 0 through 5, called the Breast Imaging Reporting and Data System:

Category 0: Assessment is incomplete and additional imaging evaluation is needed. A possible abnormality may not be completely seen or defined and requires additional evaluation including the use of spot compression, magnification views, special mammographic views, or ultrasound.

Category 1: No significant abnormality to report. The breasts are symmetrical without masses, distortion, or suspicious calcifications.

Category 2: This is a negative mammogram result that has found a benign lesion, such as benign calcifications, intramammary lymph nodes, and calcified fibroadenomas. This category ensures that other individuals viewing the mammogram do not misinterpret a benign finding as suspicious, and documents the finding for use in future mammogram assessments.

Category 3: This is a "probably benign finding," which suggests the need for a short-term follow-up. Results in this category are not expected to change. However, since the results have not been proved benign, the doctor will want to see whether the lesion changes over time. In this case, follow-up imaging is usually done every six months for a year, and then every year for two years. This schedule eliminates unnecessary biopsies but ensures that any malignancy will be detected within a short period.

Category 4: This result is a suspicious abnormality, requiring a biopsy. In this case, although the findings do not definitely appear to be cancer, there is a substantial probability of malignancy.

Category 5: These findings are characteristic of cancers, with a high probability of malignancy. Biopsy is very strongly recommended.

Mammogram Facility Certification

The U.S. Food and Drug Administration (FDA) inspects and certifies all mammogram facilities in the United States.

See also MAMMOGRAM FACILITY.

Mammography Quality Standards Act (MQSA) of 1992/1998   A federal law establishing requirements for the accreditation, certification, and inspection of MAMMOGRAPHY facilities, aiming to ensure that all women have access to high-quality mammography services. In the fall of 1998, Congress reauthorized the MQSA, extending the program to 2002. Congress enacted the law because of the understanding that the effectiveness of mammography as a breast cancer detection technique is directly related to the quality of mammography procedures.

As a result of this legislation, facilities must be certified to perform mammography lawfully and to be reimbursed by Medicare and Medicaid for mammography services. In order to be certified, the equipment, personnel, and practice of the facility must be reviewed by a U.S. Food and Drug Administration (FDA)–approved accreditation body and meet the following criteria:

- Each mammogram machine must be accredited.
- Certain personnel must meet strict standards, including radiologists, radiologic mammography technologists (the individuals who actually position women for the exam and take the mammogram pictures), and medical physicists (professionals who specialize in medical equipment and image production).
- Typical X-rays are reviewed for quality and information on radiation dose, which is required to be very low.

If the facility meets all of the appropriate standards, the FDA gives its certification. The FDA has a list of all of its certified mammography facilities, by state and Zip code, available at the FDA's Web site (http://www.fda.gov/cdrh/mammography/certified.html).

Reporting Results

In addition to certification, mammogram clinics are now required to notify women in writing of the results of their mammograms. The Mammography Quality Standards Act was recently changed in response to reports that some women were not learning soon enough they had suspicious mammogram results. Mammogram clinics are continuing to report mammogram results to the woman's doctor, who is responsible for ordering additional tests or treatments, but now clinics must mail women a separate, easy-to-understand report of their mammogram results within 30 days (sooner if the mammogram results suggest cancer is present) so that they know the results even if the doctor has not yet called to inform them.

As of April 1, 2004, there were 9,079 MQSA-certified mammography facilities operating in the United States. Facilities that fail accreditation must stop providing mammography services. However, once the deficiencies have been corrected, a facility may apply for reinstatement to resume the accreditation process. The FDA uses a state-of-the-art database that tracks certification, inspections, and accreditation information, which allows it to assess facilities' compliance with the MQSA.

mammoplasty   Plastic surgery of the breast, which includes breast augmentation, breast reduction, and BREAST RECONSTRUCTION.

MammoSite   A new method of RADIATION THERAPY that minimizes the impact on surrounding healthy tissue and cuts treatment time from weeks to days for women with early BREAST CANCER. The system, approved in 2002 by the U.S. Food and Drug Administration, delivers radiation therapy internally through a balloon implanted into a tumor's former site during a LUMPECTOMY.

In this method, the patient with breast cancer returns for a one- to five-day course of outpatient radiation treatment. No source of radiation remains in the body between treatments or after the final procedure. The balloon is deflated and the catheter removed when treatment is completed.

The treatment period is much shorter than the $6^{1}/_{2}$ weeks required for conventional radiation therapy. Because the amount of tissue and side effects are limited, women can get back to their regular activities without lingering effects. In addition, healthy breast tissue, the chest wall, the lungs, and the heart are spared unnecessary radiation, which can be a problem with standard radiation treatment.

The treatment is recommended only for early-stage cancer and for women with small tumors. Larger, more-advanced lesions require more comprehensive radiation treatment to a larger portion of the breast that the balloon could not reach.

There have been no long-term studies that assess the safety and effectiveness of the MammoSite method as a replacement for conventional radiation to the entire breast. As a result, doctors do not know what will happen 10 to 15 years after treatment. Nonetheless, studies in the *Journal of Clinical Oncology* and elsewhere have found that conventional BRACHYTHERAPY shows low local recurrence rates.

The costs for standard radiation therapy and the MammoSite method are similar.

mammotest   Another term for STEREOTACTIC BIOPSY.

Mammotome   A breast biopsy system that requires only a tiny incision of a quarter of an inch. Using an ultrasound probe or an X-ray, the doctor can then suction out abnormal tissue for examination.

manual lymphatic drainage   A very gentle technique used to treat LYMPHEDEMA that involves stimulating the skin and the underlying lymphatic vessels by hand. Also known as complex decongestive physiotherapy, the procedure is different from more traditional and vigorous massage, which concentrates on muscles and deeper tissues. That type of massage might worsen lymphedema rather than making it better.

In manual lymphatic drainage, a specially trained and certified physical, occupational, or massage therapist gently stimulates the patient's affected arm. The therapist delicately moves hands and fingers over the surface of the patient's skin in a circular motion toward the shoulder. At the end of every session, the therapist applies customized bandages to lessen the return of fluid and to reshape the affected arm to look more like the opposite one. The therapist prescribes exercises to do with the bandages in place.

Lymphedema therapy is usually performed once per day, three to five days a week for a number of weeks, depending on the extent of the swelling. Each session usually lasts one to one and a half hours. The procedure is expensive and may not be covered by medical insurance plans.

The success of manual lymphatic drainage depends on the skill and dedication of the therapist, as well as the patient's bandaging skill and dedication to a treatment program. The structure and physiological characteristics of the lymphatic system may also affect the success of treatment.

margins   The area of normal tissue that remains after a malignant breast cancer tumor has been removed. A *clear margin* means that no cancer cells are present near the borders of the tissue that was removed, and all of the cancer was removed from the site. When a surgeon is unable to obtain clear margins after a LUMPECTOMY, a second surgery to obtain a larger tissue sample and get a clear margin is necessary. Even with clear margins, additional treatment (chemotherapy or radiation therapy) may still be needed to make sure all cancer cells are killed.

marijuana (*Cannabis sativa L.*)   A member of the cannabis plant family that can relax the mind and body, ease NAUSEA, increase appetite, and heighten perception. One component of marijuana, synthetic delta-9-THC (dronabinol), is now available as the drug MARINOL to treat nausea and vomiting in chemotherapy patients. Although marijuana use is illegal in the United States, the U.S. Food and Drug Administration in 1985 approved Marinol for the treatment of nausea and vomiting associated with cancer chemotherapy in patients who did not respond to conventional antinausea treatments.

Although research has shown that THC is more quickly absorbed from marijuana smoke than from an oral preparation, any antinausea effects of smoking marijuana may not be consistent because of varying potency, depending on the source of the marijuana contained in the cigarette.

Eight states (Alaska, California, Colorado, Hawaii, Maine, Nevada, Oregon, and Washington) already allow seriously ill patients to use medical marijuana, usually through a doctor's recommendation and an independent board's certification. A similar bill that would have allowed medical marijuana in New Mexico was defeated in March of 2003.

The Marinol patient-assistance program is designed to help find potential insurance coverage for Marinol; for eligible patients with financial need, Marinol may be supplied free of charge. Information about the program is available at (800) 256-8918.

Marinol (dronabinol)   A synthetic version of MARIJUANA. It is used to treat NAUSEA and vomiting in CHEMOTHERAPY patients who do not respond to any other antinausea medication.

mastectomy   An operation to remove the breast (or as much of it as possible) as a treatment for BREAST CANCER.

In *segmental mastectomy,* the surgeon removes the cancer and a larger area of normal breast tissue around it. Occasionally some of the lining over the

chest muscles below the tumor is removed as well. Some LYMPH NODES under the arm may also be removed as a separate procedure.

In a *simple (or total) mastectomy,* the whole breast is removed; lymph nodes are not sampled.

In a *modified radical mastectomy,* the whole breast, most of the lymph nodes under the arm, and often the lining over the chest muscles are removed. The smaller of the two chest muscles is also taken out to help in removing the lymph nodes.

A *radical mastectomy* is the removal of the breast as well as the surrounding lymph nodes, muscles, fatty tissue, and skin. Formerly considered the standard surgery for breast cancer, this procedure is rarely used today. Radical mastectomy occasionally may be suggested if the cancer has spread to the chest muscles.

To perform a simple mastectomy, a surgeon makes an incision along the perimeter of the breast closest to the tumor, leaving most of the skin intact. Typically the nipple is not removed during a simple mastectomy, but the underlying tissue is gently cut free and removed. A drainage tube is inserted and the wound is then closed with stitches, tape, or clips. A mastectomy with lymph node dissection usually lasts between two and three hours; immediate breast reconstruction increases the length of surgery.

The drainage tube placed into the breast or under the arm removes blood and lymph node fluid that builds up during the healing process. Drainage tubes are usually removed within two weeks, when the drainage is reduced to less than one ounce a day.

Major soreness from mastectomy usually lasts two to three days; however, many mastectomy patients do not experience soreness after surgery. Studies have shown that many women experience phantom breast sensations after mastectomy, including sensations of unpleasant itching, pins and needles, pressure, or throbbing. This pain probably occurs as the result of damage to nerves in the area. Women who experience breast pain before mastectomy are most likely to have sensations of pain in the breast area after surgery. EXERCISE or breast massage may help ease phantom breast pain; in more severe cases, drugs may be needed. Phantom breast pain does not indicate that cancer cells are still present in the breast area or that cancer may recur.

Lymph Node Dissection

A radical mastectomy, modified radical mastectomy, or LUMPECTOMY often includes the removal of lymph nodes from the underarm (axillary node dissection). After surgery, the lymph nodes are examined to determine whether the cancer has spread past the breast.

SENTINEL-NODE BIOPSY is a new form of LYMPH NODE DISSECTION in which only one to three "sentinel" lymph nodes (the first nodes in the lymphatic chain) are removed. In this procedure, a radioactive tracer or blue dye is injected into the area near a tumor. The dye is then carried to the sentinel node (the lymph node most likely to harbor cancer cells if the disease has spread). If the sentinel node contains cancer, more lymph nodes are removed and examined, but if the sentinel node is cancer-free, additional lymph node surgery may be avoided.

Research shows that sentinel-node biopsy may eliminate the need to remove many lymph nodes and thereby reduce the probability of LYMPHEDEMA (chronic arm swelling).

Prophylactic (Preventive) Mastectomy

Preventive mastectomy is the surgical removal of one or both breasts in an effort to prevent or reduce the risk of breast cancer. The procedure of choice is a total mastectomy, in which the entire breast and nipple is removed. A subcutaneous mastectomy is recommended less often because this operation removes the breast tissue but spares the nipple, thereby increasing the risk of leaving cancerous breast tissue behind.

A woman may consider preventive mastectomy on one side if she has already had the other breast removed because of cancer. Preventive mastectomy also may be an option for women who have the cancer-causing gene *BRCA1* or *BRCA2* or who have a strong family history of breast cancer, especially if several close relatives had the disease before age 50. In addition, preventive mastectomy is sometimes considered for women who have had LOBULAR CARCINOMA IN SITU, a condition that increases their risk of breast cancer development in the same or in the opposite breast. Rarely, preventive mastectomy may be considered for women who have widespread breast microcalcifications or for women whose breast tissue is very dense. Dense breast tissue is linked to a higher risk of breast cancer and makes diagnosis of breast problems more difficult.

Although having a preventive mastectomy can reduce a woman's risk, it cannot completely protect a woman from breast cancer. Because it is impossible for a surgeon to remove all breast tissue, breast cancer can still develop in the small amount of tissue left behind.

The procedure should be considered in the context of each woman's unique risk factors and level of concern. Women who are considering a preventive mastectomy should discuss with a doctor her risk of breast cancer, the surgical procedure and her feelings about it, alternatives to surgery, and possible complications.

Breast Reconstruction

After mastectomy, many women choose to have BREAST RECONSTRUCTION using either a saline solution implant or skin, fat, and muscle from the abdomen, back, or buttocks to form a new breast. Before performing this type of procedure, the plastic surgeon carefully examines the breasts and discusses the appropriate types of reconstruction.

Women who have reconstructive surgery are followed carefully to detect complications such as infection, movement of the implant, or contracture (the formation of a firm, fibrous shell around the implant). After surgery, patients still need routine screening for breast cancer, because the risk of cancer cannot be completely eliminated.

Women who do not wish to have further surgery may be fitted with an artificial breast after healing from mastectomy. Most prostheses are made to resemble the breast's own weight and touch. Several manufacturers make special mastectomy bras that have breast pockets.

mastectomy, modified radical   The most common type of MASTECTOMY, in which the breast skin, nipple, areola, and underarm lymph nodes are removed, but the chest muscles are saved. In the past, a radical mastectomy, in which more tissue (including chest muscle) is removed, was the most frequently performed procedure for removing the entire breast. However, experts have found that a modified radical mastectomy is just as effective in most cases, and therefore, it has become more common.

See also MASTECTOMY, RADICAL.

mastectomy, partial Also called segmental mastectomy, this procedure involves the removal of a portion of the breast tissue and a margin of normal breast tissue. It usually removes less tissue than a QUADRANTECTOMY but more than a LUMPECTOMY, or wide excision.

mastectomy, prophylactic Some women at very high risk for BREAST CANCER choose to have one or both breasts removed *before* disease occurs. Although this procedure does not completely eliminate the risk (some tiny bits of breast tissue always remain), it does lower to less than 5 percent. Some people consider this a controversial and radical step to avoid breast cancer; however, some women who are at high risk believe it is worthwhile. Insurance companies may or may not cover the surgery.

mastectomy, radical (Halsted's radical) The removal of the breast as well as the surrounding LYMPH NODES, muscles, fatty tissue, and skin. Formerly the standard surgery for breast cancer, this procedure is rarely used today. In rare cases, radical mastectomy may be suggested if the cancer has spread to the chest muscles. This surgery carries a very high risk of lymphedema and leads to great deformity of the chest and shoulder.

mastectomy, segmental See MASTECTOMY, PARTIAL.

mastectomy, skin-sparing A type of MASTECTOMY in which all of the breast skin except the nipple and the areola is preserved. This procedure makes reconstruction easier and prevents scarring on the breast, allowing better results after breast reconstruction. The remaining pouch of skin provides the best shape and form to accommodate a soft tissue reconstruction or an implant. Many women believe that skin-sparing mastectomies allow the most realistic and pleasing results from breast reconstruction.

If a woman does not want to have reconstruction after a mastectomy, her surgeon will remove as much skin as is required to make the surface of the chest and the scar lie flat. However, women who think they may someday want breast reconstruction may choose a skin-sparing procedure. A skin-sparing mastectomy should not be done if the surgeon suspects that the tumor may involve the skin, such as in INFLAMMATORY BREAST CANCER.

mastectomy, subcutaneous A MASTECTOMY that is performed in a noncancer situation. The breast tissue is removed but the outer skin, areola, and nipple are left intact. This type of surgery is not suitable if there is a diagnosis of cancer.

mastectomy, total Also called a simple MASTECTOMY, this procedure includes removal of the breast with its skin and nipple, but no LYMPH NODES are removed. In some cases, a separate SENTINEL-NODE BIOPSY is performed to remove only the first one to three axillary (armpit) lymph nodes.

meat and breast cancer There are a very few studies that suggest that eating large amounts of meat increases the risk of BREAST CANCER. However, the studies are far from conclusive, and it is unclear what the reason for the increased risk might be. Possibilities include that women who eat lots of meat have more dietary fat (which is associated with obesity, a known risk factor of breast cancer). Other possibilities include the fact that processed meats have chemicals that increase risk, and that high-temperature cooking such as grilling or broiling produces chemicals that cause cancer. None of these theories has been proven, however.

A broadly varied diet high in vegetables, whole grains, and fruits and low in animal fats helps protect against heart disease and may also help protect against breast cancer.

medical oncologist See ONCOLOGIST.

Medicare A federally subsidized insurance program for citizens older than age 65 established by Congress in 1965. Medicare has two parts: Part A, which is free, pays for 80 percent of inpatient hospital care and a variety of follow-up services. Part

B, for which patients pay a monthly premium, pays 80 percent of doctors' services, outpatient hospital care, and other medical expenses. Some people also decide to buy Medigap insurance to cover the unpaid 20 percent of medical costs.

Those who are older than age 65 and have permanent kidney failure or have received Social Security Disability Income for 24 months are also eligible to enroll.

Patients with breast cancer whose disease has spread are usually considered permanently disabled and are therefore also eligible for Medicare, regardless of age. Generally, if breast cancer has spread to a major organ, such as the lung, liver, or brain, patients are accepted into the program.

Medicare/Medicaid also offers a screening program for breast and ovarian cancer for underserved women, and provides appropriate treatment if needed.

medullary carcinoma of the breast A rare type of infiltrating ductal BREAST CANCER that has a relatively well-defined, distinct boundary between tumor tissue and normal breast tissue. It also has a number of other special features, including the large size of the cancer cells and the presence of immune system cells at the edges of the tumor. Medullary carcinoma accounts for only about 5 percent of all breast cancers but has a slightly better prognosis and a slightly lower chance of spreading than invasive lobular or invasive ductal cancers of the same size.

menstruation, age at first A girl who has her first menstrual period before age 12 has a slightly higher risk of eventual development of BREAST CANCER at some point in her lifetime. Experts believe this link between early menarche and breast cancer is related to the higher exposure to ESTROGEN that occurs in women who have more menstrual periods over a lifetime.

metastasis The spread of cancer cells to other areas of the body via the LYMPHATIC SYSTEM or the bloodstream.

microcalcifications Tiny specks of calcium in the breast that may appear alone or in clusters and may or may not signal BREAST CANCER. The shape and location of microcalcifications can help a radiologist determine how likely the areas are to be malignant. In some cases, microcalcifications do not require a BIOPSY, but only a follow-up MAMMOGRAM within three to six months. In other cases, microcalcifications are suspicious and a biopsy is recommended.

microcyst A cyst in the breast that is too small to be felt but may be observed on mammography or ultrasound screening.

micrometastasis The spread of cancer outside the breast that is too small to be seen with screening tests and is therefore undetected. It is because of the possibility of micrometastasis that adjuvant CHEMOTHERAPY (chemotherapy given after the diagnosis of early-stage BREAST CANCER) is given.

mistletoe A semiparasitic plant that has been used for centuries to treat numerous human ailments; more recently, mistletoe extracts have been shown to kill cancer cells in the laboratory and to stimulate the immune system. Mistletoe for humans is used primarily in Europe, where a variety of different extracts are marketed as injectable prescription drugs. These extracts are not available commercially in the United States. Although mistletoe plants and berries are considered poisonous to humans, few serious side effects have been associated with mistletoe extract use.

The use of mistletoe as a treatment for cancer has been investigated in more than 30 clinical studies. Reports of improved survival rate or better quality of life have been common, but nearly all of the studies had major weaknesses that raise doubts about the reliability of the findings, according to federal researchers. At present, the U.S. government does not recommend the use of mistletoe to the general public.

Meanwhile, experts are investigating two components of mistletoe (viscotoxins and lectins) that they think may be responsible for certain anticancer effects. Viscotoxins are small proteins that can kill cells and possibly stimulate the immune system. Lectins are complex molecules of protein and carbohydrates that can trigger biochemical changes.

Because of mistletoe's ability to stimulate the immune system, it has been classified as a type of BIOLOGICAL RESPONSE MODIFIER (a diverse group of biological molecules that have been used to treat cancer or to lessen the side effects of anticancer drugs).

Commercially available extracts of mistletoe are marketed in Europe under a variety of brand names, including Iscador, Eurixor, Helixor, Isorel, Iscucin, Plenosol, and ABNOBAviscum. Some extracts are marketed under more than one name. For example, Iscador, Isorel, and Plenosol are also sold as Iscar, Vysorel, and Lektinol, respectively. All of these products are prepared from *Viscum album Loranthacea* (European mistletoe).

Mistletoe grows on several types of trees, and the chemical composition of extracts derived from it depends on the species of the host tree (such as apple, elm, oak, pine, poplar, and spruce), the time of year harvested, the way extracts are prepared, and the commercial producer.

At present, at least one U.S. investigator has approval to study mistletoe as a treatment for cancer.

Side Effects

Reported side effects have generally been mild, including soreness and inflammation at injection sites, headache, lymph node swelling, fever, and chills. A few cases of severe allergic reactions, including anaphylactic shock, have been reported.

However, mistletoe plants and berries are considered poisonous; they cause seizures, vomiting, and death after ingestion. The severity of the toxic effects associated with mistletoe ingestion may depend on the amount consumed and the type of mistletoe plant.

monoclonal antibodies (MOABs)   Synthetic antibodies produced by a single type of cell that are specific for a particular protein on a cell called an antigen. Researchers are examining ways to create MOABs specific to the antigens found on the surface of cancer cells.

MOABs are made by injecting human cancer cells into mice so that the immune system makes antibodies against these cancer cells. The mouse cells producing the antibodies are then removed and fused with lab-grown cells to create "hybrid" cells (hybridomas) that can produce large quantities of pure antibodies. They may be used in cancer treatment in a number of ways:

- Their reaction with specific types of cancer may enhance a patient's immune response to the cancer.
- They can be programmed to act against cell growth factors, interfering with the growth of cancer cells.
- They may be linked to anticancer drugs, radioisotopes (radioactive substances), or other toxins. When the antibodies latch onto cancer cells, they deliver these poisons directly to the tumor, helping to destroy it.
- They may help destroy cancer cells in BONE MARROW that has been removed from a patient in preparation for BONE MARROW TRANSPLANTS.
- MOABs carrying radioisotopes may also prove useful in diagnosing certain cancers, such as colorectal, ovarian, and prostate cancer.

Rituximab (Rituxan) and trastuzumab (Herceptin) are monoclonal antibodies that have been approved by the U.S. Food and Drug Administration (FDA). Herceptin is used to treat metastatic BREAST CANCER in patients who have tumors that produce excess amounts of a protein called HER-2. (About 25 percent of breast cancer tumors produce excess amounts of HER-2.) Rituxan is a monoclonal antibody used to treat lymphomas. There are several other MOABs approved for use, and clinical trials are ongoing.

mouth sores   See STOMATITIS.

mucinous carcinoma   A rare type of invasive ductal BREAST CANCER (also called colloid carcinoma) that is formed by mucus-producing cancer cells. This type of breast cancer has a slightly better prognosis and a slightly lower chance of spreading than does invasive lobular or invasive ductal cancer of the same size.

MUGA scan   Common term for "multiple-gated acquisition" scan, a noninvasive test using a radioactive isotope called technetium designed to evaluate the functioning of the heart's ventricles. MUGA scans are sometimes done to assess the health of the heart before starting treatment with certain kinds of chemotherapy, such as ADRIAMYCIN (doxorubicin), that may potentially damage the heart.

The scan takes about an hour. In this test, a small amount of radioactive material is injected into a vein, where it temporarily attaches to red blood cells. A special camera that can detect the radioactive material takes pictures of the blood flow through the beating heart.

myths about breast cancer   Although researchers have learned a lot about BREAST CANCER in recent years, there is still much to learn. What we don't know, we are often frightened about, and out of uncertainties come myths. Despite public education efforts, many women believe these falsehoods, which can prevent them from following proper precautions, thereby putting their life at risk.

MYTH: Only Those Who Have a Family History Need to Worry

It is true that FAMILY HISTORY is a significant risk factor for breast cancer—having a first-degree relative, such as a mother, sister, or daughter, who has breast cancer can double a woman's risk of development of the disease. However, women with no family history of the disease are still at risk. Only about 10 percent to 20 percent of women diagnosed with breast cancer actually have a family history of this disease. About one in eight women who lives to be 80 in the United States has breast cancer during her lifetime, according to NATIONAL CANCER INSTITUTE estimates. Even women without a family history have a high enough risk to warrant vigilance.

MYTH: A Healthy Life Can Prevent Breast Cancer

Although a healthy lifestyle may improve the odds of avoiding breast cancer, it is not a guarantee. There is some evidence linking alcohol consumption, obesity, and high-fat diet to increased breast cancer risk, but more research is needed to confirm these findings. In about two-thirds of breast cancer cases, there are no identifiable risk factors. Avoid-ing cigarettes and eating a high-fiber, low-fat DIET are good ideas, but mostly because they decrease the risk of lung cancer and coronary artery disease; experts do not know the extent to which these factors affect breast cancer.

MYTH: Bras or Antiperspirants Can Cause Breast Cancer

E-mails blaming bras or antiperspirants for the development of breast cancer pop up every so often on the Internet, but there is no truth to either claim. The bra rumor is based on the hypothesis set forth by a husband-and-wife team of anthropologists in the book *Dressed to Kill,* in which they claim that bras constrict the lymph system, causing toxins to accumulate in breast tissues that leads to cancer. They say this explains the high rate of breast cancer in Western cultures and the low rate in less-industrialized regions of the world, where women are less likely to wear bras.

However, increased pressure or a constricted lymphatic system is not what causes normal cells to become malignant. Instead, breast cancer is caused by a series of mistakes that are made in the copying of genetic material when cells divide.

The antiperspirant myth claims that antiperspirant causes breast cancer because it stops perspiration, preventing the armpits from purging toxins, which are then deposited in the lymph nodes, where they lead to cell mutations. However, experts point out that sweat is not a mechanism for eliminating toxins—that is the job of the kidney and liver. Sweat simply cools the body. Moreover, there are no toxins or carcinogens in sweat; sweat is made up of a combination of 99.9 percent water, sodium, and magnesium. In addition, people in cultures in which antiperspirant has not yet been introduced have breast cancer.

MYTH: Only Women Have Breast Cancer

Breast cancer occurs in men (although infrequently). About one of every 100 breast cancer cases strikes a man. The overall incidence of breast cancer among men is very, very low, but it does occur. Men have breast tissue, and they are exposed to some of the same hormones as women, though in much smaller amounts. They also can inherit the *BRCA* mutation, which increases their risk.

Men who have breast cancer are actually more likely to die of it than women because they are usually diagnosed at a later stage in the disease. They often are less aware of the symptoms than women, and since mammograms are not routinely recommended for men, the earliest forms of the disease are usually not detected.

MYTH: Mammograms Cause Cancer

Most experts believe that the known benefits of MAMMOGRAMS far outweigh any very small potential risk. There has been no evidence to associate any increase in breast cancer risk with routine MAMMOGRAPHY. Although having daily or weekly mammograms would not be a good idea, experts say, any tiny risk of an annual mammogram is more than offset by the 30 percent reduction in the probability of dying of breast cancer, since mammograms detect cancer so much earlier. Moreover, modern mammogram machines have much better image quality and much lower radiation dosage. The radiation dose from a mammogram is less than the radiation exposure from flying across the country.

MYTH: Breast Cancer Is Contagious

Breast cancer is not a communicable disease and cannot be spread by air particles or physical contact. Breast cancer is an abnormal increase in breast cells that causes a tumor. Changes in one woman's cells cannot affect the cells of another woman.

MYTH: If a Woman's Mother Had Breast Cancer, She Will Also Have Breast Cancer

Not necessarily: About 60 to 80 percent of women who have breast cancer have no known risk factors for the disease, including no family history of breast cancer. Although women whose mother had breast cancer are at higher-than-average risk for the disease, this risk does not guarantee that they will have breast cancer.

However, because the increased risk exists in these situations, daughters of mothers who have had breast cancer are usually closely monitored for breast cancer and should begin to have yearly screening mammograms 10 years earlier than the age at which the mother was diagnosed.

National Alliance of Breast Cancer Organizations

A network of BREAST CANCER organizations that provides information, assistance, and referrals to anyone who has questions about breast cancer and that acts as a voice for the interests and concerns of breast cancer survivors and women at risk. Services include information referrals, job discrimination–related advocacy, and professional education. For contact information, see Appendix I.

National Asian Women's Health Organization (NAWHO)

A nonprofit organization founded in 1993 to achieve health equity for Asian Americans. NAWHO's goals are to raise awareness of the health needs of Asian Americans through research and education and to support Asian Americans as decision makers via leadership development and advocacy. Through its innovative programs, NAWHO is increasing knowledge of BREAST CANCER and cervical cancer, training violence-prevention advocates, expanding access to immunizations, changing attitudes about reproductive health care, and opposing the stigma surrounding depression and mental health concerns. For contact information, see Appendix I.

National Bone Marrow Transplant Link

A national clearinghouse that provides information about a variety of BONE MARROW TRANSPLANT issues. Services include patient advocacy, research funding, referrals, and a resource guide. For contact information, see Appendix I.

National Breast and Cervical Cancer Early Detection Program (NBCCEDP)

A government program that offers free or low-cost MAMMOGRAPHY screening to uninsured, low-income, elderly, minor-ity, and Native American women. The program, which is run by the Centers for Disease Control and Prevention, was created by an act of Congress in 1990. The NBCCEDP helps low-income, uninsured, and underserved women gain access to lifesaving early-detection screening programs for breast and cervical cancers. Many deaths of these cancers—which occur disproportionately among women who are uninsured or underinsured—could be prevented by increasing cancer screening rates among all women at risk. Mammograms and Papanicolaou (Pap) tests are underused by women who have less than a high-school education, are older, live below the poverty level, or are members of certain racial and ethnic minority groups.

NBCCEDP is currently funded at $192.6 million. It provides both screening and diagnostic services, including the following:

- CLINICAL BREAST EXAMS
- Mammograms
- Pap tests
- Surgical consultation
- Diagnostic testing for women whose screening outcome is abnormal

Since its inception, the program has spread to all 50 states and 14 American Indian/Alaska Native organizations.

To date, almost 1.5 million women have been screened as part of this program, and more than 9,000 BREAST CANCERS, 48,170 precancerous cervical lesions, and 831 cervical cancers have been diagnosed.

National Breast Cancer Coalition (NBCC)

The nation's largest BREAST CANCER grassroots advocacy

group. It includes more than 600 member organizations and 70,000 members fighting breast cancer through action, advocacy, and public education. NBCC and its sister organization, the National Breast Cancer Coalition Fund, work to educate and train people to be effective activists. Services also include referrals and volunteer services. For contact information, see Appendix I.

National Cancer Institute (NCI)   A component of the National Institutes of Health, the NCI was established under the National Cancer Act of 1937 as the federal government's principal agency for cancer research and training. The National Cancer Act of 1971 broadened the scope and responsibilities of the NCI. The NCI is responsible for coordinating the National Cancer Program, which conducts and supports research, training, and health information dissemination, as well as other programs with respect to the cause, diagnosis, prevention, and treatment of cancer; rehabilitation from cancer; and continuing care of cancer patients and the families of cancer patients.

Services include the NCI's comprehensive database, which contains peer-reviewed summaries and the most current information on cancer treatment, screening, prevention, genetics, and supportive care. The NCI also maintains a registry of cancer clinical trials being conducted worldwide and directories of physicians, professionals who provide genetic counseling services, and organizations that provide care to people with cancer. For contact information, see Appendix I.

National Cancer Institute Cancer Centers Program
A program that comprises more than 50 NATIONAL CANCER INSTITUTE (NCI)–designated cancer centers engaged in multidisciplinary research to reduce cancer incidence, morbidity rate, and mortality rate. Through cancer center support grants, this program supports three types of centers:

- COMPREHENSIVE CANCER CENTERS conduct programs in all three areas of research—basic research, clinical research, and prevention and control research—as well as programs in community outreach and education.
- CLINICAL CANCER CENTERS conduct programs in

clinical research, and may also have programs in other research areas.
- CANCER CENTERS focus on basic research or cancer control research but do not have clinical oncology programs.

Several cancer centers existed in the late 1960s. Later, the National Cancer Act of 1971 strengthened the program by authorizing the establishment of 15 new cancer centers and continued support for existing ones. The passage of the act also dramatically transformed the centers' structure and broadened the scope of their mission to include all aspects of basic, clinical, and cancer-control research. Today, more than 40 cancer centers meet the NCI criteria for comprehensive status. Each type of cancer center has specific characteristics and capabilities for organizing new programs of research that can exploit important new findings and address timely research questions. All NCI-designated cancer centers are reevaluated each time their Cancer Center Support Grant is up for renewal (generally every three to five years).

Since the passage of the National Cancer Act of 1971, the Cancer Centers Program has continued to expand. Today, NCI-designated cancer centers continue to work toward creating new and innovative approaches to cancer research. Through interdisciplinary efforts, cancer centers can effectively move this research from the laboratory into clinical trials and into clinical practice. Patients who are seeking clinical oncology services (screening, diagnosis, or treatment) can obtain those services at Clinical Cancer Centers or Comprehensive Cancer Centers. They can also participate in clinical trials (research studies involving humans) at these types of cancer centers. Information about referral procedures, treatment costs, and services available to patients can be obtained from the individual cancer centers; for contact information, see Appendix II.

Comprehensive Cancer Center
To attain recognition from the NCI as a comprehensive cancer center, an institution must pass rigorous peer review. Under guidelines revised in 1997, a comprehensive cancer center must perform research in three major areas: basic research; clinical research; and cancer prevention, control, and population-based research. It must also have a

strong body of interactive research that bridges these research areas. In addition, a comprehensive cancer center must conduct activities in outreach, education, and information provision, which are directed toward and accessible to both health-care professionals and the lay community.

Clinical Cancer Centers

These centers must have active programs in clinical research and may also have programs in another area (such as basic research; or prevention, control, and population-based research). Clinical cancer centers focus on both laboratory research and clinical research within the same institutional framework. This interaction of research and clinical activities is a distinguishing characteristic of many clinical cancer centers.

Cancer Center

The general term "cancer center" refers to an organization with scientific disciplines outside the specific qualifications for a comprehensive or clinical center. Such centers may, for example, concentrate on basic research, epidemiology, and cancer-control research, or other areas of research.

National Coalition for Cancer Survivorship (NCCS) The only patient-led advocacy organization working on behalf of U.S. survivors of all types of cancer and those who care for them to ensure high-quality cancer care for all Americans. Founded in 1986, NCCS continues to lead the cancer survivorship movement. By educating all those affected by cancer and speaking out on issues related to high-quality cancer care, NCCS hopes to empower every survivor. NCCS serves a key role in policymaking in Washington, D.C., as well as providing a source of support for thousands of survivors and their families. Services include referrals, information, education, and advocacy. For contact information, see Appendix I.

National Comprehensive Cancer Network (NCCN) A nonprofit alliance of the world's leading CANCER CENTERS, established in 1995 to support member institutions in the evolving managed-care environment. The NCCN tries to strengthen the mission of member institutions by providing state-of-the-art cancer care, advance cancer prevention, screening, diagnosis, and treatment through excellence in basic and clinical research, and to enhance the effectiveness and efficiency of cancer-care delivery.

The NCCN develops programs and products that, in partnerships with managed-care companies, employers, and unions, offer people greater access to leading doctors, superior treatment, programs that continuously improve the effectiveness of treatment, and management that enhances the efficiency of cancer-care delivery. For contact information, see Appendix I.

National Family Caregivers Association A nonprofit association that provides educational and emotional support for family caregivers of cancer patients. Services include advocacy; individual, family, group, peer, and bereavement counseling; and information education. For contact information, see Appendix I.

National Hospice and Palliative Care Organization The largest nonprofit membership organization representing HOSPICE and PALLIATIVE CARE programs and professionals in the United States. The organization is committed to improving end-of-life care and expanding access to hospice care with the goal of profoundly enhancing quality of life for those who are dying and their loved ones.

Considered to be the model for high-quality, compassionate care at the end of life, hospice care involves a team-oriented approach of expert medical care, pain management, and emotional and spiritual support expressly tailored to the patient's preferences. Emotional and spiritual support is also extended to the family and loved ones. Health-care professionals who specialize in hospice and palliative care work closely with staff and volunteers to address all of the symptoms of illness, with the aim of promoting comfort and dignity. Generally, this care is provided in the patient's home or in a home-like setting operated by a hospice program. Medicare, private health insurance, and Medicaid, in most states, cover hospice care for patients who meet certain criteria. In recent years, many hospice-care programs added *palliative care* to their names to reflect that they also provide care and services to people earlier in their illness than traditional hospice programs.

Those offering palliative care seek to address not only physical pain, but also emotional, social, and spiritual pain to achieve the best possible quality of life for patients and their families. Palliative care extends the principles of hospice care to a broader population that could benefit from receiving this type of care earlier in their illness or disease process.

The National Hospice and Palliative Care Organization was founded in 1978 as the National Hospice Organization and changed its name in 2000. With headquarters in Alexandria, Virginia, the organization is an advocate for the terminally ill and their family. It also develops public and professional educational programs and materials to enhance understanding and availability of hospice and palliative care; convenes frequent meetings and symposia on emerging issues; provides technical informational resources to its membership; conducts research; monitors congressional and regulatory activities; and works closely with other organizations that share an interest in end-of-life care. For contact information, see Appendix I.

National Lymphedema Network (NLN) Nonprofit organization that provides support, education, and information on LYMPHEDEMA. This internationally recognized organization, founded in 1988, is a driving force behind the movement in the United States to standardize quality of treatment for lymphedema patients nationwide. In addition, the NLN supports research into the causes and possible alternative treatments for this often incapacitating condition. The NLN offers a toll-free recorded information line, referrals to lymphedema treatment centers, health-care professionals, training programs, and support groups; a quarterly newsletter with information about medical and scientific developments, support groups, and pen pals/net pals; educational courses; a biennial national conference on lymphedema; and an extensive computer database. For contact information, see Appendix I.

National Marrow Donor Program A national group that maintains a registry of BONE MARROW

donors, provides information on the progress of becoming a donor, and organizes donor recruitment drives. For contact information, see Appendix I.

National Patient Advocate Foundation A national network for health-care reform that supports legislation to enable cancer survivors to obtain insurance funding for medical care and participation in clinical trials. The foundation provides referrals, information, advocacy, and health insurance assistance. For contact information, see Appendix I.

National Patient Air Transport Hotline A clearinghouse used to find air transportation for patients with breast cancer who cannot afford travel for medical care. For contact information, see Appendix I.

National Surgical Adjuvant Breast and Bowel Project (NSABP) A cooperative group supported by the NATIONAL CANCER INSTITUTE that for more than 40 years has designed and conducted clinical trials in the treatment and prevention of BREAST CANCER. It was the NSABP's breast cancer studies that led to the establishment of LUMPECTOMY plus radiation rather than radical MASTECTOMY as the standard surgical treatment for breast cancer. The group was also the first to demonstrate that adjuvant therapy could increase survival rate and the first to demonstrate on a large scale that TAMOXIFEN can help prevent breast cancer.

Since its inception, the NSABP has enrolled more than 60,000 women and men in clinical trials in breast and colorectal cancer. Headquartered in Pittsburgh, the NSABP has research sites at nearly 200 major medical centers, university hospitals, large oncology practice groups, and health maintenance organizations in the United States, Canada, Puerto Rico, and Australia. At those sites and their satellites, more than 5,000 physicians, nurses, and other medical professionals conduct NSABP treatment and prevention trials. Their presence at local hospitals and medical facilities means that state-of-the-art clinical trials can be offered to patients near their homes.

Native Americans/Alaska Natives and breast cancer While Native Americans/Alaska Natives experience some of the lowest BREAST CANCER rates among all groups, they do experience higher rates of cervix and ovarian cancer. However, the Indian Health Service reports a large variability in cancer rates among this population, especially in areas such as the northern plains and Alaska.

A century ago, breast cancer in Native Americans was rare. It remains less common than in Caucasians, but the rate of death and the incidence of breast cancer has risen since the 1970s. Indeed, the five-year breast cancer relative-survival rate for Native American women is reportedly the lowest of any racial or ethnic group in the country.

Lack of access to and use of early detection services is believed to be a major contributor to this poor breast cancer survival rate. Without a doubt, greater awareness and utilization of MAMMOGRAPHY and CLINICAL BREAST EXAM screening methods could significantly reduce the mortality rate of breast cancer among Native Americans.

See also RACE AND BREAST CANCER.

natural killer cells (NK cells) White blood cells that can kill tumor cells and infected body cells. NK cells kill on contact by binding to the target cell and releasing a burst of toxic chemicals. Normal cells are not affected by NK cells, which play a major role in cancer prevention by destroying abnormal cells before they can become dangerous.

nausea Feeling sick in the stomach from CHEMOTHERAPY may occur immediately after the drug is given, or may be delayed. The pattern of nausea varies with the drug, but most often starts within one to four hours after receiving chemotherapy. The worst nausea occurs during the first 12 to 24 hours. After that, there may be occasional or unexpected episodes of mild nausea or vomiting. Fortunately, since the mid-1990s several very strong antinausea medicines that reduce or eliminate this side effect have become available.

A few chemotherapy drugs—vincristine, carboplatin, bleomycin, 5-fluorouracil (5-FU), methotrexate, and VP 16—do not usually cause nausea. Nausea also can be associated with other drugs (including antibiotics and pain medications).

Preventing Nausea

Patients should eat lightly before and for one to two days after chemotherapy, avoiding fried food, and spicy foods. Some patients have different food triggers for nausea.

Patients who are prescribed chemotherapy that is likely to cause nausea are given medicine to prevent nausea before the drugs are administered and given prescriptions for medicines to prevent nausea at home. Typical antinausea medications include prochlorperazine (COMPAZINE), lorazepam (Ativan), dexamethasone (DECADRON), ondansatron (Zofran), granisetron (KYTRIL), and dolasetron (Anzemet). All of these medications work well for nausea, but certain drugs may work better for one person than another.

Tips to Ease Nausea

Eating certain foods, such as crackers, toast, oatmeal, soft bland vegetables and fruits, clear liquids, and skinned baked chicken, can help ease nausea. Foods to be avoided include fatty, greasy, and fried foods; sweets; and hot or spicy foods. Patients should not force themselves to eat during periods of nausea because this practice may trigger aversions to favorite foods.

Patients who have nausea should sip cool liquids between meals, not during meals. Eating in a room other than the kitchen may also help if cooking smells worsen nausea.

needle biopsy See BIOPSY.

neoplasm Any abnormal growth. Neoplasms may be benign or malignant, but the term usually is used to describe a cancer.

Neupogen See GRANULOCYTE COLONY-STIMULATING FACTOR.

neutropenia A blood condition in which there are too few of a type of WHITE BLOOD CELLS called neutrophils that are important in fighting infection. About 60 percent of white blood cells are neutrophils. Because neutrophils are very important in fighting infections, low levels of these vital white blood cells make a person more likely to contract infections.

Neutropenia can be caused by CHEMOTHERAPY or RADIATION THERAPY, or by BREAST CANCER cells in BONE MARROW. All these things, as well as some infections and some medications, interfere with the production of blood cells.

Although most people with neutropenia are fine, the condition predisposes patients to infections, usually in the lungs, mouth and throat, sinuses, and skin. Painful mouth ulcers, gum infections, ear infections, and periodontal disease may occur. Severe, life-threatening infections are very rare.

In general, the blood of healthy adults contains about 1,500 to 7,000 neutrophils per cubic millimeter (children younger than age six may have a lower neutrophil count). The severity of neutropenia generally depends on the absolute neutrophil count (ANC) and is described as follows:

- Mild neutropenia: an ANC between $1,500/mm^3$ and $1,000/mm^3$
- Moderate neutropenia: an ANC between $500/mm3$ and $1,000/mm^3$
- Severe neutropenia: an ANC below $500/mm^3$

Neutropenia without fever is not usually treated. If caused by chemotherapy or radiation, it usually resolves over time. Chemotherapy may be delayed until the counts recover. If fever occurs, antibiotics are prescribed. A very sick patient may be hospitalized. If neutropenia is a problem during chemotherapy, growth factors (Neupogen) may be given after chemotherapy to prevent a fall in white blood counts.

nipple discharge   Fluid that leaks from the nipple is the third most common breast symptom for which women seek medical attention, after lumps and breast pain. Most nipple discharges are associated with benign changes in the breast, such as a hormonal imbalance or an INTRADUCTAL PAPILLOMA. However, because a small percentage of nipple discharges can indicate cancer in the breast or nipple, any persistent nipple discharge should be evaluated by a doctor.

Up to 20 percent of women may experience spontaneous milky or clear fluid nipple discharge. In fact, during a BREAST SELF-EXAM, fluid may normally be expressed from the breasts of 40 to 60 per-

cent of women. Usually a clear, milky, yellow, or green discharge from both nipples is not a symptom of breast cancer.

On the other hand, bloody or watery nipple discharge—especially if it occurs at only one breast—is considered abnormal. Only about 10 percent of abnormal discharges are caused by breast cancer.

To examine nipple discharge, a small amount of the fluid is placed on glass slides and examined under a microscope to determine whether cancer cells are present. Radiologic studies including a mammogram or a ductogram may be done. Sometimes if one duct is abnormal it is surgically removed.

nodularity   Increased density of breast tissue (usually caused by hormonal changes) that causes the breast to feel lumpy. Also called normal nodularity, it usually occurs symmetrically in the breasts.

Nolvadex   See TAMOXIFEN.

noninvasive carcinomas   BREAST CANCER is often discovered at an early stage, when the tumor has not yet grown into the surrounding tissues, remaining instead within the borders of a duct or lobule. These tumors are known as noninvasive, in situ tumors (tumors that remain "in the site" of origin). In situ tumors are usually too small to have formed a lump, so they usually are not felt or noticed during a physical exam; they are often discovered by MAMMOGRAPHY. Noninvasive carcinomas include DUCTAL CARCINOMA IN SITU and LOBULAR CARCINOMA IN SITU.

noninvasive ductal carcinoma   See DUCTAL CARCINOMA IN SITU.

nonsteroidal anti-inflammatory drugs (NSAIDs)   Regular use of ibuprofen and aspirin inhibits the formation and growth of BREAST CANCER, according to data from the NATIONAL CANCER INSTITUTE'S Women's Health Initiative (WHI) Observational Study. These results suggest that even women at high risk for breast cancer may be protected by taking NSAIDs. However, experts note that before usage guidelines for NSAIDs can be implemented, additional studies are needed, especially since not all studies have shown similar benefits.

The WHI enrolled 80,741 postmenopausal women between 50 and 79 years of age with no reported history of cancer, other than non-melanoma skin cancer. Almost 1,400 of these women were later diagnosed with breast cancer.

The study found that women who took two or more NSAIDs per week for five to nine years reduced their risk of breast cancer by 21 percent. Extending the use to 10 or more years resulted in an even greater reduction of 28 percent. The probability of development of breast cancer was estimated and adjusted for age and other BREAST CANCER RISK FACTORS (such as body mass, ESTROGEN use, FAMILY HISTORY, and EXERCISE).

Researchers observed that ibuprofen was more effective than aspirin in preventing breast cancer (49 percent versus 21 percent). Regular use of low-dose (less than 100-mg) aspirin had no effect.

Studies have shown that NSAIDs potentially limit breast cancer development by interfering with cyclooxygenose-2 (COX-2), which is found in most human breast cancers. Recent studies indicate that COX-2—an enzyme that generates prostaglandins—may be implicated in several biological events throughout the process of tumor development.

Nurses' Health Study (NHS)

One of the largest prospective investigations into the risk factors for major chronic diseases in women, sponsored by Brigham and Women's Hospital in Boston. The study indicates the dietary and health records of more than 100,000 female nurses across the country and has provided important information about the development of BREAST CANCER, heart disease and other health issues.

The NHS was established in 1976, and a second study of younger nurses—the NHS II—was established in 1989. The studies have grown to include a team of clinicians, epidemiologists, and statisticians at the Channing Laboratory, along with collaborating investigators and consultants in the surrounding medical community of the Harvard Medical School, Harvard School of Public Health, Brigham and Women's Hospital, Dana Farber Cancer Institute, Boston Children's Hospital, and Beth Israel Hospital.

The primary motivation in starting the first NHS was to investigate the potential long-term consequences of the use of birth control pills, a potent drug that was being prescribed to hundreds of millions of healthy women. Registered nurses were selected to be followed because experts believed their nursing education would allow them to respond accurately to brief, technically worded questionnaires. The first study included 122,000 nurses who are contacted every two years to answer a follow-up questionnaire regarding diseases and health-related topics such as smoking, hormone use, and menopausal status.

Because researchers recognized that DIET and nutrition would play important roles in the development of chronic diseases, in 1980 the first food-frequency questionnaire was collected. Subsequent diet questionnaires were collected in 1984, 1986, and every four years since. At the request of some of the nurses and with the addition of investigators to the research team interested in quality-of-life issues, questions related to quality-of-life were added in 1992 and repeated every four years. Because certain aspects of diet cannot be measured by questionnaire (especially minerals that become incorporated in food from the soil in which it is grown), the nurses submitted 68,000 sets of toenail samples between the 1982 and 1984 questionnaires.

To identify potential biomarkers such as hormone levels and GENETIC MARKERS, 33,000 blood samples were collected in 1989. These samples are stored and used in case/control analyses. A second blood collection from those who previously gave a sample was conducted in 2000/2001.

Nurses' Health Study II

The primary motivation for developing the NHS II was to study oral contraceptives, diet, and lifestyle risk factors in a population younger than that of the original study. This younger generation included women who started using oral contraceptives during adolescence and who were therefore exposed to these hormones during their early reproductive life. Several studies, suggesting such exposures might be associated with substantial increases in risk of breast cancer, provided a strong justification for investment in this large cohort. In addition, researchers planned to collect detailed information on the type of oral contraceptive used, which was not obtained in the original Nurses' Health Study.

The initial target population included women between the ages of 25 and 42 years in 1989; the upper age was to correspond with the lowest age group in the NHS. A total of 116,686 women remain in the second NHS.

Every two years, nurses receive a follow-up questionnaire with questions about diseases and health-related topics including SMOKING, HORMONE use, pregnancy history, and menopausal status. In 1991, the first food-frequency questionnaire was collected, and subsequent food-frequency questionnaires are administered at four-year intervals. A two-page quality-of-life supplement was included in the first mailing of the 1993 and 1997 questionnaires. Blood and urine samples from approximately 30,000 nurses were collected in the late 1990s.

nutrition and cancer treatment   Although good nutrition may not cure BREAST CANCER, dietary factors do play an important role in cancer treatment. A patient who is battling a severe disease such as breast cancer needs adequate nutrition to maintain strength and overall well-being, keep the immune system functioning, prevent the breakdown of body tissue, and help the body heal. A well-nourished person is better able to tolerate treatment side effects and may be able to handle more aggressive treatments.

However, nutrition can be a problem for women who have breast cancer for several reasons. If the breast cancer has spread, it may interfere with eating and digestion through problems chewing and swallowing, gastrointestinal tract blockages, or interference with digestive enzymes and hormones. In addition, breast cancer treatment such as RADIATION THERAPY and CHEMOTHERAPY can cause NAUSEA, vomiting, swallowing problems, painful mouth sores and sore throat, and dry mouth. Treatment may alter a patient's ability to taste or smell. Depression and lack of energy may make a person unwilling to eat, and appetite and metabolism may change.

Loss of appetite can be caused by the cancer itself, cancer treatment, or depression. CACHEXIA is the medical term for the wasting and dramatic weight loss seen in some cancer patients. Although this effect may not be preventable, attention to eating and good nutrition allows a better quality of life, helps the body tolerate treatment, and can contribute to improved resistance to infection.

Improving Nutrition

There are a number of lifestyle changes that patients with breast cancer can make to try to improve their nutrition. These include the following:

- *Relaxation:* Patients should choose a quiet place to eat, listen to soothing music, and lessen distractions.
- *Presentation:* Patients can try to make eating a more pleasurable experience by preparing and presenting food in appetizing, attractive ways.
- *Spontaneous mealtimes:* Patients should eat when they are hungry and not wait for mealtime. Because nausea or lack of appetite may come and go, patients should eat whenever they feel they can.
- *Small meals:* It is often better to eat many small meals throughout the day than to load the stomach with three big meals.
- *Snacks:* Patients should keep snacks nearby and eat between meals.
- *Favorite foods:* Patients with breast cancer should concentrate on having favorite foods available, because their availability sometimes helps improve appetite.
- *Change of diet:* Sometimes eating a different type of food can stimulate the appetite.
- *Watching temperature:* Patients should pay attention to the temperature of the food they eat and notice what works better. Some patients find that warm or room-temperature food is better tolerated; others find that cold foods are more soothing. In general, hot and spicy foods are not well tolerated by most patients.
- *Avoiding strong smells:* Patients should avoid cooking foods with unpleasant smells. It may be better to eat food with little or no smell, such as cottage cheese or crackers.
- *Loading calories:* Patients can get extra calories by adding dry milk, honey, jam, or brown sugar to food whenever possible.

Nausea Tips

Patients who feel nauseated should call their doctor for antinausea medication. Taken as directed, it is often quite effective. Patients who are vomiting should not try to eat or drink until the vomiting has stopped. Good diet choices for nausea include crackers, toast, oatmeal, soft bland vegetables and fruits, clear liquids, and skinned baked chicken. Foods to be avoided are fatty, greasy, or fried foods; sweets; and hot or spicy foods. Patients should not force themselves to eat during periods of nausea because eating may trigger aversions to favorite foods.

Patients who have nausea should drink liquids between meals, not during meals. Eating in a room other than the kitchen may help if cooking smells worsen nausea.

Physical Eating Problems

Some patients may have trouble with eating due to physical problems related to the spread of breast cancer or to the effects of chemotherapy. If this is the case, patients should

- Avoid foods that may irritate the mouth, such as spicy, acidic, citrus, or salty foods.
- Take very small bites of food.
- Cook foods until they are very tender.
- Puree foods in a blender or food processor.
- Mix foods with broth, sauces, or thin gravies to make them easier to swallow.
- Drink through a straw.

obesity and breast cancer   Weight gain and body mass have long been known to be risk factors for BREAST CANCER. In fact, weight contributes to between one-third and one-half of all breast cancer deaths among older women, according to the AMERICAN CANCER SOCIETY. In fact, the amount of weight a woman gains after age 18 is a strong signal as to whether she will get breast cancer later in life, according to research released in 2004 by the Society.

Older women who gained 20 to 30 pounds after high school graduation were 40 percent more likely to get breast cancer than women who did not, according to findings in one of the largest studies of weight and breast cancer ever done. The risk doubled if a woman gained more than 70 pounds, but even modest amounts of weight gain lead to a significantly increased risk of breast cancer.

Obesity is strongly linked to breast cancer because fat tissue produces ESTROGEN, and estrogen can help breast cancer grow. The more fat cells a woman has, the heavier she is and the higher her estrogen levels. Researchers believe there is no question that estrogen is the common denominator of most of a woman's risk factors for breast cancer.

Weight gain also is the second leading cause of all cancers, according to research published in 2003 in the *New England Journal of Medicine*. The 2004 research specifically examines the link between weight gain amounts and breast cancer—and for the first time, did so in a large group. The 2004 study included 1,934 breast cancer cases among 62,756 women involved in a separate long-term cancer prevention study. Post-menopausal women ages 50 to 74 were asked their weight when the study began in 1992 and their weight when they were 18 years old. Surveys were sent to the women in 1997, 1999, and 2001 to inquire about any new cancers. Women taking estrogen hormones were not included in the study. Lean postmenopausal women not taking hormone replacement therapy produce very little estrogen and had the lowest cancer risk in the study.

oncogenes   Genes that may trigger or allow cancer to grow. Normally these genes—when not damaged—are responsible for helping cells to grow and spread. When damaged in some way, these genes can cause cells to become malignant. BREAST CANCER SUSCEPTIBILITY GENES include *ATM*, *BRCA1*, and *BRCA2*, *LKB1*, *p53*, and *P-TEN*.

oncologist   A physician whose primary interest and training is cancer. Clinical oncologists are the physicians who treat patients with BREAST CANCER. In most cases, when a woman is diagnosed with breast cancer, a clinical oncologist takes charge of her overall care through all phases of the disease. Within the field of clinical oncology there are three primary disciplines: medical oncology, surgical oncology, and radiation oncology.

- *Medical oncologists* are physicians who specialize in treating cancer with medicine/chemotherapy.
- *Surgical oncologists* are physicians who specialize in surgical aspects of cancer including BIOPSY, staging, and surgical resection of tumors.
- *Radiation oncologists* are physicians who specialize in treating cancer with therapeutic radiation.

Education and Training

Clinical oncologists complete between four and seven years of postgraduate medical education, depending on their primary discipline. In order to become practicing cancer specialists, medical oncologists usually take board exams administered by the American Board of Internal Medicine, and radiation oncologists usually take board exams administered by the American Board of Radiology. Surgical oncologists do not have an equivalent specialty board, but general surgeons are certified by the American Board of Surgery; those surgeons who choose to specialize further in oncology receive a *certificate of special competence* once they have completed their oncology training program.

Regardless of their own particular discipline, medical, radiation, and surgical oncologists are broadly trained in all three areas of oncology and are knowledgeable about the appropriate use of each treatment approach.

oncologist, medical　　See ONCOLOGIST.

oncologist, radiation　　See ONCOLOGIST.

oncologist, surgical　　See ONCOLOGIST.

oncology　　The branch of medicine that deals with the study of cancerous tumors.

oncology clinical nurse specialist (CNS)　　An advanced practice nurse with a master's degree who has received extensive education in the needs of cancer patients. A CNS specializing in oncology works primarily in hospitals to provide and supervise care for cancer patients. Oncology CNSs monitor their patients' physical condition, prescribe medication, and manage symptoms. They are trained to apply nursing theory and research to clinical practice and may function as researchers, administrators, consultants, and educators in this field.

The CNS can help women who are trying to deal with their diagnosis and/or treatment regimen. Managing symptoms, maintaining health and wellness during treatment, and coping with information about breast cancer and its treatment are all areas of expertise that the clinical nurse specialist can share with patients and families. The oncology CNS works closely with the entire health-care team to ensure that a patient's plan of care is comprehensive, identifies the patient's

needs, and is clear and manageable for the patient and family.

one-step procedure　　A procedure in which a surgical biopsy is performed with general anesthesia and, if BREAST CANCER is found, a MASTECTOMY or LUMPECTOMY is done immediately as part of the same operation.

organochlorines　　A group of chlorinated hydrocarbons that include the banned pesticide dichlorodiphenyltrichloroethane (DDT). DDT was once widely used in agriculture and malarial control programs around the world. Although DDT was effectively banned for use as a pesticide in the United States in 1972 (almost 30 years after it was introduced), it can remain active in tissues for up to 50 years. It was banned because it is toxic in animals and because it does not disperse in the environment, but instead builds up in biological systems, where it cannot be metabolized. Eating animals that have consumed DDT—or eating animals that have eaten animals tainted with DDT—may poison anyone who eats the meat.

Multiple studies looking at the effect of DDT and its residue in the blood have reached different conclusions about a possible link to breast cancer. Some studies (including a large Belgian study) have indicated an increased risk of breast cancer with DDT residue. Other studies have not found a link. Whether DDT is related to breast cancer remains controversial.

ovarian cancer–breast cancer link　　Most known genetic mutations that increase BREAST CANCER risk also appear to increase risk of ovarian cancer. In 1994, two BREAST CANCER SUSCEPTIBILITY GENES were identified: *BRCA1* on chromosome 17 and *BRCA2* on chromosome 13. When a woman carries a mutation in either *BRCA1* or *BRCA2*, she is at an increased risk of being diagnosed with breast cancer (and, to a lesser extent, ovarian cancer) at some point in her life. Experts estimate that for women in the general population the lifetime risk for ovarian cancer is 1.7 percent, whereas for women with altered *BRCA1* or *BRCA2* genes, the risk is 16 to 60 percent.

BRCA1 or *BRCA2* normally help to suppress cell growth. A person who inherits either gene in an altered form has a higher risk of getting breast or ovarian cancers. In fact, experts believe that inherited alterations in the *BRCA1* or *BRCA2* genes are responsible for nearly all cases of familial ovarian cancer and about half of all cases of familial breast cancer.

The likelihood that breast and/or ovarian cancer is associated with *BRCA1* or *BRCA2* is highest in families who have

- A history of multiple cases of breast cancer (especially if diagnosed at a young age)
- Cases of both breast and ovarian cancer
- One or more family members who have two primary cancers (original tumors at different sites)
- An Ashkenazi (Eastern European) Jewish background

However, not every woman in such families carries an alteration in *BRCA1* or *BRCA2*, and not every cancer in such families is linked to alterations in these genes.

Genes are small pieces of DNA, the material that acts as a master blueprint for all the cells in the body. A person's genes determine such traits as hair and eye color, height, or skin color. Any mistakes in a gene that interfere with its job can lead to disease.

Both men and women carry two copies of each *BRCA* gene in their cells. One copy of the *BRCA1* gene is present on each of a person's two chromosome 17s, and one copy of the *BRCA2* gene is present on each of a person's two chromosome 13s. People inherit one copy of each of their genes from their mother and another copy of each gene from their father. If one parent has a defective *BRCA1* or *BRCA2* gene, there is a 50 percent chance the child may inherit this defective copy and a 50 percent chance the child may inherit the normal copy. If a person inherits a defective *BRCA1* or *BRCA2* gene, then each of that person's children likewise has a 50 percent chance of inheriting it.

The *BRCA1* and *BRCA2* genes produce a chemical substance that helps the body prevent cancer. Most women have two normal copies of both the *BRCA1* and *BRCA2* genes, both of which produce this cancer-preventing substance. However, some women have a genetic defect in one copy of their two *BRCA1* and *BRCA2* genes; as a result, their body does not produce a normal amount of this cancer-fighting substance. These women are at very high risk of breast or ovarian cancer.

Women who have an inherited alteration in one of these genes have an increased risk of development of ovarian or breast cancer at a young age (before menopause) and often have multiple close relatives who have the disease.

Some evidence suggests that there are slight differences in patterns of cancer between people who have *BRCA1* alterations and people who have *BRCA2* alterations, and even between people who have different alterations in the same gene. For example, one study found that alterations in a certain part of the *BRCA2* gene were associated with a higher risk for ovarian cancer than alterations in other areas of *BRCA2.*

Most research related to *BRCA1* and *BRCA2* has been done on large families of many affected individuals. Estimates of breast and ovarian cancer risk associated with *BRCA1* and *BRCA2* alterations have been calculated from studies of these families. Because family members share a proportion of their genes and, often, their environment, it is possible that the large number of cancer cases seen in these families may be partly due to other genetic or environmental factors. Therefore, risk estimates that are based on families with many affected members may not accurately reflect the levels of risk in the general population.

If a patient tests positive for altered *BRCA1* or *BRCA2* genes, there are several possible approaches to take. Careful monitoring for symptoms of cancer may result in a diagnosis of disease at an early stage, when treatment is more effective. Surveillance methods for breast cancer may include mammography and clinical breast exams. For ovarian cancer, surveillance methods in these high-risk women may include transvaginal ultrasound, CA 125 blood testing, and clinical exams.

Patients may also choose prophylactic surgery, in which the doctor removes as much of the at-risk tissue as possible in order to reduce the probability of development of cancer. Preventive MASTECTOMY (removal of healthy breasts) and preventive salpingo-oophorectomy (removal of healthy fallopian tubes and ovaries) are no guarantee against developing these cancers, although in each case they lower risk dramatically.

p53 A TUMOR-SUPPRESSOR GENE that, when mutated, has been linked to some cases of BREAST CANCER. A test for the mutation can be done on tumor tissue. An inherited inborn or spontaneous defect in the *p53* gene causes LI-FRAUMENI SYN-DROME (LFS), an extremely rare condition associated with a higher risk of many cancers, including breast cancer. The *p53* mutations were reported first in 1990; subsequent studies have shown that more than two-thirds of families who have LFS have inherited mutations of one of the two copies of the *p53* tumor-suppressor gene; the second copy is normal. Mutations in certain areas of the gene cause more aggressive cancers than mutations in others.

Paget's disease of the breast An uncommon change in the nipple that occurs in 1 to 4 percent of all women who have BREAST CANCER, and is sometimes called mammary Paget's disease.

This finding was named after Sir James Paget, a scientist who noted an association between changes in the appearance of the nipple and underlying breast cancer. A number of other diseases have also been named after Paget, including Paget's disease of the bone, which makes bones dense and more fragile.

Cause

Two major theories have been proposed to explain the development of this type of breast cancer. According to one theory, cancer cells called Paget cells break off from a tumor in the breast and move through the milk ducts in the breast to the surface of the nipple. In the other theory, the skin cells of the nipple spontaneously become cancerous Paget cells.

Symptoms

Symptoms of Paget's disease of the breast include itching, burning, redness, and scaling skin on the nipple and the areola surrounding the nipple. The changes may resemble eczema. There may be a bloody discharge from the nipple, and the nipple may appear flattened against the breast. Almost half of all women who have Paget's disease of the breast also have a lump in the breast that can be felt at the time of diagnosis.

Diagnosis

If a doctor suspects Paget's disease, a nipple BIOPSY is performed to look for large, malignant-appearing cells in the skin overlying the nipple.

Because most women who have Paget's disease of the breast also have an underlying breast tumor, a MAMMOGRAM will be ordered. If a mass is felt most women have invasive breast cancer in addition to Paget's disease. In women without a palpable mass, most women have DUCTAL CARCINOMA IN SITU, although a significant minority have INVASIVE BREAST CANCER. Only rarely are the changes seen in the nipple the only changes in the whole breast.

Treatment

Modified radical MASTECTOMY is the usual treatment for Paget's disease when the woman has an underlying breast cancer or when the cancer has spread beyond the central portion of the breast behind the nipple. In this operation, the surgeon removes the breast, some of the lymph nodes under the arm, and the lining over the chest muscles. The surgeon may also remove part of the chest wall muscles.

Breast-conserving therapy can be done if no cancer is found and no lump is felt. However, most of the time there is a cancer and the breast-conserving therapy must remove both the nipple/areolar complex and the cancer within the breast, followed by radiation.

Adjuvant CHEMOTHERAPY or HORMONAL THERAPY will be determined by characteristics of the invasive cancer, not by the Paget's disease.

pain control   Controlling BREAST CANCER pain is a key component of any overall treatment plan; the most successful methods combine multiple therapies to prevent pain. When pain does break through, the proper dose of pain reliever should be taken immediately. Many patients have a tendency to wait until the pain is excruciating before seeking relief, but waiting too long often results in use of more pills and less effective pain control.

Estimates of persistent pain among patients with breast cancer range from about 14 percent to almost 100 percent. The most common estimates found that pain was poorly controlled in 26 to 41 percent of all cancer patients.

One obstacle to measuring the scope of the problem is that patients themselves often give their doctors poor insight into their pain; some believe that pain is just part of the breast cancer experience and must be tolerated. Other patients have an unrealistic fear of opiates and often choose to suffer instead of asking for the drugs.

The best pain treatment depends on the level of pain and its cause. Mild pain often can be treated with acetaminophen, aspirin, or nonsteroidal anti-inflammatory drugs (NSAIDs). Ibuprofen and naproxen are two NSAIDs frequently used for mild cancer pain. Moderate to severe pain usually requires an opioid, usually beginning with codeine and progressing to other options such as oxycodone, morphine, and hydromorphone.

Long-acting narcotics, such as methadone and sustained-release morphine sulfate, are used when breakthrough pain is a problem. For patients who have trouble swallowing pills, options include liquid morphine and a fentanyl skin patch.

Although pain is not always a prominent feature of cancer, it is one of the most feared symptoms. Today there is no reason why most patients who have cancer pain cannot be made comfortable. The first step in managing cancer pain is proper evaluation. There are various types of pain in cancer, whether it is caused by injury of tissues around the tumor (nociceptive pain), the tumor's stimulation of nerves (neuropathic pain), or individual mental responses to sensation from the tumor (psychogenic pain).

Not surprisingly, self-reporting by the patient is the most important way to assess pain. A full history, physical exam, and appropriate lab and imaging studies (X-ray, computed tomography, MAGNETIC RESONANCE IMAGING) should reveal how the disease process is producing pain. But the pain's intensity, its features, and the factors that affect it are all important in determining the best strategy for treatment.

Acute Pain

Certain procedures involved in breast cancer diagnosis or treatment can sometimes produce acute pain; they include bone marrow biopsy, NEEDLE ASPIRATION, CHEMOTHERAPY (especially by injection), immunotherapy (pain in the joints or muscles), and radiation. Such attacks can usually be managed with adequate doses of nonmorphine painkillers.

Chronic Pain

The most common chronic breast cancer pain occurs when the cancer spreads to the bone. Experts do not know why some bone metastases are painless and others are terribly painful. If the spine is involved, there may be damage to the spinal cord or nerve roots, which can cause severe radiating nerve pain.

Other types of chronic pain conditions include POSTMASTECTOMY PAIN SYNDROME, caused by nerve damage after surgery, SENTINEL-NODE BIOPSY, or radiation. Chemotherapy can sometimes cause persistent nerve pain, which usually decreases over time after the drug is discontinued.

Opioid Drugs

The most typical way to ease severe pain in women with breast cancer is to use derivatives of morphine, the opioid derivatives. The choice of drug depends on the woman's age, presence of coexisting liver or kidney disease, and possible interactions with other medications. Although taking drugs by mouth is usually preferred, other methods (such as the transdermal skin patch) can be used if there is difficulty in swallowing or severe gastrointestinal upset.

For continuous or frequently recurring pain, it is usually best to have a fixed dosage schedule (such as every four hours) rather than administration of the drug "as needed." Starting at a low dose, the dosage is increased until pain stops or side effects prevent an increase. If pain "breaks through" the schedule, a rescue dose can be added immediately; rescue dose levels are typically 5 to 15 percent of the total daily dose of the drug.

Oral doses can be given more often, if necessary, with as little as two hours between doses; the minimal interval between intravenous administrations can be as short as 10 to 15 minutes. It is important to know that there is no "correct" or "maximum" dosage for patients with breast cancer—the correct dosage is simply whatever prevents pain.

In many cases, the development of side effects does not prevent further increase in dosage; the treating physician can prescribe medications or other therapies to counteract the most common problems that occur with opioids, such as nausea, vomiting, and constipation.

Nonopioid Analgesics

Acetaminophen and NSAIDs are good painkillers, but they have a maximal dose level above which no more benefit can be expected. These medications are most useful to people who have bone pain, or inflammatory pain in which the affected area is warm, red, and swollen. A newer type of NSAID, cyclooxygenase-2 (COX-2) inhibitors, may be superior in preventing possible stomach or kidney toxicity.

In addition, certain types of cancer may do well with a particular drug directed at the tissue involved, such as treating bone pain with bisphosphonates.

Adjuvant Drugs

Adjuvant medications are drugs that help analgesics work more effectively. Some drugs that are not primarily painkillers may have pain-relieving activity as well as their main effect. For instance, steroids, antidepressants, some anesthetics, antiepilepsy drugs, and major tranquilizers may be helpful for various types of nerve pain. They are usually along with other pain medications. Adjuvant drugs include the following:

- *Tricyclic antidepressants* such as amitriptyline and doxepin, which can improve the action of opioids and can treat nerve pain
- *Benzodiazepines* such as lorazepam and diazepam, which control anxiety to help reduce dosage of pain pills
- *Selective serotonin reuptake inhibitors* and other antidepressants, which improve mood
- *Nerve-pain modulators,* such as gabapentin, which help control nerve pain

Radiation Therapy and Chemotherapy

In addition to its main use as a way of destroying cancer cells, radiation therapy is often used to control pain, chiefly in managing the spread of cancer from the breast to the bone. Chemotherapy can provide pain relief in cancer by shrinking a tumor, but there is often a problem of balancing this sort of improvement against the toxic effects that chemotherapy can produce.

Nondrug Therapy

There are many alternative treatments for patients with breast cancer whose pain is not adequately controlled by medication, provided primarily by specialists in hospital settings. A cancer treatment center or pain clinic is the best place for getting information and advice on these therapeutic approaches, if the patient's cancer-management team does not offer them. The most common are the following:

- Acupuncture
- Exercise
- Heat or cold treatment
- Massage
- Breathing exercises
- Relaxation techniques
- Hypnosis
- Individual, group, or family psychological therapy

palliative treatment Medical treatment used to treat pain and symptoms and improve quality of life when a cure is not possible. This can be achieved by using medications, radiation, or surgery. For example, irradiating BREAST CANCER that has spread to the bone may not cure the cancer in the bone but can ease pain.

See also HOSPICE.

palpation   A procedure of using the hands to examine the breast. A palpable mass is a lump in the breast that can be felt with the hands.

Patient Advocate Foundation   A national network advocating health-care reform. Its primary function is to support legislation that enables cancer survivors to obtain insurance funding for medical care and participation in clinical trials. The group also serves as an active liaison between the patient and insurers, employers, and/or creditors. In doing so, they resolve insurance, job retention, and/or debt crisis matters related to the patient's diagnosis. Other services include referrals, information, advocacy, and health insurance assistance. For contact information, see Appendix I.

pectoralis muscles   Muscular tissues under the breast that are attached to the front of the chest wall and extend to the upper arms. They are divided into the pectoralis major and the pectoralis minor muscles.

peg procedure   A new type of breast reconstruction designed to reduce a patient's MASTECTOMY scar. The peg procedures can recreate both the shape and the size of the breast as well as of the nipple and areola.

In one type of peg procedure, the traditional straight-line mastectomy scar is replaced with a circular scar hidden within the border of the newly created nipple. The breast is reconstructed using a muscle flap from the back which is used to create the breast mound itself, as well as the nipple areolar complex. The results have been cosmetically excellent.

personality and breast cancer   Although the idea has been popular for a long time, there is no scientific evidence for the belief that there is such a thing as a "cancer personality." It is certainly possible that women who have been diagnosed with

breast cancer are anxious and depressed, but this does not mean that these uncomfortable emotions caused the malignancy.

Most recently, a 2003 Japanese study found that personality type does not appear to be associated with the risk of cancer. In this study, researchers examined the incidence of cancer among more than 30,000 people in Japan who had completed personality questionnaires with four personality subscales: extroversion (sociability, liveliness), neuroticism (emotional instability, anxiousness), psychoticism (tough-mindedness, aggressiveness, coldness), and social naivete or conformity. During seven years of follow-up, there were 986 cases of cancer but no association between any personality subscales and risk of breast cancer. Although higher levels of neuroticism were associated with cancers diagnosed in the first three years of follow-up, this finding could indicate that neuroticism may be a consequence of cancer rather than a cause.

A few earlier studies had found links between cancer and certain personality types, such as being extroverted, having a "type 1" personality, and lacking emotion. However, these studies had various weaknesses, tending to focus on small numbers of subjects and often failing to include a control for important breast cancer risk factors.

pesticides   Chemicals used to protect crops by killing organisms that eat them. Farmers may use them to prevent crop damage by insects, rodents, and molds or to prolong the storage life of food crops after harvest. Pesticides also may be used on animal farms to control insect pests. Herbicides are related chemicals used to kill weeds.

Use of some pesticides is no longer permitted because of toxic effects or cancer-causing potential. Unfortunately, some pesticide residues are still found in food long after the pesticides were banned, because long-lasting pesticides can remain in the environment many years after use. Small amounts of these residues are sometimes found in food crops grown on contaminated soil or in fish that live in polluted waters.

PET scans   A type of scan in which a small amount of a harmless radioactive substance tagged to a natural body compound, often glucose, is injected into a vein to enable a scanner to produce detailed pictures of the parts of the body where active cells take up the glucose. In areas that are actively growing (such as in cancers), a PET scan can reveal visible dark spots. PET scans are sometimes used in the staging of breast cancer. They are also being investigated in screening for breast cancer.

However, the ability of the tests to detect very early cancers such as ductal carcinoma in situ (DCIS), and to differentiate benign from malignant tumors, is still preliminary. In the future it may become an important screening test.

Peutz-Jeghers syndrome (PJS) An early-onset disorder characterized by colored lesions on the lips and mouth and multiple gastrointestinal polyps—as well as a high risk of development of BREAST CANCER, among other malignancies. Mutations in the *STK11* gene at chromosome 19p13.3, which appears to function as a TUMOR SUPPRESSOR GENE, have been identified as one cause of PJS.

In one study, scientists estimated that for someone with PJS the risk of development of cancer (other than skin cancer) between the age of 15 to 64 is 93 percent. The highest cumulative risk in these patients was for breast cancer (54 percent) and ovarian cancer (21 percent)—estimates that are similar to those observed in women carrying *BRCA1* or *BRCA2* mutations.

phantom breast pain More than a third of women who have had a MASTECTOMY experience phantom breast sensations after surgery, whether or not breast reconstruction was performed.

Symptoms of phantom breast pain may include itching, pins-and-needles sensation, pressure, or throbbing. Physicians believe that phantom breast pain occurs after mastectomy for the same reason it appears after limb amputations. During a mastectomy, small nerves between the breast tissue and skin are severed, causing the neural connections in the brain to reorganize. This process, as well as the spontaneous firing of electrical signals from the ends of cut or injured nerves, causes phantom sensations.

Women who experience breast pain before mastectomy are most likely to have sensations of pain in the breast area afterward. Patients who experience phantom sensations in the breast area after surgery should report their symptoms to their doctors immediately so that the pain can be properly managed.

In some cases, EXERCISE or breast MASSAGE may help alleviate phantom breast pain, although patients should first discuss these options with their physicians. In more severe cases, medications may be prescribed to reduce pain. Phantom breast pain does not indicate that cancer cells are still present in the breast area or that cancer may recur.

Phase I trial A study in which researchers test a new drug or treatment in a small group of people (between 20 and 80 subjects) for the first time to evaluate its safety, determine a safe dosage range, and identify side effects.

See also CLINICAL TRIALS; PHASE II TRIAL; PHASE III TRIAL; PHASE IV TRIAL.

Phase II trial A clinical study in which researchers test a drug or treatment with a larger group of people (between 100 and 300 subjects) than participated in a PHASE I TRIAL to see whether a drug or treatment is effective and to evaluate its safety further.

See also CLINICAL TRIALS; PHASE I TRIAL; PHASE III TRIAL; PHASE IV TRIAL.

Phase III trial A clinical study in which researchers test a drug or treatment with a larger group of people (between 1,000 and 3,000 subjects) than participated in a Phase I or II trial to confirm effectiveness, monitor side effects, compare the treatment to commonly used methods, and collect safety information.

See also CLINICAL TRIALS; PHASE I TRIAL; PHASE II TRIAL; PHASE IV TRIAL.

Phase IV trial A postmarketing study that provides more information about a drug or treatment, including the treatment's risks, benefits, and optimal use.

See also CLINICAL TRIALS; PHASE I TRIAL; PHASE II TRIAL; PHASE III TRIAL.

phenolics A category of more than 2,000 PHYTOCHEMICALS, or plant chemicals. The chemical structure of these phytochemicals gives them the ability to mop up many FREE RADICALS as they circulate through the bloodstream. For this reason, phenolics are considered to be some of the most powerful antioxidants and are studied for their ability to interfere with tumors.

phyllodes tumor   A type of benign tumor (also spelled *phylloides*) that occurs in the glandular and connective breast tissue and is far less common than a FIBROADENOMA. Phyllodes tumors are usually benign, but on very rare occasions, they may be malignant and spread.

Treatment of phyllodes tumors involves removing the mass and a one-inch margin of surrounding breast tissue. Cancerous phyllodes tumors are surgically removed by either LUMPECTOMY or MASTECTOMY but do not typically respond well to CHEMOTHERAPY or RADIATION THERAPY.

Physician's Data Query (PDQ)   A comprehensive cancer database maintained by the NATIONAL CANCER INSTITUTE. It has been distributed since 1984 to physicians and the public and is now available in multiple forms including fax, e-mail, conventional mail, and the Internet, in both English and Spanish.

The PDQ contains peer-reviewed summaries of cancer treatment, screening, prevention, genetics, and supportive care and directories of physicians, professionals who provide genetics services, and organizations that provide cancer care.

The PDQ also contains the world's most comprehensive cancer clinical trial database, with about 1,800 abstracts of trials that are open and accepting patients, including trials for cancer treatment, genetics, diagnosis, supportive care, screening, and prevention. In addition, there is access to about 12,000 abstracts of clinical trials that have been completed or are no longer accepting patients.

The PDQ cancer-information summaries are peer reviewed and updated monthly by six editorial boards composed of specialists in adult treatment, pediatric treatment, complementary and alternative medicine, supportive care, screening and prevention, and genetics. The boards review current literature from more than 70 biomedical journals, evaluate its relevance, and synthesize it into clear summaries.

phytochemicals   Natural compounds found only in plants that protect them from effects of sunlight and environmental threats. Many of these compounds are currently under investigation for their role in blocking the formation of some cancers. They may also protect against some forms of heart disease, arthritis, and other degenerative diseases.

While phytochemicals can be found in varying amounts in all fruits, vegetables, grains, oils, nuts, and seeds, some of these foods have higher levels of phytochemicals. Some of these phytochemicals are currently being studied for their potential to prevent BREAST CANCER.

Many studies have already provided evidence that eating more fruits and vegetables decreases the risk of breast cancer. In fact, phytochemical research helped prompt the NATIONAL CANCER INSTITUTE to initiate its "5-a-Day" program for healthy eating, in which consumers are urged to eat more foods such as garlic, broccoli, onions, and soy products.

Phytochemicals, which include thousands of different components in plant foods, differ from vitamins and minerals in that they are not considered essential nutrients. Yet a diet that includes phytochemicals from a wide range of fruits and vegetables has been associated with improved health. Since different phytochemicals are present in different foods, eating a varied diet is important to ensure that a person receives all the protection possible.

The specific phytochemical content of different fruits and vegetables tends to vary by color, and each has particular functions. Some phytochemicals act as ANTIOXIDANTS, some protect and regenerate essential nutrients, and others work to deactivate cancer-causing substances.

Allium compounds   Allium compounds such as allyl sulfides may help detoxify and rid the body of some carcinogenic compounds. Food sources include onions, garlic, scallions, and chives.

Carotenoids   Carotenoids such as alpha-carotene, beta-carotene, cryptoxanthin, LYCOPENE, and LUTEIN work as antioxidants, helping to offset harm caused by environmental pollutants such as pesticides and smoking. Food sources include dark green, orange, or red fruits and vegetables, especially carrots, sweet potatoes, tomatoes, spinach, broccoli, cantaloupe, and apricots.

Glucosinolates   Glucosinolates such as glucobrassicin are metabolized to produce two other phytochemicals, isothiocyanates and INDOLES, which trigger production of enzymes that block cell damage due to carcinogens. Food sources include cruciferous vegetables such as broccoli, cabbage, and brussels sprouts.

Polyphenols Polyphenols such as ellagic acid and ferulic acid are thought to prevent conversion of substances into carcinogens and to inhibit mutations. Food sources include oats, soybeans, and fruits and nuts—especially strawberries, raspberries, blackberries, walnuts, and pecans.

Flavonoids Flavonoids include more than 2,000 powerful antioxidants from sources such as coffee, tea, cola, berries, tomatoes, potatoes, broad beans, broccoli, Italian squash, onions, and citrus fruits.

In the Future

Someday, scientists may develop "superbreeds" of certain foods with an extra dose of beneficial phytochemicals. Seed catalogues already offer home gardeners the opportunity to buy seeds for several of these supervegetables. For example, sulforaphane has been identified as a potent inducer of detoxifying enzymes (broccoli is a good source, and three-day-old broccoli sprouts are even better—they have between 20 and 50 times more sulforaphane than do mature broccoli). In one study, rats fed sulforaphane had fewer malignant tumors, and those tumors developed at a slower rate.

In addition to high-sulforaphane broccoli sprouts, consumers can now also buy high-lycopene tomatoes and high-beta-carotene cauliflower. Soon, some package labels may even list the amounts of dominant protective substances, just as food labels today list the amount of calories or carbohydrates.

See also PHYTOCHEMICALS.

plastic surgeon A surgeon specializing in plastic surgery who is certified by the American Board of Plastic Surgery (ABPS) and has completed a minimum of five years of surgical training after medical school, including a plastic surgery residency program. After training, a surgeon must pass comprehensive oral and written exams before being granted certification.

Any woman contemplating BREAST RECONSTRUCTION should discuss her options with a plastic surgeon. It is important to make sure that the plastic surgeon is certified by the American Society of Plastic Surgeons (ASPS) and has experience with breast reconstruction. ASPS members are certified by the ABPS and required to attend continuing medical education courses regularly and adhere to a strict code of ethics. Women may contact the ASPS at (800) 635-0635 to find out whether a plastic surgeon is board certified. The ASPS Web site also allows women to search for a plastic surgeon by name, city, state, or zip code.

pleural effusion A buildup of fluid in the space between the lungs and the interior walls of the chest (the pleural cavity) that can be caused by cancers, infections, blood clots, or other diseases.

port Also called a life port or port-a-cath, this is a permanent IV surgically implanted under the skin (usually on the chest) to enter a large blood vessel. It is used to deliver medication, chemotherapy, blood products and to obtain blood samples. A port is usually inserted if the veins in a woman's arm are difficult to use for treatment, or if certain types of chemotherapy drugs need to be administered, especially if they need to be administered 24 hours a day.

postmastectomy pain syndrome Discomfort that begins either immediately or soon after a LUMPECTOMY or MASTECTOMY. The burning, stabbing pain usually affects the front or sides of the chest in the area of the surgery, and sometimes even the upper arm.

Postmastectomy pain syndrome is a fairly common problem after breast surgery, affecting as many as 30 percent of patients.

Patients who have postmastectomy pain often describe it as burning and intensified by light touch or pressure; it can sometimes be so severe that it disrupts the person's daily life. The pain usually results from irritation of one or more of the nerves in the chest wall, which may have been trapped by scar tissue or cut during surgery. In some cases, a painful bundle of nerves (neuroma) grows at the stump of a severed nerve.

Diagnosis

Some patients report that a diagnosis of their condition was difficult to obtain. Diagnosing postmastectomy pain syndrome quickly is a problem because the pain may take some days to become apparent. In only a small percentage of patients, pain as well as paresthesia (a tingling nerve sensation) are present immediately after surgery. Another common time for the syndrome to appear is after postsurgical RADIATION THERAPY. LYMPHEDEMA can be a side effect of radiation and perhaps aggravates the syndrome; or there may be other, underreported radiation side effects that contribute to pain. Few long-term studies have been done on this condition.

Doctors can use a physical exam to confirm that there is a painful or sensitive spot near the surgical scar; computed tomography (CT) scans are sometimes used to determine whether a recurrent tumor may be causing the symptoms. Doctors may use a nerve block injection or anesthetic around the painful structures or along the path of the nerves involved to help confirm the diagnosis.

Treatment

Some patients benefit from oral nonsteroidal anti-inflammatory drugs plus additional pain medications. The use of topical ointments (such as nonprescription treatments for sunburn) can sometimes reduce the pain.

Generally, opiates and narcotics such as paracetamol and morphine have not worked well against this syndrome. Among the drugs that have proved helpful are amitriptyline (Elavil), venlafaxine (Effexor), gabapentin (Neurontin), mirtazapine (Remeron), clonidine, anticonvulsants, muscle relaxants, and antiarrhythmic heart medications.

Long-term relief can sometimes be obtained with the use of therapeutic nerve block injections containing anesthetic and anti-inflammatory medications. Injections can be given into a neuroma or along the path of the nerves involved in postmastectomy pain syndrome. Nerve block treatments are usually given in a short series, which can be repeated intermittently as needed. Nerve stimulation procedures can sometimes help chest wall pain that persists. For patients who find that the pain is interfering significantly with their physical functions, physical therapy exercises are used to help them resume normal daily activity.

Some patients have found relief in physical therapies such as acupuncture, biofeedback, compressions on the surgery sites, moist heat treatment, ice bags, osteopathy, and phantom limb massage. In certain extreme cases, repeat surgeries to clean out scar tissue and tighten loose skin have been effective.

Among the last resorts are spinal cord stimulators, intracathal drug pumps, and various neurolytic procedures in which the nerves themselves are sacrificed or modified to reduce the pain. These procedures require the services of an interventional pain specialist, preferably one certified by either the American Board of Anesthesiology or the American Board of Pain Medicine.

poverty and cancer   Research confirms that the poor are more likely than the socially advantaged to die of BREAST CANCER. This is a reversal from the 1950s, when the rate of death was nearly 50 percent higher among those who were socially advantaged.

pregnancy   BREAST CANCER occurs about once in every 3,000 pregnancies. It may be difficult to detect early in pregnant or nursing women because often their breasts are tender and swollen. Because of the problems in detecting tumors in these women, cancers are often found at a later stage. For this reason, pregnant women with breast cancer may have lower survival rates than nonpregnant women who have breast cancer. However, breast cancer in the mother does not appear to harm the fetus, and breast cancer cells do not seem to pass from the mother to the unborn child.

Diagnosis

To detect breast cancer, experts recommend that pregnant and nursing women examine their own breasts in addition to having CLINICAL BREAST EXAMINATIONS during their routine prenatal and postnatal checkups. If anything abnormal is noticed, ultrasounds or biopsies may be used to evaluate a problem.

Staging

If breast cancer is found, doctors must decide how advanced the cancer is (a procedure called STAGING). Methods used to stage breast cancer can be changed so that the fetus is exposed to less radiation. CAT scans are usually avoided, but X-rays of the chest and blood tests may be ordered to make sure the lungs and liver are healthy.

Treatment

Treatment options for pregnant women depend on the stage of the disease and the age of the fetus. Treatment may include some surgery and/or chemotherapy. Radiation is almost never used during pregnancy, but can be delayed until after the baby is delivered. During the first trimester the baby is at greatest risk and chemotherapy should not be given. General anesthesia is safe, but if it can be postponed until the second trimester it is probably better.

Ending the pregnancy does not seem to improve the mother's chance of survival. If the cancer must be treated with chemotherapy and radiation therapy, which may harm the fetus, ending the pregnancy is sometimes considered. This difficult decision also may depend on the stage of cancer and the mother's chance of survival.

Pregnancy after Breast Cancer

Pregnancy does not seem to affect the survival rate of women who have had breast cancer in the past. Some doctors recommend that a woman wait two years after treatment for breast cancer before planning to have a baby, so that any early recurrence of the cancer can be detected. This recommendation may affect a woman's decision to become pregnant.

Likewise, a baby does not seem to be affected by the mother's previous breast cancer. However, effects of certain cancer treatments on later pregnancies are not known. In particular, the effects on later pregnancies of treatment with HIGH-DOSE CHEMOTHERAPY and BONE MARROW TRANSPLANT are not known.

prepuberty growth   Factors such as height and weight before puberty may influence a girl's eventual risk of BREAST CANCER when she grows up, according to British research on twins. A girl's risk of breast cancer as an adult increased by 44 percent if she was thinner than her twin sister before age 10, and by 27 percent if she was the taller of the two at that age. Moreover, her risk increased by 53 percent if her breasts developed earlier, and by 79 percent if she had a smaller waist-to-hip ratio at age 20 than her twin. The researchers note, however, that these associations were stronger in fraternal twins than in identical twins, and stronger in twins without a family history of breast cancer than in twins with a genetic predisposition.

prevention of breast cancer   Some risk factors, such as family history, genetic patterns, and age of menstruation and childbirth, cannot be altered. Things can be changed, however, that may affect a woman's chances of developing the disease. Steps that can be taken to reduce risk include choosing to breast-feed, eating a healthy diet, getting plenty of EXERCISE, preventing excessive weight gain, taking preventive drugs such as TAMOXIFEN, and avoiding excess ALCOHOL and HORMONE REPLACEMENT THERAPY. Women at risk of inheriting a BREAST CANCER SUSCEPTIBILITY GENE can consider being tested to find out whether they definitely have the gene; if they do, they may consider preventive surgery or more frequent mammograms and exams.

Exercise

Recent studies suggest that regular exercise may decrease breast cancer risk in younger women and may decrease the chance of cancer recurrence in women who have breast cancer. Other studies have found that women who have cancer who exercise live longer than those who do not.

Diet

Some evidence suggests a link between diet and breast cancer. Ongoing studies are looking at ways to prevent breast cancer through changes in diet or dietary supplements, but whether specific dietary changes actually prevent breast cancer is not yet known. A high-calorie, high-fat diet may lead to obesity, which is a known risk factor in postmenopausal women.

BRCA Genes

Research has led to the identification of mutations in certain genes that increase the risk of breast cancer development. Women who have a strong family history of breast cancer may choose to have a blood test to see whether they have inherited a change in the *BRCA1* or *BRCA2* gene. If they have inherited the gene, some women choose preventive surgery or medications to lower their risk more frequent screenings, which may include MRIs and pelvic ultrasounds.

Preventive Drugs

Scientists are studying drugs that may prevent the development of breast cancer. Tamoxifen, an antiestrogen, is approved to reduce the risk of breast cancer in women at higher risk for the disease. A current study is comparing raloxifene to tamoxifen.

Prophylactic Mastectomy

Some women at very high risk for breast cancer choose to have one or both breasts removed *before* disease occurs. Although this surgery does not completely eliminate the risk (some tiny bits of breast tissue always remain), it does lower the risk considerably, to less than 5 percent. Some people consider this a controversial and radical step to avoid breast cancer; some women who are at high risk consider it a worthwhile step. Insurance companies may or may not cover the surgery.

primary site   The original site where a tumor, such as a BREAST CANCER tumor, first appeared. If a patient with breast cancer has cancer that has spread to other organs, the breast is the primary site and cancers in other organs are secondary.

See also SECONDARY BONE CANCER; SECONDARY BRAIN CANCER; SECONDARY LIVER CANCER; SECONDARY LUNG CANCER; SECONDARY SITE.

progesterone   A female HORMONE that stimulates the growth of normal breast cells as well as some BREAST CANCER cells. If breast cancer cells are found on a BIOPSY, the lab performs a PROGESTERONE RECEPTOR ASSAY to check for PROGESTERONE receptors on the malignant cells. The presence of progesterone receptors suggests that the tumor depends on progesterone to grow. Women who have these receptors may benefit from HORMONE THERAPY, which blocks these receptors and starves breast cancer cells of the progesterone they need to grow. Women who have progesterone receptor cells have a better prognosis because they are most likely to respond to hormone therapy.

progesterone receptor assay (PRA)   A test that is done on BREAST CANCER tissue to see whether the tumor is dependent on the hormone PROGESTERONE

for its growth. Breast cancer cells that are progesterone receptor positive respond favorably to hormonal therapy.

Project Survive   An Internet support network for women with BREAST CANCER that offers patients an alternative to conventional support groups. Despite research showing the effectiveness of support groups in aiding recovery, only 10 to 15 percent of patients with breast cancer take part in a conventional support group. Providing a support group over the Internet allows the network to reach patients for whom the stress of coping with treatments makes it impractical to attend a support group in person.

See also Appendix I.

prolactin   A HORMONE that normally stimulates breast-tissue growth and differentiation during puberty, pregnancy, and breast-feeding. It is unclear whether prolactin is important in BREAST CANCER development or whether prolactin-blocking medications could be developed to treat breast cancer. Recent studies have shown a prolactin receptor on many breast cancer cells, but it has not been made clear that higher levels of prolactin in the body predispose to breast cancer development.

protocol   A treatment plan for therapy that also includes details on drug administration, dosage, and duration, together with type and method of radiation. *Protocol* may refer to either a standardized treatment program or experimental programs.

***P-TEN* gene**   Mutations in the *P-TEN* gene can increase a woman's risk of breast cancer. The *P-TEN* gene, also called *MMAC1,* is located on chromosome 10. The role of this chromosome in the development of various sporadic cancers has been investigated for nearly a decade. Experts believe that the *P-TEN* mutation is responsible for the increase in thyroid and breast cancers seen in patients with COWDEN'S DISEASE.

See also BREAST CANCER SUSCEPTIBILITY GENES.

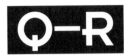

quadrantectomy   Removal of a quarter of the breast, including the skin and connective tissues. The surgeon may also perform a separate procedure to remove some or all of the LYMPH NODES in the armpit (either an axillary node dissection or a SENTINEL NODE BIOPSY).

R. A. Bloch Cancer Foundation, Inc.   A nonprofit foundation that offers a toll-free cancer hotline, home volunteers who have diagnoses similar to those of clients, support groups, educational and special-interest presentations, and a list of medical multidisciplinary second-opinion boards. For contact information, see Appendix I.

race and breast cancer   There are striking racial differences among women who have BREAST CANCER, which affect both the risk of development of breast cancer and the survival rate of whose who are diagnosed.

The age-adjusted incidence of invasive breast cancer indicates that white, Hawaiian, and black women have the highest rates in the United States. The lowest rates occur among Korean, Native American, and Vietnamese women. White non-Hispanic women have a risk of breast cancer four times that of Korean women.

Although IN SITU breast cancer (noninvasive breast cancer) occurs at much lower rates than invasive breast cancer, it has a similar racial–ethnic pattern. White non-Hispanic women have the highest rates—more than twice the rate of Hispanic women. (Rates for in situ breast cancers could not be calculated for Alaskan Native, Native American, Korean, or Vietnamese women because of the small number of cases.)

Mortality rates are much lower than incidence rates for breast cancer, ranging from just 15 percent of the incidence rate for Japanese women to 33 percent for African-American women.

Racial differences in breast cancer survival rates have worsened since 1980, but the disparity cannot be attributed entirely to inequalities in access to health care, according to results of a study of women in the Department of Defense (DoD) health-care system. In the study of the DoD system, between 1980 and 1984, African-American women who have breast cancer were 1.3 times more likely to die than Caucasian women with breast cancer were. Between 1995 and 1999, African-American women were 1.8 times more likely to die than Caucasian women. Over the 20 years of the review, Caucasians showed greater improvement in overall survival rate than African Americans. Moreover, there was a greater shift toward diagnosis at an earlier stage in Caucasians than in African Americans.

Some evidence suggests that the different outcomes among African-American and Caucasian women may be due to differences in the tumors themselves or to environmental and behavioral factors such as obesity. Other studies support the theory that inequality in access to physicians, screening MAMMOGRAMS, and treatment explain the differences. It is also possible that the higher breast cancer death rate among African-American women is related to the fact that a larger percentage of their breast cancers are diagnosed at a later, less treatable stage.

It may be, therefore, that differences in biology explain the variable mortality across cultures. Differences in health-care decisions also may affect outcome.

radiation and breast cancer   Young women who received high dosages of chest radiation to treat

Hodgkin's disease face up to an eight times higher risk of BREAST CANCER.

Hodgkin's disease is a type of cancer involving the LYMPH NODES. Unlike most other cancers, it strikes young people about as often as it does older ones. Researchers estimate that in 83 of 1,000 women breast cancer may develop after 25 years if they were treated for Hodgkin's disease with high-dose chest radiation alone when they were 30 or younger. Nonetheless, the benefits of Hodgkin's disease treatment far outweigh the risks; 50 years ago, the typical patient survived only a few years. Today, treatment including radiation and CHEMOTHERAPY has boosted the five-year survival rate to 85 percent.

Moreover, lower targeted dosages of radiation have been given to patients with Hodgkin's disease during the past decade, and these women may not face as high a risk of breast cancer as their predecessors.

However, if radiation to the pelvis was used, destroying ovarian function, or if chemotherapy caused premature menopause, the risk of breast cancer actually decreased.

The AMERICAN CANCER SOCIETY suggests that women who have had such radiation treatment consider starting yearly MAMMOGRAMS at age 30 instead of age 40.

Radiation on the Job

Likewise, women who worked as radiation technologists before 1950 have a higher risk of death of breast cancer than those who began the job in more recent years. The safeguards were not as good as they are now, and these women were exposed to high-dose radiation.

A study of female medical radiation workers in China suggested that the earlier these women had been first employed, the more their breast cancer risk increased. In the United States, most medical radiation workers are women.

After adjusting for age of menopause, age at first birth, and family history of breast cancer, the study authors found that women who began working as radiologic technologists before 1940 were nearly three times more likely to die of breast cancer than those first employed in 1960 or later. They also found that women who began working between 1940 and 1949 were about two and a half times more likely to die of breast cancer than those who

started working in 1960 or later. Moreover, technologists who first performed fluoroscopy (an X-ray technique) and multifilm procedures before 1950 had statistically significant higher risks than technologists who first performed these procedures in 1960 or later. The decline in risk over time probably reflects necessary reductions in the recommended radiation exposure limit.

radiation oncologist See ONCOLOGIST.

radiation therapy Treatment for BREAST CANCER in which a beam of radiation is directed to the breast to kill any remaining cancer cells in the breast. Women who have had a LUMPECTOMY almost always have radiation therapy. The radiation may be directed at the breast by a machine (external radiation) or may be administered by radioactive material in thin plastic tubes that are placed directly into the breast (implant radiation). Some women have both kinds of radiation therapy.

In external radiation therapy, the patient usually goes to the treatment center five days a week for several weeks. For implant radiation, a woman stays in the hospital for several days while the implants remain in place; they are removed before the woman goes home. This procedure is less frequently used.

During radiation therapy women may be tired, especially toward the end of the treatments. This feeling may continue for a while after treatment is over. Resting is important, but research has suggested that trying to stay reasonably active can help fend off fatigue.

It is also common for the skin in the treated area to become red, dry, tender, and itchy, and the breast may temporarily feel heavy and hard. Toward the end of treatment, the skin may become moist; exposing this area to air as much as possible helps the skin heal. These effects of radiation therapy on the skin are temporary, and the area gradually heals once treatment ends. However, there may be a permanent change in the color of the skin of the breast, and the breast texture, size, and density may be altered.

radiologist A medical doctor who has specialized in radiology and who diagnoses diseases of the human body by using X-rays, ultrasound, radio waves, and radioactive materials. To become a radiologist, a student must attend medical school and then usually spend four additional years as an intern and resident in radiology.

radiotherapy   See RADIATION THERAPY.

radio wave–ablation therapy   An experimental technique that destroys BREAST CANCER cells without surgery. Instead of cutting out a tumor, the experimental technique uses radio wave energy to kill cancer cells deep inside the breast. Because the therapy is still experimental, in the ongoing California study of this technique, all of the women have a conventional LUMPECTOMY or MASTECTOMY after the radio wave treatment. After this conventional surgery, researchers carefully examine the excised breast tissue to confirm that the radio wave treatment eradicated all the cancer.

If the pilot trial finds radio wave treatment effective in killing the tumor cells, the technique could offer advantages over lumpectomy. For one thing, a large incision does not have to be made, and the technique kills only the tumor and a thin layer of tissue surrounding it. In a lumpectomy, much more tissue is removed. With the radio wave technique, the cosmetic results should be much better.

Radio wave therapy, also known as radio-frequency ablation, has been used for many years to treat liver and bone cancers; other researchers around the country are studying the therapy as a treatment for lung and prostate cancers.

However, radio wave therapy is showing particular potential in treating breast cancer. Over the last few years, the therapy has been tested in a small number of patients with breast cancer at Stanford University, the University of Texas M. D. Anderson Cancer Center in Houston, and the Weill Cornell Breast Center in New York, all with favorable results.

Technique

To perform radiofrequency ablation, doctors first locate the tumor with ultrasound and then introduce a thin metal probe into the tumor through the skin. Tiny wires at the tip of the probe vibrate, generating a frictional heat that kills all of the cells

touched by the probe. Patients walk away after the procedure with only a tiny cut visible on the skin. The killed cancer cells eventually form a scar inside the breast.

Reach to Recovery   A program sponsored by the AMERICAN CANCER SOCIETY in which volunteers who have survived BREAST CANCER and gone on to live normal, productive lives offer understanding, support, and hope to newly diagnosed patients and their family. Through face-to-face visits or by phone, Reach to Recovery volunteers provide support for anyone newly diagnosed or facing recurrence.

Volunteers are trained to provide support and up-to-date information, including literature for spouses, children, friends, and other loved ones. Volunteers can also, when appropriate, provide patients with breast cancer with a temporary breast form and information on types of permanent prostheses as well as lists of where those items are available within a patient's community. (No products are endorsed.)

Reach to Recovery works with carefully selected and trained volunteers who have fully adjusted to their breast cancer treatment. All volunteers complete initial training and participate in ongoing continuing education sessions. For contact information, see Appendix I.

reconstruction of breast   See BREAST RECONSTRUCTION.

reconstructive surgeon   A physician (also called a plastic and reconstructive surgeon) who uses specific techniques to repair visible skin defects and problems in underlying tissue caused by surgery or in some cases BREAST CANCER itself.

A reconstructive surgeon can use grafts of the skin, bone, and cartilage to repair defects and can transfer tissue from one part of the body to another. In these techniques, the surgeon carefully prepares the patient's skin and tissues by using precise cutting and suturing techniques to minimize scarring.

Recent advances in the development of miniaturized instruments, new materials for artificial limbs and body parts, and improved surgical techniques have expanded the range of reconstructive operations that can be performed. Most breast reconstructive surgery involves a stay in the hospital and general anesthesia.

The risks associated with reconstructive surgery include the postoperative complications that can occur with any surgical operation with anesthesia, such as infection, internal bleeding, pneumonia, and reactions to the anesthesia. In addition to these general risks, reconstructive surgery carries specific risks:

• Undesirable scar tissue
• Persistent pain, redness, or swelling
• Infection
• Anemia or fat embolisms from liposuction
• Rejection of skin grafts or tissue transplants
• Loss of normal feeling or function in the area of the operation
• Complications resulting from unforeseen technological problems

recurrence The return of cancer after treatment. There are three types of BREAST CANCER recurrence: local, regional, and distant.

In a local recurrence, cancerous tumor cells remain in the original site and grow back over time.

A regional recurrence of breast cancer is more serious than a local recurrence, because it usually indicates that the cancer has spread past the breast and the underarm LYMPH NODES.

A distant breast cancer recurrence (also known as a METASTASIS) is the most dangerous type of recurrence. In this case, breast cancer spreads to distant regions of the body, such as the bone, lung, liver, or brain.

Treatment depends on the type and severity of the breast cancer recurrence. Breast cancer recurrences may be treated with additional surgery, CHEMOTHERAPY, radiation, or other drug therapies (such as TAMOXIFEN).

red blood cell A type of blood cell that carries oxygen from the lungs to other parts of the body. Red blood cells contain hemoglobin, an iron-rich protein that is responsible for absorbing oxygen in the lungs and later releasing it to the body's tissues. CHEMOTHERAPY drugs kill rapidly dividing cells, including red blood cells. This is why many chemotherapy patients eventually develop a deficiency of red blood cells called ANEMIA, which if untreated, may lead to FATIGUE, dizziness, headaches, and shortness of breath.

During chemotherapy treatment patients have regular blood tests to check the number of red cells in the blood; the next chemotherapy treatment may be postponed, and a blood transfusion given, if the counts are very low. Other treatments for anemia include injections of ERYTHROPOIETIN (Procrit or Aranesp), which can boost red blood cell count.

Erythropoietin is the major blood growth factor that encourages the bone marrow to produce more red blood cells. Although it is a naturally occurring substance, it can now be made in the laboratory in much larger quantities than patients normally produce on their own. This drug is given by injection under the skin and helps boost red cells in patients on chemotherapy. Erythropoietin can cause side effects, including flu symptoms, rashes, and high blood pressure.

relapse See RECURRENCE.

Relief Band A patented watchlike electronic medical device that provides drug-free, noninvasive relief from NAUSEA and vomiting. It relieves symptoms by gently stimulating nerves on the underside of the wrist. When activated, the device emits a low-level electrical current across two small electrodes on its underside. It is available by prescription for the treatment of nausea and vomiting caused by CHEMOTHERAPY, but it can also be obtained over the counter for nausea caused by motion sickness. The band is the only medical device to be approved by the U.S. Food and Drug Administration for use in hospitals and doctors' offices for the treatment of nausea and vomiting caused by chemotherapy.

remission The complete or partial disappearance of signs and symptoms of a disease in response to treatment; the period in which a disease is under control. Remission of a BREAST CANCER does not necessarily indicate cure.

retraction The process of skin's pulling in toward breast tissue, often referred to as dimpling.

risk factors See BREAST CANCER RISK FACTORS.

saline implants   A breast implant inserted after a MASTECTOMY to reconstruct the breast. Saline implants have a silicone rubber shell that is inflated by the physician to the desired size with sterile saline solution. Most implants have a valve that is sealable by the surgeon.

There are two types of saline solution–filled implants: One is a fixed-volume implant filled with the entire volume of saline solution at implantation. The second type is an adjustable-volume implant, which is filled intraoperatively and has the potential for further postoperative adjustment.

Before 1992, two types of breast implants were available—silicone and saline solution, both with an outer silicone shell. In 1992, the U.S. Food and Drug Administration (FDA) restricted the use of silicone-gel-filled implants because the agency was concerned that silicone gel leakage into the body could be harmful and because manufacturers were unable to provide adequate safety data on their implants. As a result of the FDA's decision, silicone-gel implants can now be used only in controlled clinical studies of reconstruction after MASTECTOMY, correction of congenital deformities, or replacement of ruptured silicone-gel implants that were used for augmentation.

Experts believe that saline solution–filled implants are safer than silicone implants because rupture or leakage releases only salt water into the body.

Risks

Though the FDA believes that the saline implants on the market are reasonably safe, there still are risks. Breast implants are artificial medical devices that can rupture, ripple, harden, change shape, and shift position, causing infection, pain, and loss of feeling in the nipple or tissue of the breast.

Moreover, many of the changes to the breast after implantation are irreversible. If a woman later chooses to have her implant removed, she may experience dimpling, puckering, wrinkling, or other changes of the breast.

Capsular contracture   One of the most common complications reported for saline solution–filled breast implants is capsular contracture. Because the implant is a foreign object, the body usually forms scar tissue around it. The tightening and squeezing of this scar tissue are called capsular contracture; it can cause breast tissue hardening, skin rippling, and breast shape changes. It also may cause pain that can be so severe that surgery may be needed to remove the scar tissue or replace the implant itself.

Implant rupture or deflation   Breast implants have a limited life, and a rupture can occur at any time. Once the implant ruptures, surgery is required to remove or replace it.

Other complications   Surgery also may be necessary if the implant area becomes infected, shifts, or causes calcium to form in the surrounding tissue. Another potential complication of implant surgery is nerve damage that may cause a change in sensation or loss of feeling in nipples and breast tissue. These symptoms may disappear eventually but can be permanent in some patients.

Breast cancer risks   The physical and cosmetic results of breast implants may be affected by chemotherapy, radiation therapy, or any factor that significantly alters the healing process. Skin cell death may occur because circulation to the remaining tissue has been changed by a mastectomy.

Implant Procedure

The breast reconstruction process may begin at the time of the mastectomy (immediate reconstruction) or weeks to years afterward (delayed reconstruction). Immediate reconstruction may help some women psychologically. In addition, it is often cheaper to combine the mastectomy procedure with the first stage of the reconstruction. However, there may be a higher risk of complications (such as deflation) with immediate reconstruction, and the initial surgery time and recuperation time may be longer.

One advantage of delayed reconstruction is that a woman can delay her reconstruction decision and surgery until radiation therapy and chemotherapy are completed. Delayed reconstruction also may be recommended if the surgeon anticipates healing problems with the mastectomy or if a woman needs more time to consider her options.

Breast reconstruction with implants can be a one-stage procedure, but more often it is done in two stages. This is because achieving the best cosmetic outcome usually takes more than one operation, especially if the reconstruction procedure includes building a new nipple. In the one-stage procedure, after the general surgeon removes the breast tissue, the plastic surgeon inserts a breast implant.

In a two-stage procedure, the plastic surgeon implants a breast tissue expander and replaces it several months later with the breast implant. The tissue expander placement may be done at the time of a mastectomy, or it may be delayed until months or years later.

During a mastectomy, the surgical oncologist often removes skin as well as breast tissue, leaving the chest tissues flat and tight. To create a breast-shaped space for the breast implant, the plastic surgeon places the tissue expander under the remaining chest tissues. The tissue expander is a balloonlike device made from elastic silicone rubber. It is inserted unfilled, and over time, sterile saline fluid is added by inserting a small needle through the skin to a filling port in the device. As the tissue expander fills, the skin over the expander begins to stretch, creating a new breast-shaped pocket for a breast implant. Tissue expanders are usually implanted with general anesthesia during one- to two-hour surgery. Typically, a woman can resume normal daily activity after two to three weeks. Because the chest skin is usually numb from the mastectomy surgery, a

woman may not experience pain from the placement of the tissue expander. However, she may feel pressure or discomfort after each filling of the expander, which subsides as the tissue expands. Tissue expansion typically takes four to six months.

Once the skin has expanded sufficiently, the plastic surgeon performs a second surgery to remove the tissue expander and place the permanent breast implant into the pocket. The surgery to replace the tissue expander with a breast implant is usually done with general anesthesia in an operating room. It may require a brief hospital stay or be done on an outpatient basis.

Silicone Implants

Silicone implants have a silicone rubber shell that is filled with silicone gel. Silicone implants vary in shell surface (smooth or textured), shape, profile, volume, shell thickness, and number of shell lumens. Most silicone-gel-filled implants are not adjustable.

For some years controversy has existed over silicone implants used for breast augmentation or replacement after mastectomy. Adverse effects of their use have been widely reported in the media, and conflicting information has been published in the medical literature. In the early 1990s it was reported that silicone breast implants were responsible for connective tissue diseases in some women. After a comprehensive evaluation of the evidence on health effects of silicone breast implants, the Institute of Medicine issued a statement declaring there was no definitive evidence linking breast implants to cancer, neurological diseases, neurological problems or other systemic diseases. However, the controversy and the resulting publicity prompted the FDA first to ban any use of these implants and then to permit only limited use, mainly as replacements after mastectomy. Silicone implants are not available to the general U.S. public, although they are still widely used in Europe.

However, they are still available in the United States in a few research cases: women seeking breast reconstruction or revision of an existing breast implant, women who have had breast cancer surgery, a severe injury to the breast, a birth defect that affects the breast, or a medical condition that causes a severe breast abnormality.

sarcoma of the breast A very rare type of BREAST CANCER that originates in the connective tissue. If the tissue of origin is known, it is designated by a prefix, as in *angiosarcoma, fibrosarcoma,* or *liposarcoma.* In contrast to carcinomas, sarcomas typically spread through the bloodstream, not the lymphatic system. Sarcomas of the breast are usually oval, round, or lobular on MAMMOGRAPHY. On ULTRASOUND, sarcomas are usually clearly outlined, lesions that may have cystlike spaces.

secondary bone cancer Cancer in the bone that has spread from the breast or other cancer sites. This is also called a METASTASIS or recurrence of BREAST CANCER.

The bone is the most common site of secondary cancer from the breast; those areas most commonly affected are the spine, skull, pelvis, hipbones, and upper bones of the arms and legs.

Bone contains two types of living cells—*osteoclasts,* which destroy and remove small amounts of old bone, and *osteoblasts,* which help build up new bone. In secondary bone cancer, the cancer cells that have spread to the bone produce chemicals that prompt the osteoclasts to become overactive and destroy more bone than can be replaced. This process can lead to some of the symptoms of secondary bone cancer.

Symptoms

Secondary bone cancer can cause a number of symptoms, including pain, presence of calcium in the blood, fractures, or anemia.

Pain Pain in the affected bone can range from mild to severe. Some bone pain may cause a dull ache over the affected area or a burning or stabbing pain that may be either persistent or worse at night. Certain movements may affect the pain, and there may be tenderness at the site. Bone pain can almost always be relieved or controlled, and a number of effective pain relievers are available. A mild painkiller such as a nonsteroidal anti-inflammatory drug (for example, ibuprofen) may be tried first. If this is not enough to relieve the pain, a stronger painkiller such as hydrocodeine may be used. In cases in which pain is severe, a morphine-based drug is often prescribed. Sometimes a combination of drugs may be needed. Patients should take these medications at specified times rather than wait until the pain is unbearable.

In some cases, these drugs may not control the pain fully. The patient may need to be admitted to a hospital or into a hospice for an assessment by a palliative-care pain team.

Hypercalcemia Sometimes, secondary bone cancer can alter the bone structure so that calcium is released into the bloodstream. If the calcium level is too high, it may cause nausea, vomiting, constipation, or drowsiness. In more severe cases, a woman may be very thirsty, weak, or confused. Symptoms can be relieved by drinking plenty of water or having intravenous (IV) fluids to flush the calcium out of the body. Bisphosphonates such as Aredia is used to treat severe hypercalcemia, and can prevent it in women with bone metastases.

Fractures Secondary bone cancer may weaken the bone, thereby increasing the risk of fracture. Radiation treatment can help prevent a weak bone from fracturing. Alternatively, an orthopedic surgeon can try to prevent fractures by securing the bone with a metal screw or plate or replacing a joint. The implants that are used are designed to last indefinitely.

If a bone has already fractured, the orthopedic surgeon tries to repair the fracture by using a metal screw or pin or joint replacement. In rare cases, a whole section of bone can be replaced (endoprosthesis).

If an area of vertebra fractures or collapses, it can cause pressure on the spinal cord that may require emergency surgery. If the symptoms appear gradually, radiation treatment may be recommended first. With either treatment, steroids are given to help reduce inflammation. Sometimes a combination of all three treatments may be used.

Anemia In rare cases, the secondary breast cancer cells may invade the bone marrow, where blood cells are made. This may lower the level of white cells, platelets, and red cells, causing anemia, bleeding tendencies and risk of infection. A bone marrow test may be needed to make this diagnosis.

Diagnosis

Secondary bone cancer can be diagnosed with X-rays or a BONE SCAN that can detect small areas of breast cancer cells that have migrated to the bones.

Bone X-ray A bone X-ray can reveal certain changes in the bone, although it may not identify small areas of secondary bone cancers.

Bone scan A bone scan is a more sensitive test than an X-ray and can highlight any abnormal areas of bone more clearly. A bone scan reveals the entire skeleton, whereas X-rays highlight only one particular area. A small amount of a weak, harmless radioactive substance is injected into a patient's vein a few hours before the scan. Any areas of bone cancer show up as an increased uptake of the radioactive substance in the affected area. A scan is not painful, but the patient must lie flat and still for about half an hour. It is important to remember that people who have other bone conditions such as osteoporosis and arthritis also may have abnormal bone scan findings without having secondary bone cancer. For this reason, abnormal areas need to be looked at with plain X-rays as well.

Magnetic resonance imaging (MRI) This scan uses magnetism instead of X-rays to provide a detailed picture of an area of bone. As with a bone scan, the MRI is not painful, but it does require patients to lie flat and still.

Treatment

Secondary bone cancer can be treated and pain eased, but the cancer cannot be cured. The aim is to relieve symptoms and improve a woman's quality of life by controlling the growth of the cancer. Treatments may include hormone therapy, chemotherapy, radiation therapy, or surgery, either alone or in combination. The treatment offered depends on a number of factors, including symptoms, extent of the cancer spread in the bones, whether a woman is postmenopausal, the type of breast tumor, and the woman's general health.

Hormone therapy This may be the first choice of treatment for secondary bone cancer. A number of hormone therapies are available; the drugs most commonly used first are the AROMATASE INHIBITORS or TAMOXIFEN. Women who are already taking tamoxifen when they have secondary bone cancer may be given aromatase inhibitors. This treatment is only effective if the cancer has estrogen or progesterone inhibitors.

Chemotherapy If the secondary bone cancer does not respond to hormone treatment or has stopped responding to it, chemotherapy drugs may be tried next. These may be given alone or in combination. Secondary bone cancer can be slow to respond to chemotherapy, however, and a woman may need several weeks or months of therapy before any benefit can be seen.

Radiation therapy The aim of radiation treatment is to improve quality of life by improving mobility, decreasing pain, and preventing possible fractures. Radiation therapy for secondary bone cancer can be given in a single dose, or in divided doses over a few days to weeks, so side effects will be mild.

Radiation therapy may also be given internally, by injecting a radioisotope into a vein. The radioisotope travels through the bloodstream and delivers radiotherapy to the bones affected by the cancer cells. It is sometimes useful when the secondary cancer is widespread, although it is not commonly used for secondary bone cancer from the breast.

Bisphosphonates These drugs target the parts of the skeleton where there is high bone turnover. Although they do not treat the cancer directly, they may help reduce the breakdown of the bone by restricting the action of the osteoclasts. When given to women with secondary bone cancer, they help decrease pain and reduce risk of fractures, and need for surgery or radiation. They also reduce the risk of hypercalcemia.

secondary brain tumor Cancer in the brain that has spread from a different primary site such as the breast. This also may be described as a metastasis or recurrence of BREAST CANCER in the brain.

Symptoms

Symptoms that breast cancer has spread to the brain depend on the area of the brain affected. Women who have this condition may have some of these symptoms, but it is unlikely they would experience all of them.

The most common symptom of secondary brain cancer is a headache different from other headaches. It is generally worse in the morning, gradually receding during the day, or it may be continuous and worsen over time. The headache may occur with NAUSEA, vomiting, or FATIGUE. Other possible symptoms include general weakness or weakness down one side of the body, unsteadiness, seizures, or double vision. Less common symptoms include behavior changes, confusion, and speech problems. Although these symptoms can begin suddenly, they more typically develop slowly.

Diagnosis

During a physical exam, the physician may check the eyes for swelling caused by pressure from the brain; examine the arms and legs for changes in sensation, strength, and changes in reflexes; and may look at the woman's balance and walking ability.

Radiologic tests include MRIs or CAT scans. A MAGNETIC RESONANCE IMAGING (MRI) scan uses magnetic waves instead of X-rays and is an effective way of diagnosing brain tumors. On rare occasions BIOPSY of the tumor to confirm the diagnosis may be necessary.

Treatment

Breast cancer that has spread to the brain cannot be cured, so any treatment tries to control the symptoms to improve quality of life. Treatments may include RADIATION THERAPY, administration of steroid drugs, surgery, or, in some cases, CHEMOTHERAPY.

Radiation This is the most commonly used treatment for secondary brain cancer. It is given in daily doses over about five days. Fatigue is a common side effect of radiation therapy, especially radiation therapy given to the brain. Hair loss is another common side effect. If a brain cancer recurs as a single dominant area, stereotactic radiosurgery (a very localized type of radiation) sometimes may be used.

Steroids Steroid drugs are used to reduce the inflammation and pressure around the brain tumor and can relieve symptoms such as headache and nausea. They are often prescribed before any investigations to confirm the diagnosis of a secondary brain tumor.

Steroids for secondary brain cancer are given in high doses at first and can usually be reduced once other treatments such as radiation therapy are given. Some of the more common side effects of steroids in high doses are indigestion, thrush in the mouth, increased appetite and weight gain, muscle weakness, and sleeplessness.

Surgery Surgery is rarely possible for secondary brain cancer, since there are usually a number of small tumors rather than a single area that can be removed. If surgery is an option, the doctor and the patient should consider the patient's general health and fitness in deciding whether the procedure would improve her quality of life.

Chemotherapy While chemotherapy is not usually used to treat cancer in the brain, some drugs are able to penetrate brain tissue and shrink cancers. The ability of drugs to get into the brain is increased after radiation, so these agents may be used when a secondary brain cancer recurs.

secondary liver cancer A type of cancer that occurs when malignant cells spread from the breast (or another primary site) through the bloodstream and settle in the liver. It also may be called liver metastasis or a recurrence of BREAST CANCER. The cells that have settled in the liver are breast cancer cells; this condition is not the same as cancer that originates in the liver.

The liver is a very important organ in the body, made up of different sections called lobes and surrounded by a capsule. It is in the right upper abdomen, near several other organs, including the bowel, the diaphragm, and the right kidney. The liver converts food into heat and energy, stores glucose and vitamins, and produces bile to help digest food. The liver also breaks down harmful substances such as alcohol and drugs and produces important proteins needed to help blood clot. Because the liver is a large organ, it may be able to keep working even if part is affected by cancer.

Symptoms

Secondary liver cancer may not cause any symptoms, or it may cause a number of problems such as weakness, APPETITE LOSS, NAUSEA, hiccups, ascites, pain, or jaundice.

Pain Secondary liver cancer can stimulate the liver to grow, stretching its capsule and causing mild discomfort or pain under the ribs or in the right shoulder. The enlarged liver may also press on the nerves that lead to the right shoulder, causing referred pain there. It can usually be helped with painkillers such as anti-inflammatory drugs (for example, ibuprofen). Liver pain also responds well to morphine-based drugs. Sometimes steroid drugs can help reduce swelling around the liver, reducing pain. In some cases radiotherapy or chemotherapy may be used to help relieve pain by shrinking the enlarged liver.

Nausea A woman may feel nausea because the enlarged liver puts pressure on the stomach or because toxins are building up in the body from liver damage. Some women lose their appetite as a result of the nausea, which may trigger weight loss. The best way the symptoms is to treat the cancer itself with chemotherapy or hormone therapy.

Hiccups Hiccups may occur as the enlarged liver presses on the diaphragm, triggering spasms. Women may find that sitting upright and drinking small amounts frequently are helpful.

Ascites This buildup of abdominal fluid can occur if the blood or lymphatic flow through the liver is blocked, causing bloating that may make a woman feel uncomfortable and sometimes breathless. This bloating develops over weeks or months. Diuretics may help reduce the amount of fluid in the abdomen, but insertion of a drain into the abdomen to remove the extra fluid (paracentesis) may be necessary. It is usually done with local anesthesia and can be repeated if the fluid builds up again.

Fatigue Many women find that they tire more easily; it may be possible to treat the cause of the tiredness. In some cases, steroid drugs can help to boost energy levels.

Jaundice Jaundice can occur when the bile duct becomes blocked, tinting the skin and the whites of the eyes yellow. In some cases, urine may become darker and stools may become pale. Patients may need to have a stent inserted into the bile duct to drain the bile. Jaundice can cause itching, which may be worse at night. Alcohol can make the itching worse, as can soaps and heavily perfumed products. Antihistamine tablets or cream may help.

Diagnosis

Because secondary liver cancer causes an enlarged liver, the doctor may be able to feel it on examina-

tion. Next, blood tests may be ordered, since damaged liver cells release certain substances that can be detected in the blood. Blood tests can measure these substances and may also help to show how effective any treatment has been.

In most cases a specialist can tell whether the cancer cells in the liver are from the breast. If there is any doubt, a small piece of tissue from the liver is biopsied.

An ultrasound, magnetic resonance imaging (MRI), or CT scan can reveal any abnormalities of the liver.

Treatment

Secondary liver cancer can be treated, although it cannot be cured. The aim is to relieve the patient's symptoms and improve quality of life by slowing the growth of the cancer. Treatments may include chemotherapy, hormone therapy, or rarely, radiation therapy.

Chemotherapy CHEMOTHERAPY is the first choice for treatment of breast cancer when it has spread to the liver. There are many possible drugs and excellent responses are often seen.

Hormone therapies Hormone therapies are typically used to treat breast cancers that are sensitive to estrogen (estrogen receptor positive). If a woman was already taking a hormone drug such as TAMOXIFEN when secondary liver cancer developed, she might be given a different hormone drug.

Monoclonal antibodies These new drugs are used to treat secondary breast cancer. When the cancer expresses the H_2N antigen. Only about 20 percent of breast cancers have this antigen, but when it is present HERCEPTIN alone or in combination with chemotherapy can be very helpful.

secondary lung cancer A type of cancer that occurs when malignant cells spread from the breast (or another primary site) through the bloodstream and settle in the lungs. This type of spread may also be described as a metastasis or a recurrence of breast cancer. The cells in the lungs are BREAST CANCER cells, not primary lung cancer cells.

Symptoms

Secondary lung cancer may cause a number of different symptoms ranging from mild to severe, depending on how advanced the metastases are. They may include shortness of breath, cough, pain, pleural effusion, APPETITE LOSS, weight loss, and FATIGUE.

The most common symptom of secondary lung cancer are shortness of breath (dyspnea). Relaxation techniques can be very helpful in easing breathing, and medicines such as morphine can help ease the feeling of breathlessness and the anxiety that it can cause. If the tumor narrows or blocks the bronchial tubes, a bronchodilator such as albuterol sulfate (Ventolin) can be given through either an inhaler or a nebulizer. If the tumor causes swelling or inflammation, steroid drugs such as dexamethasone or prednisolone can help.

A cough is another common symptom that may be caused by an infection or by the cancer itself. Cough medicine may control coughing and loosen phlegm; breathing salt water through a nebulizer can also loosen the phlegm, making it easier to expel. If the cough is very difficult to control, a medication such as morphine may help.

The tumor or excessive coughing also may cause pain in the chest, shoulder, or back area. Painkillers may be used.

Another cause of shortness of breath is *pleural effusion*, which is a buildup of extra fluid around the lung, causing breathlessness. This can be treated by drawing off the extra fluid; drugs also can be injected to stop the fluid from building up.

Appetite or weight loss may occur because of the cancer, symptoms, or the side effects of treatment. Nutritional supplements such as high-calorie drinks may help. Secondary lung cancer also may cause fatigue.

Diagnosis

A chest X-ray is usually the first test ordered if secondary lung cancer is suspected. However, if a tumor is small, it may not always show up on an X-ray. If the X-rays are not clear, patients may need a CT scan.

If the diagnosis is still uncertain, the doctor may order a BIOPSY of the lungs. With local anesthesia, a tube is inserted through the mouth and down into the lungs so that a small piece of lung tissue can be removed.

Treatment

Secondary lung cancer can be treated, although it cannot be cured. The aim is to ease symptoms and improve quality of life by slowing or shrinking the cancer. Treatments may include chemotherapy, hormone therapy, and radiotherapy, either alone or in combination.

secondary tumor   A tumor that develops when cancer cells spread beyond their original site.

See also SECONDARY BONE CANCER; SECONDARY BRAIN CANCER; SECONDARY LIVER CANCER; SECONDARY LUNG CANCER.

selective estrogen-receptor modulators (SERMs) A group of drugs that cause estrogenlike responses in certain tissues while preventing estrogenlike responses in other parts of the body. Specifically, SERMs block the actions of ESTROGEN in breast tissues and certain other tissues by occupying the estrogen receptors on cells. When a SERM is in the estrogen receptor, there is no place for the real estrogen to attach. Although the SERM fits in the estrogen receptor, it does not send messages to the cell nucleus to grow and divide. Three of the best-known SERMs are TAMOXIFEN (Nolvadex), raloxifene (Evista), and toremifene (Fareston).

However, SERMs do send estrogenlike signals when they attach to bone cells, liver cells, and elsewhere in the body; therefore, SERMs seem to help prevent or slow osteoporosis in postmenopausal women and may help lower cholesterol level. This dual effect—blocking estrogen in some places and imitating estrogen in other places—allows SERMs to have multiple beneficial effects in many women who have breast cancer.

Tamoxifen

Tamoxifen has been used for more than 20 years and was the first of the SERM antiestrogen medications available. In appropriately selected cases, it is a powerful weapon against breast cancer. Many large studies show that tamoxifen can reduce the probability of cancer recurrence, progression, or development for women who have many risk factors. Side effects include hot flashes, vaginal dryness or discharge, irregular periods, nausea, and leg cramps. Rare side effects include blood clots and an increased risk of ENDOMETRIAL CANCER. Tamoxifen may be recommended for both pre- and post-menopausal women at all stages of disease.

Toremifene

This relatively new antiestrogen SERM has properties and side effects similar to those of tamoxifen, but unlike tamoxifen, toremifene does not seem to increase the risk of endometrial cancer. On the basis of research available to date, the U.S. Food and Drug Administration (FDA) has restricted the use of toremifene to postmenopausal women whose breast cancer has spread.

Raloxifene

The antiestrogen SERM medication raloxifene strengthens bones and is FDA-approved for osteoporosis treating or preventing in postmenopausal women. Raloxifene was found to lower the risk of breast cancer in these women who have osteoporosis, but testing has not been completed on women with breast cancer. So far, only tamoxifen has been approved by the FDA for treatment of breast cancer and reduction of breast cancer risk in women at high risk. The Study of Tamoxifen and Raloxifene (STAR) is now comparing tamoxifen to raloxifene for breast cancer prevention in high-risk women.

Side effects are similar to those of tamoxifen, including hot flashes, vaginal changes, and, rarely, blood clots, stroke, and pulmonary embolism. Raloxifene does not seem to increase the risk of endometrial cancer.

sentinel node The first LYMPH NODE that filters fluid coming from the breast, and the first place to which BREAST CANCER cells are likely to spread. In some cases, there can be more than one sentinel node.

In breast cancer, the sentinel node is usually located in the axillary nodes (the group of lymph nodes under the arm); however, in a small percentage of cases, the sentinel node is found elsewhere in the lymphatic system of the breast.

See also SENTINEL-NODE BIOPSY.

sentinel-node biopsy A new surgical technique used for BREAST CANCER that is an alternative to standard axillary lymph-node dissection, sparing many women more invasive surgery and side effects. However, the sentinel-node procedure is not appropriate for everyone. It has limitations and drawbacks and must be performed by a surgeon who has significant experience with the technique.

The "sentinel" lymph node is the first node that filters fluid from the breast. If cancer cells are breaking away from a tumor and traveling away from the breast, the sentinel node is more likely than other lymph nodes to contain cancerous cells. In some cases there is more than one sentinel node.

Instead of removing 10 or more lymph nodes and analyzing all of them to look for cancer, as a surgeon does during a standard axillary-node dissection, a sentinel-node biopsy procedure removes only the single node most likely to have malignant cells. If this node has no malignant cells, chances are the other nodes have not been affected. (In practice, the surgeon usually removes a cluster of two or three nodes—the sentinel node and those closest to it—during a sentinel-node biopsy.)

Sentinel-node dissection is a good option for women who have early-stage invasive breast cancer who have a low to moderate risk of lymph-node involvement. In these women, it is critical to find out whether the cancer has moved beyond the breast.

However, a sentinel-node biopsy is not warranted if the surgeon has good reason to believe that a woman's lymph nodes are involved; in this case, a standard axillary lymph-node dissection with removal of multiple nodes makes most sense. This is because the surgeon does not want to miss a significant amount of cancer that may be in the nodes. If the lymph nodes are involved, it is also important to know how many nodes are involved, because researchers have found that the more nodes that are involved, the more serious the disease and the more aggressive treatment should be.

In general, sentinel-node dissection is *not* appropriate for the following women:

• Anyone who is likely to have cancer in the lymph nodes

- Women with any prior surgery or treatment that could have altered the normal pattern of lymph drainage
- Women who had chemotherapy before surgery to reduce the size of a large cancer or to treat many involved lymph nodes (lymphatic flow may be altered by the inflammation and scar tissue that occur as the body and the chemotherapy battle the tumor)
- Women with large, multifocal, or inflammatory breast cancer

In the operating room, the surgeon injects a radioactive liquid, a blue dye, or both into the area around the tumor and then watches to see where the dye travels and seems to concentrate. This injection can be painful, but the burning lasts for only a few minutes.

The process illuminates the pathway by which the lymph travels when it drains away from the part of the breast with the tumor, indicating which lymph node is the "sentinel node" for a particular tumor. If a radioactive substance is used, the doctor locates the radioactive substance in these sentinel nodes with a scanner. The surgeon makes a small incision and removes only the nodes with radioactive substance or blue dye.

After the sentinel node and one or two nodes closest to it are removed, the surgeon looks at them and feels them in the operating room to see whether they seem to be affected by cancer. Next, the nodes are sent to the pathology lab for analysis under a microscope.

If the sentinel node does *not* show any cancer, probably no other axillary lymph nodes contain cancer; that means that the chance is good that the cancer has not spread beyond the breast. Treatment decisions can be made with this important information in mind.

If the sentinel node *does* contain cancer, another treatment step may be needed. During surgery, if a surgeon suspects that the sentinel node just removed is affected by cancer, he or she may decide to remove more nodes for evaluation (an axillary dissection) during the same operation. If the laboratory finds significant cancer present in the sentinel node (or nodes) after surgery, the surgeon may recommend another operation (an axillary

dissection) to remove and analyze more lymph nodes from the armpit.

Alternatively, the medical team may recommend radiation treatment of surrounding lymph nodes as the best way to treat cancer that may have spread there. The need for additional treatment (surgery, radiation, or both) if the sentinel node is involved represents a key limitation of the sentinel lymph-node approach. For this reason, many doctors favor the traditional lymph-node approach.

When a surgeon has to remove only one lymph node or a small cluster of two or three nodes to know whether breast cancer has spread, the other lymph nodes remain intact. This prevents uncomfortable temporary side effects, such as lymph backup in the armpit, which often occurs after traditional lymph-node removal. Traditional surgery also can cause other lingering side effects, including discomfort and numbness in the armpit and the upper arm and swelling of the arm on the side of the affected breast (LYMPHEDEMA). Finally, the more surgery a woman has in the breast and armpit area, the more potential for numbness, heightened sensitivity, and discomfort.

If sentinel lymph-node biopsy proves to be as effective as the standard axillary lymph-node dissection, the new procedure could decrease the risk of lymphedema.

Some surgeons already perform sentinel-node biopsies in patients who have breast cancer, although it is still considered an investigational procedure. The concept of mapping the sentinel node was first reported in 1977 by a researcher who was studying cancer of the penis. The technique was later used to study drainage patterns of melanoma and was first reported for breast cancer in 1993. Since then, researchers have improved methods for finding the sentinel node, and several studies have shown that when the sentinel node finding is negative, the remaining node findings are also negative in a majority of cases. These studies were done in a small number of centers and overall survival rate was not examined in these trials.

Side effects of sentinel-node biopsy can include minor pain or bruising at the biopsy site and the rare possibility of an allergic reaction to the blue dye used in finding the sentinel node. Some women experience POSTMASTECTOMY PAIN SYNDROME caused by temporary nerve damage in the area where the dye was injected.

shift work   Working nights may increase a woman's risk of BREAST CANCER, according to two recent studies. Experts caution that women who work nights do not need to change jobs, but they should follow the same precautions advised for all women, including having regular breast cancer screenings.

The larger of the two studies concluded that nurses who worked rotating night shifts for 30 years or more had a 36 percent higher risk of breast cancer than those who did not work nights. This study used data from more than 78,000 women in the long-term national NURSES' HEALTH STUDY, which is based at Harvard Medical School. The other study, by researchers at the University of Washington and the University of Connecticut, looked at the effect of sleep habits and bedroom lighting on breast cancer. Two groups of women were found more likely than others to have breast cancer: women who often did not sleep in the middle of the night (specifically, between 1 A.M. and 2 A.M.) and women who worked from 11 P.M. to 7 A.M. This study was much smaller, with about 1,400 participants.

The conclusions are consistent with those of earlier small studies that show a pattern of more breast cancers among women who work nights. Researchers believe the link is related to the supply of melatonin, a hormone that helps to regulate the body's natural clock. Melatonin also prevents tumor growth, and light exposure during night work reduces melatonin production.

A 1999 Finnish study of breast cancer risk among visually impaired women also indirectly supports this idea. Women who are completely blind have a higher-than-average production of melatonin, and they are only half as likely as sighted women to have breast cancer.

In the Nurses' Health Study, women were asked how many years they had worked rotating shifts that included at least three night shifts per month. Only among women who worked 30 years or more of such shifts did the researchers find an increased risk that was too high to be explained by chance. Because the nurses were not asked whether they had worked permanent night shifts, researchers do not know to what extent permanent night work might affect breast cancer risk. One theory hypothesizes that the body may be able to adapt to permanent night work, but the overall melatonin level should be lower, exposing the worker to some risks.

Although the number of jobs requiring night work is increasing, the number of women working many years of such shifts is not high enough to produce a significant public health concern. Experts suggest that women who work nights and are concerned about breast cancer risk should make a point of controlling whatever risk factors they can, such as by drinking alcohol moderately (not more than one drink a day), maintaining reasonable weight, getting lots of exercise, and not using birth-control pills or hormone-replacement therapy for long periods. Women are also advised to have regular screenings for breast cancer.

silicone breast implants and cancer   There is no association between breast implants and subsequent risk of BREAST CANCER, according to one of the largest studies on the long-term health effects of silicone breast implants. Breast implants first appeared on the market in 1962, but since the beginning there have been a number of reports of connective-tissue disorders and cancers among implant patients. In 1992, because of the lack of sufficient evidence on the long-term safety of implants, the U.S. Food and Drug Administration restricted the use of silicone breast implants to women who were seeking breast reconstruction in controlled clinical trials, and Congress directed the National Institutes of Health to undertake a large follow-up study to evaluate the long-term health effects of the implants.

Researchers from the NATIONAL CANCER INSTITUTE reported that after the first part of the analysis, scientists found no change in breast cancer risk among women followed for more than 10 years. However, the results do not confirm the findings, from several other studies, that exposure to implants reduces a woman's risk for breast cancer. This finding may relate to the longer follow-up in this study than in most others.

This study did not assess women who were undergoing breast reconstruction after breast cancer surgery, so predicting whether similar results would be found for this population is not possible.

The majority of the previous studies have also focused on women who received implants for cosmetic reasons. It is estimated that between 1.5 million and 2 million U.S. women have had breast implants since they first appeared on the market. Future analyses of the data will evaluate the risk of other cancers, connective-tissue disorders, and causes of death.

Sisters Network, Inc.   The first national BREAST CANCER survivors support group organized for African-American women. Services include community education and awareness programs, person-to-person support, a speaker bureau, and a national newsletter. Sisters Network is committed to increasing local and national attention to the devastating impact of breast cancer in the African-American community. It has more than 2,000 members. For contact information, see Appendix I.

smokers, teenage girl   Teen girls almost double their risk of BREAST CANCER if they start smoking within five years of their first menstrual period, according to a Canadian study. Even if they quit in their early 20s, the damage may already be done.

There is a critical period in which adolescent girls have an increased susceptibility to cancer-causing agents that have the breast as the target. In the study, Canadian scientists interviewed 318 premenopausal women and 700 postmenopausal women who had been treated for breast cancer and compared them with a control group of women who had not had the disease. Women who started smoking regularly within five years of starting their periods were 70 percent more likely to have breast cancer before age 50 than nonsmokers.

Although there is never a "good" time to start smoking, for women the five years after they have their first menstrual period is the most dangerous. The theory is that during puberty, the cells that make up the breast are developing so rapidly they are more susceptible to damage caused by the carcinogens in tobacco smoke.

smoking and breast cancer   Tobacco is highly addictive and has been linked to 20 percent of all deaths in the United States because of its cancer-causing chemicals and the corrosive effect of ciga-

rette smoke on the lungs. Although most experts believe that tobacco smoking has little or no association with breast cancer risk, newer studies have challenged this conclusion. More investigation is needed to resolve these issues.

Understanding the potential association of active and passive smoking with breast cancer risk is important, because unlike the case with many other breast cancer risk factors, women have some control over their exposure to tobacco smoke.

Four small studies compared women who smoked to women who had no exposure to tobacco smoke (they had neither smoked nor ever been passively exposed to tobacco smoke). Three of the studies reported that smokers had a statistically significant increased breast cancer risk of two to four times that of the other women.

However, this is an area of research with considerable controversy. A recent review of these studies by the International Agency for Research on Cancer (IARC) dismissed a linkage between smoking and breast cancer risk. Because a large number of women smoke or have smoked, final answers to this question are important.

Regarding passive exposure to tobacco smoke, most, but not all, studies have reported an association between passive smoking and breast cancer. Only two of these studies showed a *dose relationship*, in which an increase in breast cancer risk was related to an increase in tobacco-smoke exposure. Other studies, which compared the risk of breast cancer among women exposed to passive smoke to that of women whose passive-smoke exposure was less clearly defined (nonsmokers or those who have never smoked), have had conflicting results. Some studies reported increases in risk for passive smokers, some reported decreases in risk, and some reported no association with risk. All of these studies were also recently reviewed by the IARC. The agency found that it was unlikely that passive smoking increased breast cancer risk.

The tobacco smoke that a smoker inhales is different from the smoke inhaled by those nearby. The major source of passive smoke is the burning of the cigarette rather than what is exhaled by smokers. Both types of smoke contain thousands of similar chemicals, although the concentrations of the chemicals are different. Toxic chemicals are found in higher concentrations in tobacco smoke leaving the cigarette than in inhaled smoke; in some cases, the concentrations are far higher. Smoke that leaves the cigarette is largely produced from the lower-temperature burning of cigarettes between inhalations, and the chemicals are less degraded than in the smokers' inhalations. However, many factors, such as room size and air flow, can affect the dilution of the smoke, and the resulting exposure can differ greatly.

Passive exposure to tobacco smoke is very common. The most recent studies of the number of nonsmokers in the United States who are exposed to tobacco smoke were conducted in 1991. These studies used a breakdown product of nicotine, cotinine, in the blood of nonsmokers as a marker for tobacco smoke exposure. They reported that 90 percent of nonsmokers older than age four had measurable levels of cotinine. Because of changes in smoking policies since 1991, the prevalence of environmental tobacco smoke exposure may have decreased. Measurements made in 1999 of the typical levels of this marker in nonsmokers' blood indicated that levels substantially lower than those reported in 1991. Because the typical levels of cotinine have decreased, it is also likely that a smaller percentage of people have detectable levels.

How Smoke Affects the Breast

It is biologically possible for active cigarette smoking or passive exposure to tobacco smoke to affect a woman's breast cancer risk. There is direct documentation that breasts of active smokers are exposed to chemicals within tobacco smoke. Among women who smoke, study of breast fluid, found in the ducts, has shown the presence of tobacco chemicals at higher concentrations than were found in blood. Women passively exposed to tobacco smoke have tobacco chemicals in their blood, too, but examinations of their breast fluid have not been carried out.

Exposure to tobacco smoke at a young age, either by smoking or by being around people who smoke, may be related to an increased breast cancer risk. Sixteen studies have compared women who smoked at a young age to women who had never smoked or who were not current smokers. Most studies reported a small increase in breast cancer risk associated with starting smoking before

age 17. Two studies found about a doubling of breast cancer risk among women who smoked at a young age; one of the studies reported this effect only for premenopausal breast cancer.

The association of exposure to passive smoke at a young age with breast cancer risk has been examined in five studies. These studies typically looked at exposure up to age 19. Four of these studies, which used women with no exposure to tobacco smoke as controls, reported approximately a doubling of breast cancer risk among women who were exposed to passive smoke. The remaining study used women who never smoked as the comparison and found no association between tobacco smoke exposure and breast cancer risk.

The breast undergoes a major period of development during adolescence, and studies in animals have demonstrated that this is a period of great susceptibility to cancer-causing agents.

Increases in breast cancer risk were linked, in several studies, to the amount of time a woman has smoked or the number of cigarettes she smoked a day. However, the relationship between breast cancer and the level of smoking exposure is not as clear as it is for lung cancer. People who smoke the least (or for the shortest time) have the lowest risk of lung cancer; people who smoke the most (or for the longest time) have the highest risk. People who smoke amounts between these two extremes have risks that fall between the two extremes.

Most breast cancer studies have not seen a dose relationship between smoking and breast cancer risk. It could be that a woman would have to exceed a certain exposure level for risk to increase.

The clarity of these studies' results is also affected by the very complicated relationship between tobacco smoke exposure and breast cancer risk, which could support associations with either increased or decreased risk. On one hand, tobacco smoke contains chemicals that can cause breast cancer in animals and could thus be associated with an increase in breast cancer risk. On the other hand, smoking has been shown to have many effects that counter the effects of estrogen, which could decrease breast cancer risk.

Quitting smoking, therefore, may lead to a temporary increase in the risk of breast cancer. Most of the studies that have examined the breast cancer risk of women who have quit smoking have supported this finding. In many of these studies, breast cancer risk was highest shortly after the women stopped smoking and gradually decreased over five to 20 years, depending on the study. The interplay between the effects of the cancer-causing chemicals and the apparent opposition of estrogen is critical to breast cancer risk. The nature of this interplay is poorly understood.

The increase in breast cancer risk associated with quitting smoking should be considered in the context of overall health. After quitting smoking, a woman's risk of breast cancer temporarily increases by 25 to 450 percent (depending on the study examined). This increase is in sharp contrast to the high risks for other health problems associated with continued smoking. For example, there is a well-established 1,000 to 2,000 percent increase in lung cancer risk associated with smoking. Without question, the effects of quitting smoking on overall health are beneficial.

Marijuana Smoking and Breast Cancer

The relationship between smoking marijuana and breast cancer risk has not been studied. However, marijuana smoke has been shown to contain many of the toxic substances found in tobacco smoke. Unfortunately, there have not been enough studies to evaluate a possible link of marijuana smoking with breast cancer.

Smoking and Breast Cancer Survival Rate

The effect of smoking on the survival rate of women who have breast cancer is unclear. Some studies have reported an association between smoking and an increase in the risk of death; others found no association with the risk of death of breast cancer. Smokers may be at increased risk for the spread of cancer. Two studies have reported an increase in the spread of tumors from the breast to the lungs in women who smoked. The survival rate of women with breast cancer who stopped smoking has been examined in one study. Their survival rate was found to be similar to that of women with breast cancer who never smoked.

Experts believe that quitting smoking and avoiding passive exposure to tobacco smoke make good sense. Although it is unclear whether smok-

ing and passive exposure to tobacco smoke are associated with breast cancer risk, women can control their exposure to these potential risk factors. There are also many other health benefits to be gained by decreasing or eliminating either of these exposures.

Quitting smoking is difficult, but a number of drug and behavioral programs have been shown to increase the likelihood of success. Quitting smoking not only makes one ultimately feel better, but decreases the risk of many diseases, including heart disease, stroke, many respiratory diseases, and cancer.

The effects of passive exposure to tobacco smoke are just beginning to be understood. Until more is known, decreasing exposure is desirable. Minimizing tobacco smoke exposure is particularly important for children, who appear to be more sensitive to its toxic effects.

See also SMOKERS, TEENAGE GIRL.

Social Security Disability Insurance (SSDI) A government social program that pays benefits to a person who is insured, meaning that the person has worked long enough to be eligible and paid Social Security taxes. If a person becomes disabled and expects the condition to continue for at least six months, he or she may be eligible for SSDI. Often the government accepts as a disability cancer that has spread (such as metastatic BREAST CANCER).

soy products Foods (such as tofu and miso) that contain proteins and substances called ISOFLAVONES. Isoflavones may provide certain health benefits, including relief from symptoms of menopause and reduced risk of heart disease and bone loss. Studies show that the risk of BREAST CANCER is six times higher for American women than for women who live in Asian countries, where soy foods are commonly eaten. However, the effects of soy on cancer are not fully understood, especially on cancer fueled by ESTROGEN. So, right now it is impossible to say whether soy prevents or promotes breast cancer.

Current advice for eating soy ranges from eating none to eating soy foods (not soy pills and powder) several times a week as a low-fat replacement for animal protein. Patients should seek medical advice regarding soy for their individual needs. Soy can be obtained by eating

- Tofu (a curd made from cooked, pureed soybeans)
- Miso (a mixture of fermented soybean paste and a grain such as rice or barley)
- Dried soybeans
- Roasted soybeans or nuts (soybeans that are soaked in water and baked)
- Edamame and natto (steamed whole green beans and fermented, cooked whole beans)
- Tempeh (a combination of whole, cooked soy beans and grains cultured with an edible mold)
- Soy milk (the liquid expressed from cooked, pureed soybeans)

The ability of the body to use the nutrients in soy foods varies with the food and the way it is made. In general, soy that has been processed least (such as tofu, tempeh, and mature, green, and roasted soybeans) contains most protein and naturally occurring isoflavones. Soy germ is the source highest in isoflavones.

Isoflavones are a type of PHYTOESTROGEN, a type of naturally occurring plant estrogen that may offer women some of the benefits of estrogen without increasing the risk of breast cancer.

Isoflavones have become so popular that they are now available as diet supplements. But research on the effectiveness and safety of isoflavone supplements is contradictory. Some studies suggest that taking isoflavone supplements may help prevent breast cancer. Other studies suggest that consuming a type of isoflavone called genistein may carry some risk of actually promoting breast cancer. Soy foods have been eaten safely for centuries and can help improve cholesterol levels and promote heart health. But for now, no one knows how beneficial or safe it is to use isoflavones as a diet supplement.

S-phase   A test performed to determine how fast a tumor is growing. A high S-phase level would indicate that the tumor is aggressive. S-phase tests are sometimes used in conjunction with other lab findings to determine a prognosis and course of therapy for BREAST CANCER.

spot view   Also called a compression MAMMO-GRAM, cone view, or focal compression view, this procedure compresses a specific area of breast tissue by using a small plate or cone. The procedure allows for better tissue separation and better visualization of the area in question.

A spot compression view can reveal the borders of an abnormality or questionable area better than standard mammography views. Some areas that look unusual on standard MAMMOGRAPHY images are often revealed as completely normal tissue on spot views. In addition, true abnormalities usually appear more prominently.

staging   A medical attempt to find out whether a patient's BREAST CANCER has spread and, if so, to what parts of the body. A doctor stages cancer by studying information obtained during the physical exam, surgery, X-rays and other imaging procedures, and lab tests. Knowing the stage of the disease helps the doctor plan treatment.

Typically, breast cancer stages are numbered from I through IV (IV is the most severe); Roman numerals also are divided into subcategories.

STAR   See STUDY OF TAMOXIFEN AND RALOXIFENE.

statistics in cancer   There are more than 200,000 new cases of BREAST CANCER diagnosed in men and women each year, and about 40,000 yearly deaths. Women with early stage breast cancer are not likely to die; women with stage IV metastatic cancer have an average life expectancy of 18 months.

These cancer statistics are often cited in medical stories and can be helpful for a broad perspective; they are less helpful to understanding one person's specific outlook.

For example, many people have heard that a woman's lifetime risk of development of breast cancer is one in eight. These are frightening odds for women who misinterpret that statistic to mean that at any time, at any moment, they have a one in eight chance of having breast cancer. In fact, the *actual* probability of breast cancer development changes throughout a woman's life, so that a 20-year-old woman has a *current* risk of only one in 2,500 of the disease within the next 10 years; a 50-

year-old woman has a current risk of about one in 39. Moreover, heredity, ethnicity, reproductive history, lifestyle, and other risk factors all contribute to a person's overall breast cancer risk.

Incidence

Incidence is the number of new cases of cancer in a specific population group within a set period—usually one year. Incidence rate is the number of new cases in a population. The incidence usually is expressed in terms of the number of cases per 100,000 people.

Prevalence

Prevalence is the total number of people who have breast cancer or a particular risk factor for breast cancer at a particular moment in time in the entire population. For large groups of people, prevalence is estimated by collecting information from a smaller subset of people and then extrapolating that information to the general population.

For example, by collecting DNA information from patients with breast cancer, scientists have estimated that the prevalence of the *BRCA1* gene in the total population is between 0.04 percent and 0.2 percent, meaning that many fewer women than 1 percent of the total population have this BREAST CANCER SUSCEPTIBILITY GENE.

Morbidity and Mortality

Morbidity is a state of illness. For instance, experts may comment that smoking is a major cause of morbidity in the United States. *Mortality* pertains to death. The *mortality rate* is the number of people in a population group who die of cancer within a set period (usually one year). A breast cancer mortality rate is usually expressed in terms of deaths per 100,000 people.

Prognosis

Prognosis is the prediction of the outcome of a disease, usually including the chance for recovery. Physicians may base a prognosis on statistical precedents; however, each patient's prognosis is affected by many factors, including the patient's age and general health, the type and stage of breast cancer, and the effectiveness of the particular treatment used. Therefore, although a prognosis may help explain the severity of a disorder or guide treatment decisions, it cannot be used to predict disease outcomes for an individual.

Survival Rate

Survival rate is the number of people who have breast cancer and survive over a period. Scientists commonly use five-year survival rate as the standard statistical basis for defining when breast cancer has been successfully treated.

The five-year survival rate includes anyone who is living five years after a cancer diagnosis, including those who are cured, those who are in remission, and those who still have cancer and are having treatment. The overall five-year survival rate measures everyone who has ever been diagnosed with a particular cancer equally and therefore may lead to distorted statistics. For example, a 90-year-old woman and a 30-year-old woman who have breast cancer are grouped together. The 90-year-old may die of other causes within the five-year period because of normal life expectancy, and this difference can skew the data.

A more statistically accurate view of survival is the *relative five-year survival rate,* which compares a cancer patient's survival rate with the survival rate of the general population, taking into account differences in age, gender, race, and other factors. In this case, the 30-year-old and the 90-year-old would be treated as statistically different.

Risk

Risk is the chance that an individual will contract a disease. *High-risk* is a probability of having breast cancer that is higher than the probability for the general population. For example, women whose mother and sisters have been diagnosed with breast cancer have a higher risk of development of breast cancer than women who have no breast cancer in their family.

A *risk factor* is anything that has been identified as increasing a person's chance of having a disease. It can be controllable or uncontrollable, personal or environmental. For example, risk factors for breast cancer development include having a hereditary predisposition to the disease (uncontrollable) and getting too little exercise (controllable). *Relative risk* is a measure of how much a particular risk factor increases the risk of development of a specific cancer. For example, the risk for breast cancer development increases for a woman whose mother and sister both had breast cancer. The relative risk of development of breast cancer if a woman's mother or sister has the disease is 14, meaning she has 14 times the risk of cancer of a woman without a family history.

Attributable risk is a measure of how much of the total incidence of disease is caused by that risk factor. For example, even though the relative risk of development of breast cancer for a woman who has the *BRCA1* gene is high, most cases of breast cancer are not caused by the *BRCA1* gene, since the prevalence of the *BRCA1* gene is low.

Lifetime risk is the probability of having or dying of cancer during one's lifetime. A woman has a lifetime risk of one in eight of development breast cancer, meaning that for every eight women in the population, one eventually will develop cancer.

stellate A star-shaped mass that appears on a MAMMOGRAM. It is caused by irregular growth of cells into surrounding tissue. It may be associated with a malignancy or some benign conditions.

stem cell A common cell found in BONE MARROW that, in its most primitive state, has the ability to develop into a wide variety of cells. In a recent animal study at the University of Michigan Comprehensive Cancer Center, scientists discovered tumor-inducing BREAST CANCER cells that have many of the properties of stem cells. They make copies of themselves and produce all the other kinds of cells in the original tumor. Although similar cells had been identified in human leukemia, these were the first to be found in solid tumors.

The discovery of the breast cancer stem cells could explain current treatment failures and help researchers zero in on the most dangerous cancer cells. The goal of current breast cancer treatment has been to kill as many cells within the tumor as possible. The Michigan study suggests that the current model may be targeting the wrong cells with the wrong treatments. Instead, doctors may need to develop drugs targeted at the tumor's stem cells. If there is to be a real cure for advanced breast cancer, it will be necessary to eliminate these cells.

What this means for women who have cancer is that for the first time, doctors can identify cells that

determine whether the cancer will recur or be cured.

In the study, scientists found that as few as 100 to 200 of the breast cancer stem cells, isolated from eight of nine tumors in the study, easily formed tumors in mice, while tens of thousands of the other cancer cells from the original tumor failed to do so.

stereotactic needle biopsy A new type of BIOPSY that combines standard MAMMOGRAPHY and biopsy methods with digital imaging and computer technology. The technique can pinpoint breast lumps better than ever before. Biopsies are obtained either with a hollow needle (core needle biopsy) or with a vacuum device (MAMMOTOME) biopsy.

Either is performed while the breast is compressed during mammography. The sophisticated equipment produces three-dimensional images and performs precise needle biopsies. A computer-generated grid automatically helps the radiologist pinpoint the lesion and position the biopsy needle accordingly. A needle is inserted into the lump, and a piece of tissue is removed and sent to the lab for analysis. A local anesthetic is used, and most patients can resume normal activities within hours. Biopsy results are typically available in 24 hours.

Experts recommend stereotactic biopsy for women whose mammograms show small, nonpalpable, suspicious masses or for patients who have already been treated for breast cancer and have suspicious changes in their mammogram findings. The new procedure is designed to detect abnormalities that are easily accessible and probably benign.

By removing just enough tissue for complete evaluation, stereotactic needle biopsy can eliminate the need for a more costly and extensive biopsy, such as an excisional biopsy. This can spare a previously treated women from the disfigurement that can occur during invasive biopsy of a breast that has already had surgery or radiation therapy.

stomatitis Inflammation of the soft tissues of the mouth that often occurs as a side effect of CHEMOTHERAPY and radiation therapy. Stomatitis can cause dry mouth, soreness, burning sensations, swelling, redness, and taste changes. In a patient with breast cancer, this can lead to serious problems of malnutrition, which can further lead to infections. Patients should take medication to ease symptoms and ought to avoid

- Hot, spicy food
- Highly acidic fruits and juices such as tomato or orange
- Carbonated drinks
- Salty food
- Toothpaste or mouthwash that contains salt or alcohol

Instead, patients should eat soft, unseasoned food; rinse the mouth and teeth with warm water or a rinse of baking soda and warm water; and use lip balm on lips.

stress and breast cancer The complex relationship between physical health and psychological health is not completely understood. Scientists do know that many types of stress activate the body's endocrine system, which can affect the immune system, although it has not been shown that stress-induced changes in the immune system cause breast cancer.

The relationship between BREAST CANCER and stress has received particular attention, since some studies of women who have breast cancer have shown significantly higher rates of this disease among those who experienced traumatic life events and losses within several years of their diagnosis. Although studies have shown that stress factors (such as death of a spouse, social isolation, and medical-school examinations) alter the way the immune system functions, they have not provided scientific evidence of a direct cause-and-effect relationship between these immune system changes and the development of cancer.

One area currently being studied is the effect of stress on women already diagnosed with breast cancer to discover whether stress reduction can improve the immune response and possibly slow cancer progression. Researchers are investigating this by determining whether women who have breast cancer who are in support groups have a better survival rate than those who are not in support groups.

stroma The fatty tissue and connective tissue surrounding the ducts, lobules, blood vessels, and lymphatic vessels in the breast.

Study of Tamoxifen and Raloxifene (STAR) One of the largest BREAST CANCER prevention studies ever begun, recruiting 22,000 postmenopausal women who are at least 35 years old and are at increased risk for development of breast cancer. The study will determine whether RALOXIFENE is as effective as TAMOXIFEN in reducing the risk of breast cancer in women who have not had the disease and whether the drug has benefits over tamoxifen, such as fewer side effects. As with tamoxifen, most of the side effects of raloxifene are mild or moderate, but women who take raloxifene are also at increased risk for pulmonary embolism and deep vein thrombosis.

The study also will evaluate the effects of tamoxifen and raloxifene on the incidence of INTRADUCTAL CARCINOMA IN SITU, LOBULAR CARCINOMA IN SITU, endometrial cancer, ischemic heart disease, fractures of the hip and spine, and fractures of the wrist. Finally, the study will evaluate the toxic effects of these drugs and their effect on the quality of life of participants.

Study Criteria

The study is open to postmenopausal women at increased risk for development invasive breast cancer who are at a greater risk than 1.66 percent over five years and meet one of the following criteria:

- At least 12 months since spontaneous menstrual bleeding
- Prior documented hysterectomy and bilateral salpingo-oophorectomy
- At least 55 years of age with prior hysterectomy, with or without oophorectomy
- Less than 55 years of age with a prior hysterectomy without oophorectomy or in whom status of ovaries is unknown, with documented follicle-stimulating HORMONE level demonstrating elevation in postmenopausal range
- No clinical evidence of malignancy on physical exam within 180 days
- No evidence of suspicious or malignant disease on bilateral mammogram within the past year

- No bilateral or unilateral prophylactic mastectomy
- No prior invasive breast cancer or intraductal carcinoma in situ (women with lobular carcinoma in situ are allowed to participate).

For women in the United States interested in joining the study, information on STAR is available from the NATIONAL CANCER INSTITUTE's Cancer Information Service at (800) 4-CANCER (800-422-6237); people in Canada may call the Canadian Cancer Society's Cancer Information Service toll-free at (888) 939-3333. Information about this study is also available at http://cancer.gov/star on the Internet.

support groups   Groups that give people affected by a condition or illness, such as breast cancer, an opportunity to meet and discuss ways to cope. Women diagnosed with breast cancer, and their families, face challenges that may lead to feelings of being overwhelmed, afraid, and alone. Cancer support groups can help people affected by breast cancer feel less alone and can improve their ability to deal with the uncertainties and challenges that breast cancer creates.

People who have been diagnosed with breast cancer sometimes find they need help coping with the emotional as well as the practical aspects of their disease. In fact, attention to the emotional burden of breast cancer is sometimes part of a patient's treatment plan. Breast cancer support groups are designed to provide a confidential atmosphere in which patients or breast cancer survivors can discuss the challenges that accompany the illness with others who may have experienced the same challenges. Support groups have helped thousands of women cope with similar situations.

However, not only the patient with breast cancer may need a support group. Family and friends are affected when cancer touches someone they love, and they may need help in dealing with stresses such as family disruptions, financial worries, and changing roles within relationships. To help meet these needs, some support groups are designed just for family members of people diagnosed with breast cancer; other groups encourage families and friends to participate along with the patient or breast cancer survivor.

Several kinds of support groups are available to meet the individual needs of people at all stages of cancer treatment, from diagnosis through aftercare. Some groups are general breast cancer support groups; more specialized groups work with teens or young adults or family members. Support groups may be led by a professional, such as a psychiatrist, psychologist, or social worker, or by patients with breast cancer or survivors. In addition, support groups can vary in approach, size, and frequency with which they meet. Many groups are free, but some require a fee (insurance may cover the cost).

Locating a Group
Many organizations offer support groups for people diagnosed with breast cancer and their family members or friends. Oncology health-care workers may have information about support groups, and hospital social service departments can also provide information about breast cancer support programs. The local office of the AMERICAN CANCER SOCIETY can provide lists of support groups. Additionally, many newspapers carry a special health supplement containing information about where to find this type of help.

suppressor genes   See TUMOR SUPPRESSOR GENES.

supraclavicular nodes   Lymph nodes located above the collarbone. When breast cancer spreads to these nodes it is a regional cancer, which is more serious than a locally confined cancer.

surgical margins   See MARGINS.

Surveillance, Epidemiology, and End Results (SEER)   A program of the NATIONAL CANCER INSTITUTE (NCI) that is the most authoritative source of information on breast cancer incidence and survival rate in the United States. The NCI's SEER cancer registry program has been expanded to cover more of the racial, ethnic, and socioeconomic diversity of the United States, allowing better description and tracking of trends in health disparities. Methodological studies are seeking better ways to measure socioeconomic factors and determine their relationship to cancer incidence, survival, and mortality rates.

Additionally, the NCI supports a growing body of research to examine the environmental, sociocultural, behavioral, and genetic cause of breast cancer in different populations and apply these discoveries through interventions in clinical and community settings. These interventions cover topics such as dietary modification, exercise, and adherence to screening practices.

survival rate   The percentage of patients in a given population who are still alive a specified time after diagnosis with a particular disease. For instance, the five-year survival rate for the following stages of breast cancer is

- *Stage 0:* 100 percent
- *Stage 1:* 98 percent
- *Stage 2a:* 88 percent
- *Stage 2b:* 76 percent
- *Stage 3a:* 56 percent
- *Stage 3b:* 49 percent
- *Stage 4:* 16 percent

Because the survival rate at five years includes patients who are living with metastatic disease, survival rates at 10 years are lower. Breast cancer can recur at any time, although the highest risk is during the first five years. It is important to remember that these survival rates can give an individual only a general idea of her likely longevity. Some women with advanced breast cancer live significantly longer than seven years, and some women with early stage breast cancer live less than five years. Researchers are constantly developing new treatment alternatives to prolong breast cancer survival rate.

Susan G. Komen Breast Cancer Foundation   A leader in the field of BREAST CANCER education, screening, and treatment and the largest private funding source in the world for breast cancer research and community-outreach programs.

The foundation was started in 1982 by Nancy Goodman Brinker, two years after her sister Susan Goodman Komen died from breast cancer. By the end of 2000, the Komen Foundation and its affiliates had raised more than $300 million. Key to its success is the Komen Race for the Cure, the largest series of 5K runs/fitness walks in the world. This event, created by Nancy Brinker, has grown from one local race with 800 participants to a national series of more than 100 races with more than 1 million participants.

As a result of her efforts, Nancy Brinker has expanded her role, serving under three U.S. presidents on the National Cancer Advisory Board and testifying before Congress in 2000. She has also participated in the International Women's Forum, and is a collaborating partner for the National Dialogue on Cancer. For contact information, see Appendix 1.

symptoms of breast cancer   Early BREAST CANCER usually does not cause pain or any other symptoms, but as it grows it can cause the following changes:

- A lump or thickening in or near the breast or in the underarm area
- A change in the size or shape of the breast
- Nipple discharge or tenderness
- Inversion of the nipple into the breast
- Ridges or pitting of the breast (the skin resembles the skin of an orange)
- A change in the appearance or feel of the skin of the breast, areola, or nipple

tamoxifen (Nolvadex) A drug taken as a pill that has been used for more than 20 years to treat patients with BREAST CANCER. Tamoxifen works against breast cancer in part by interfering with the activity of ESTROGEN, a female hormone that promotes the growth of breast cancer cells.

In October 1998, on the basis of the results of the Breast Cancer Prevention Trial (BCPT), the U.S. Food and Drug Administration approved tamoxifen to reduce the incidence of breast cancer in women at high risk for the disease. The BCPT was a study of more than 13,000 pre- and postmenopausal high-risk women ages 35 and older who took either tamoxifen or a placebo for up to five years. The study showed that in addition to reducing the number of these women who had breast cancer, tamoxifen works as estrogen does to preserve bone strength, decreasing fractures of the hip, wrist, and spine.

Risks

However, there are risks involved in taking tamoxifen. The drug increases the risk of endometrial cancer, which begins in the lining of the uterus, and uterine sarcoma, which develops in the muscular wall of the uterus. Like all cancers, endometrial cancer and uterine sarcoma are potentially life threatening. Women who have had a hysterectomy and are taking tamoxifen are not at increased risk for these cancers.

In the BCPT, women who took tamoxifen had more than twice the probability of endometrial cancer development of women who took a placebo—the same as the risk in postmenopausal women who have estrogen replacement therapy. This risk is about two cases of endometrial cancer per every 1,000 women who take tamoxifen each year. Most of the endometrial cancers that have occurred in women taking tamoxifen have been found in the early stages, and treatment has usually been effective. However, for some patients with breast cancer who had endometrial cancer while taking tamoxifen, the disease was life threatening.

Of greater concern was the finding that tamoxifen also was linked to an increased risk of a rare type of cancer known as uterine sarcoma. In the BCPT, there were about two cases of this disease per 10,000 women who used tamoxifen each year. Research so far suggests that uterine sarcomas are more likely to be diagnosed at later stages than endometrial cancers and may therefore be harder to control and more life threatening. Because of this risk, a "black box" warning about the risk for uterine sarcoma was added to the labeling of tamoxifen. Black boxes are used to draw attention to problems that are serious and potentially life threatening. Doctors emphasized that the new warning was directed only at women who have not had breast cancer but are at high risk. The warning does not tell those women not to take tamoxifen, but it does urge them to talk to their doctors about its benefits and risks.

The warning does not apply to women who have already had breast cancer and who take tamoxifen to prevent a recurrence. For those women, the benefits far outweigh the risks.

Abnormal vaginal bleeding and pelvic pain are symptoms of both endometrial cancer and uterine sarcoma. Women who are taking tamoxifen should have regular pelvic examinations and should be checked promptly if they have any abnormal vaginal bleeding or pelvic pain between scheduled exams.

Tamoxifen received additional approval in June 2000 for use in women who have DUCTAL CARCINOMA IN SITU, after breast surgery and radiation. It is also approved to reduce the risk of invasive breast cancer.

taxanes A group of drugs that includes paclitaxel (Taxol) and docetaxel (Taxotere), which are used in the treatment of breast and other cancers. Taxanes have a unique way of preventing the growth of cancer cells, affecting cell structures called microtubules that play an important role in cell functions.

In normal cell growth, microtubules are formed when a cell starts dividing. Once the cell stops dividing, the microtubules are broken down or destroyed. Taxanes stop the microtubules from breaking down; cancer cells become so clogged with microtubules that they cannot grow and divide.

Taxol and Taxotere are both very active in treating breast cancer. Studies comparing them note differences in side effects: Taxol causes more nerve damage, and Taxotere causes more fluid retention. They both can cause low blood counts and allergic reactions and hair loss.

thermal imaging A new way of diagnosing breast problems, by measuring and mapping the heat from the breast with the use of a special camera. A computer looks for "hot spots" or differences in heat, then analyzes the images. The theory is that an area of increased heat may indicate an increase in blood vessel formation due to cancer. However, studies have not proved this to be an effective screening tool for early diagnosis of breast cancer and it is not a replacement for mammograms.

Although thermography has been approved by the U.S. Food and Drug Administration as safe, it is not approved as a stand-alone screening test for breast cancer. It is not a reliable diagnostic test, since it can miss some cancers and can have a high false-positive rate.

See also DIGITAL MAMMOGRAPHY; DUCTOGRAM; MAMMOGRAPHY.

three-dimensional mammography See FULL-FIELD DIGITAL TOMOSYNTHESIS.

thrombocytopenia A drop in the number of platelets (blood cells responsible for clotting) that is

often a side effect of radiation therapy or chemotherapy. Certain types of cancer also may directly destroy platelets in the blood. Severe cases of thrombocytopenia can have grave consequences because minor injuries can result in serious blood loss. The condition can be treated with transfusions of platelets, intravenous gamma-globulin, removal of the spleen, and medications to boost the platelet count. When radiation therapy or chemotherapy is stopped, the platelet count should return to normal.

TRAM flap See TRANSVERSE RECTUS ABDOMINIS MYOCUTANEOUS FLAP.

transillumination The inspection of a breast by passing a light through the tissues. In this procedure, transmitted light is photographed by a video camera that sends the image to a TV monitor while recording images on videotape or disk.

Because different tissues have different patterns of light absorption, cysts appear different from solid lumps. Although some large cancers can be detected with this procedure, its ability to identify the very small, curable cancers that can often be seen with MAMMOGRAPHY has yet to be proved. Experts caution that at its present state of development, transillumination is not an appropriate imaging technique for breast cancer screening.

transverse rectus abdominis myocutaneous flap (TRAM flap) The most common type of procedure using a patient's own tissue flap to reconstruct a breast after MASTECTOMY. In the transverse rectus abdominis myocutaneous (TRAM) flap procedure, a section of skin, fat, and muscle from the abdomen is surgically moved to the chest area. The tissue flap may be left attached to the blood supply and moved to the breast area through a tunnel under the skin (a pedicled flap), or it may be removed completely and reattached to the breast area by microsurgical techniques (a free flap). A pedicle TRAM flap procedure typically takes three to six hours of surgery with general anesthesia; a free TRAM flap procedure generally takes longer because of the microsurgical requirements.

Flap surgery requires a hospital stay of several days and generally has a longer recovery time than breast reconstruction using SALINE IMPLANTS. Flap surgery also creates scars at the site where the flap was taken in addition to the scars on the reconstructed breast.

However, flap surgery has the advantage of using the woman's own tissue to replace the breast. Saline solution implants eventually need to be replaced; TRAM flaps do not. This procedure may be useful when the chest tissues have been damaged and are not suitable for tissue expansion. Another advantage of flap procedures over saline implants is that alteration of the unaffected breast is generally not needed to improve symmetry.

The TRAM flap procedure is a major operation and more extensive than a mastectomy operation, requiring good general health and strong emotional motivation. Women who are very overweight, smoke cigarettes, have had previous surgery at the flap site, or have any circulatory problem may not be good candidates for a tissue flap procedure. Also, women who are very thin may not have enough tissue in the abdomen to create a breast mound with this method.

The TRAM flap is sometimes referred to as a tummy tuck reconstruction because it may leave the stomach area flatter. The TRAM procedure may require a blood transfusion. Typically, the hospital stay is two to five days, and the patient can resume normal daily activity after six to eight weeks. Some women, however, report that resuming normal activities takes up to one year.

Because there may be temporary or permanent muscle weakness in the abdominal area, women who are considering pregnancy after reconstruction should discuss this with the surgeon.

treatments   BREAST CANCER may be treated with local or systemic (bodywide) therapy; many patients have both kinds of treatment. Local therapy (surgery and RADIATION THERAPY) is used to remove or destroy breast cancer in a specific area. When breast cancer has spread to other parts of the body, systemic therapy is usually used.

Systemic treatments are used to destroy or control cancer throughout the body. CHEMOTHERAPY, hormonal therapy, and biological therapy are systemic treatments. Some patients have systemic therapy to shrink a tumor before local therapy.

Others have systemic therapy after local therapy to prevent cancer recurrence or to treat cancer that has spread.

Surgery

Surgery is the most common treatment for breast cancer and can range from a simple removal of the tumor (LUMPECTOMY) to a total removal of the breast and lymph nodes (MASTECTOMY). At diagnosis, the woman's doctor explains each type of surgery, discusses and compares benefits and risks, and describes how each affects a woman's appearance. Surgery causes short-term pain and tenderness in the area of the operation, so women may need to talk with their doctor about pain management as well.

Breast-conserving surgery   An operation to remove the cancer but not the breast is called breast-sparing surgery or breast-conserving surgery. Lumpectomy (also called segmental mastectomy or partial mastectomy) is a type of breast-sparing surgery.

In a lumpectomy, the surgeon removes the breast cancer and some normal tissue around it. (Sometimes an EXCISIONAL BIOPSY serves as a lumpectomy.) Often, some of the lymph nodes under the arm are removed.

After breast-sparing surgery, most women receive radiation therapy to destroy cancer cells that remain in the area.

Mastectomy   A mastectomy is an operation to remove the breast (or as much of the breast as possible), sometimes followed by BREAST RECONSTRUCTION, performed either at the same time as the mastectomy or in a later surgery. Women considering reconstruction should discuss this with a plastic surgeon before having a mastectomy.

After surgery, the skin over the surgical area may be tight, and the muscles of the arm and shoulder may feel stiff. Because nerves may be injured or cut during surgery, a woman may have numbness and tingling in the chest, underarm, shoulder, and upper arm (POSTMASTECTOMY PAIN SYNDROME). These sensations usually end within a few weeks or months, but some women have permanent numbness. Some women have some permanent loss of strength in these muscles, but for most women, reduced strength and limited movement are temporary. The doctor, nurse, or physical therapist can recommend exercises to help a woman regain movement and strength in her arm and shoulder.

In *segmental mastectomy,* the surgeon removes the cancer and a larger area of normal breast tissue around it. Occasionally, some of the lining over the chest muscles below the tumor is removed as well.

Simple (or total) mastectomy is the removal of the whole breast.

In a *modified radical mastectomy,* the whole breast, most of the lymph nodes under the arm, and often the lining over the chest muscles are removed. The smaller of the two chest muscles is also taken out to aid removal of the lymph nodes.

Radical mastectomy is the removal of the breast as well as the surrounding lymph nodes, muscles, fatty tissue, and skin. Formerly considered the standard for breast cancer, it is rarely used today. In rare cases, radical mastectomy may be suggested if the cancer has spread to the chest muscles.

Axillary lymph-node dissection In most cases, the surgeon removes lymph nodes under the arm to help determine whether cancer cells have entered the lymphatic system. This is called an axillary lymph node dissection and may result in fluid building up in the arm and hand and cause swelling (LYMPHEDEMA). To prevent this, women need to protect the arm and hand on the treated side from injury or pressure, even years after surgery. Women should not have blood pressure taken or injections given on the affected side, and they should contact their doctor if an infection develops in that arm or hand. Doctors can discuss how a woman should handle any cuts, scratches, insect bites, or other injuries to the arm or hand.

A *sentinel-node biopsy* is offered at some cancer centers. This procedure reduces the number of lymph nodes that must be removed during breast cancer surgery, which decreases the risk of lymphedema and arm numbness. Before surgery, the doctor injects a radioactive substance or blue dye near the tumor; it then flows through the lymphatic system to the first lymph nodes where cancer cells are likely to have spread (the sentinel nodes). This injection can be momentarily quite painful, but the burning lasts for only a few minutes. The doctor uses a scanner to locate the radioactive substance in these sentinel nodes. The surgeon makes a small incision and removes only the nodes with radioactive substance or blue dye. A pathologist checks the sentinel lymph nodes for cancer cells; if no cancer cells are detected, removal of additional nodes may not be necessary. If sentinel-node biopsy proves to be as effective as the standard axillary lymph node dissection, the new procedure could spare patients the risk of lymphedema.

Radiation Therapy

Women who have had a lumpectomy almost always have radiation therapy after the surgical wound has healed. Doctors use radiation to kill any remaining cancer cells. The radiation may be directed at the breast by an external machine or may originate from radioactive material in thin plastic tubes that are placed directly into the breast (implant radiation). Some women have both kinds of radiation therapy.

In external radiation therapy, the patient usually goes to the hospital five days a week for several weeks. For implant radiation, a woman stays in the hospital for several days while the implants remain in place; they are removed before the woman goes home.

Radiation therapy is also sometimes used before surgery to destroy cancer cells and shrink tumors. It may be used alone or with chemotherapy or hormonal therapy. This approach is most often used in cases in which the breast tumor is large or not easily removed by surgery.

After several radiation therapy treatments, a woman is likely to become extremely tired. This feeling may continue for a while after treatment. Resting is important, but research has suggested that trying to stay reasonably active can help fend off fatigue.

It is also common for the skin in the treated area to become red, dry, tender, and itchy, and the breast may temporarily feel heavy and hard. Toward the end of treatment, the skin may become moist; exposing this area to air as much as possible helps the skin heal. These effects of radiation therapy on the skin are temporary, and the area gradually heals once treatment ends. However, there may be a permanent change in the color of the skin.

Chemotherapy

Often, after surgery to remove the breast cancer, a doctor recommends chemotherapy drugs to kill any remaining cancer cells that may have been missed during surgery. CHEMOTHERAPY for breast cancer is usually a combination of drugs that may be given in a pill or by injection on an outpatient basis over several months.

The type of drug and dosage vary from patient to patient, depending on the medical situation. Chemotherapy drugs most often used to treat breast cancer include the following:

- Adriamycin (doxorubicin)
- Cytoxan (cyclophosphamide)
- Ellence (epirubicin)
- Nolvadex (tamoxifen)
- Taxol (paclitaxel)
- Taxotere (docetaxel)
- Xeloda (capecitabine)

Other drugs are used to treat metastatic breast cancer.

Very often, a doctor prescribes a combination of chemotherapy drugs to treat breast cancer. Common combinations include the following:

- CMF: cyclophosphamide, methotrexate, and fluorouracil
- CAF: cyclophosphamide, doxorubicin (Adriamycin), and fluorouracil
- AC: doxorubicin (Adriamycin) and cyclophosphamide
- Doxorubicin and cyclophosphamide with paclitaxel
- Doxorubicin followed by CMF
- Cyclophosphamide, epirubicin, and fluorouracil

Side effects caused by chemotherapy drugs vary a great deal, depending on several factors, including the types of drugs used, their dosages, and the length of treatment. The benefits of treating cancer with chemotherapy drugs outweigh the risk of complications for most women, and effects are often tolerable with proper care and rest.

Women who are still menstruating may be able to become pregnant during treatment. Because the effects of chemotherapy on an unborn child are not known, a woman should talk with her doctor about birth control before treatment begins. After treatment, some women regain their ability to become pregnant, but in women older than age 40, infertility may be permanent.

Hormonal Therapy

Hormone therapy treatment prevents cancer cells from receiving the hormones they need to grow by blocking hormone receptors or by preventing formation of hormones. Blocking the ovaries with medicine or removing them surgically is another type of hormone therapy. The side effects of hormonal therapy depend on the kind of drug or treatment.

The drug TAMOXIFEN is the most common hormonal treatment, which blocks the cancer cells' use of estrogen but does not stop estrogen production. Tamoxifen may cause hot flashes, vaginal discharge or irritation, nausea, and irregular periods. Women who are still menstruating and having irregular periods may become pregnant more easily when taking tamoxifen.

The drug slightly increases the risk for blood clots in the veins, stroke, and cancer of the uterine lining. Any unusual vaginal bleeding should be reported to the doctor.

Young women whose ovaries are removed to deprive cancer cells of estrogen experience menopause immediately, and their symptoms are likely to be more severe than those associated with natural menopause.

Biological Therapy

This treatment method is designed to enhance the body's natural defenses against cancer. The monoclonal antibody trastuzumab (HERCEPTIN) is an example. It targets breast cancer cells that have too much of a protein known as human epidermal growth factor receptor-2 (HER-2). By blocking HER-2, Herceptin slows or stops the growth of these cells. Herceptin may be administered alone or with chemotherapy.

The side effects of biological therapy depend on the types of substances used. Rashes or swelling at the injection site are common, and flulike symptoms also may occur. Herceptin may cause these and other side effects, but effects generally become less severe after the first treatment. Less commonly, Herceptin can also cause damage to the heart that can lead to heart failure. It can also affect the lungs, causing breathing problems that require immediate medical attention. For these reasons, women are checked carefully for heart and lung problems before Herceptin is prescribed.

Treatment Options

A woman's treatment options depend on a number of factors. These factors include her age and menopausal status, her general health, the size and location of the tumor and the stage of the cancer, the results of lab tests, and the size of her breast. Certain features of the tumor cells (such as whether they depend on hormones to grow) are also considered before settling on a particular treatment.

Women who have early stage breast cancer (stages 0 through II) may have breast-sparing surgery followed by radiation therapy to the breast, or they may have a mastectomy, with or without breast reconstruction. Sometimes radiation therapy is also given after mastectomy. Breast-sparing surgery and mastectomy are equally effective. The choice depends mostly on the size and location of the tumor, the size of the woman's breast, certain features of the cancer, and the woman's preferences about preserving her breast.

In either approach, lymph nodes under the arm usually are removed. Many women who have stage I and most who have stage II breast cancer have chemotherapy and/or hormonal therapy after primary treatment with surgery or surgery and radiation therapy. This added treatment is called ADJUVANT TREATMENT, and is given to destroy any cancer cells remaining in the body. This decreases the chance that breast cancer will return.

Chemotherapy may also be given to shrink a tumor before surgery, a technique called neoadjuvant therapy.

Patients who have stage III breast cancer usually have both local and systemic treatments. The local treatment may include surgery and/or radiation therapy to the breast and underarm to remove or destroy the cancer in the breast. It is followed by chemotherapy or hormonal therapy to stop the disease from spreading. Chemotherapy may also be given before local therapy to shrink the tumor.

Women who have stage IV breast cancer receive chemotherapy and/or hormonal therapy to destroy cancer cells and control the disease. They may have surgery or radiation therapy to control the cancer in the breast. Radiation may also be useful to control tumors in other parts of the body.

Rehabilitation

Rehabilitation is an important part of breast cancer treatment. Women recover differently, depending on the extent of the disease, type of treatment, and other factors.

Exercising the arm and shoulder after surgery can help a woman regain motion and strength in these areas and can also reduce pain and stiffness in the neck and back. Carefully planned exercises should be started as soon as the doctor says the woman is ready, often within a day or so after surgery. Exercising begins slowly and gently and can even be done in bed. Gradually, exercising can be more active, and regular exercise becomes part of a woman's normal routine. (Women who have a mastectomy followed by immediate breast reconstruction need special exercises, which the doctor or nurse can explain.)

Often, LYMPHEDEMA after surgery can be prevented or reduced with certain exercises and by resting with the arm propped up on a pillow. If lymphedema occurs, the doctor may suggest exercises and other ways to deal with this problem. For example, some women who have lymphedema wear an elastic sleeve or use an elastic cuff to improve lymph circulation. The doctor also may suggest other approaches, such as medication, manual lymph drainage, or use of a machine that gently compresses the arm.

Regular follow-up exams are important after breast cancer treatment. A woman who has had cancer in one breast should immediately report to her doctor any changes in the treated area or in the other breast. Because a woman who has had cancer in one breast is at risk of having the disease in the opposite breast, mammograms are an important part of follow-up care.

tubular carcinoma A type of infiltrating ductal BREAST CANCER that makes up only about 2 percent of all breast cancers. These tumors have a slightly better prognosis and a slightly lower chance of spreading than invasive lobular or invasive ductal cancers of the same size.

Women tend to be diagnosed with tubular carcinoma in the early sixth decade, usually by the appearance of a mass on a screening MAMMOGRAM as opposed to the appearance of a palpable breast lump. Not infrequently, tubular carcinomas are discovered incidentally in biopsies performed for unrelated reasons.

Pure tubular carcinomas are typically small, with an average diameter of less than one centimeter. Tubular carcinomas detected by screening mammography are typically smaller than palpable lesions, and pure tumors are smaller, on average, than tumors made of mixtures of tubular carcinomas and other types.

As with other types of breast cancer, however, the size of the tumor strongly influences the likelihood of its spread into the axillary nodes. About 67 percent of tubular carcinomas that spread were larger than one centimeter. The relative infrequency of LYMPH NODE spread in women who have small tubular carcinomas has led some investigators to advocate abandoning axillary lymph-node dissection in these patients.

Even patients whose cancer had spread to the lymph nodes had a relatively good prognosis. In such an event, the cancer usually spreads to no more than three nodes. Researchers also concluded that even when this cancer does spread to the nodes, it does not affect ultimate survival rates for these patients.

No differences were found in local recurrence rates when using conservative surgery and radiation therapy compared to those in patients who had invasive ductal carcinoma.

tumor-suppressor genes Genes that suppress the growth of tumors. Both *BRCA1* and *BRCA2* genes are considered to be tumor-suppressor genes. Mutations in these genes impair their ability to block the development of cancer.

See also BREAST CANCER SUSCEPTIBILITY GENES; ONCOGENES.

ultrasound scan Also called sonography, this diagnostic technique uses high-frequency sound waves to produce images of structures inside the body. An ultrasound is sometimes used to determine whether a mass discovered on a MAMMOGRAM is a fluid-filled CYST or a solid tumor; solid tumors are more likely to be malignant.

Results of a new study show that breast ultrasound is more accurate than MAMMOGRAPHY for women 45 years old or younger who have symptoms of breast cancer and may be an appropriate initial imaging test for investigating these women. Each test is good at detecting certain types of problems but may miss others. For example, mammograms are excellent at finding calcium deposits, which can be an early sign of BREAST CANCER—but mammograms can be hard to read in younger women, because higher estrogen levels make their breasts lumpy and dense. On the other hand, ultrasound is excellent at identifying cysts, which are a common cause of benign breast lumps in young women, but may miss breast cancer in older women.

Doctors have begun to rely more on ultrasound when they are worried about a breast lump in premenopausal women. This study confirms that an ultrasound is slightly better than a mammogram at identifying breast cancer in women 45 and younger. In fact, an ultrasound was just as good as a mammogram for women up to age 55—although ultrasound became less accurate as women aged. Experts suggest that a combination of both tests is probably the best approach for many women, especially in the years right around menopause.

In younger women—particularly those who have not gone through menopause—a mammogram or ultrasound is not always needed when a lump in the breast appears. Many breast lumps are just benign, fluid-filled cysts that recede spontaneously. A doctor may ask the patient to return in one or two months for a repeat examination; if the lump persists or grows, then further tests are needed.

In older, postmenopausal women, a new breast lump is more worrisome. In addition to an examination, the doctor will almost certainly recommend either an ultrasound, mammogram, or aspiration, in which a small needle is used to draw fluid out of the lump. On the basis of the results of these tests, additional follow-up may be needed, but noncancerous lumps are much more common than breast cancer.

A normal mammogram or ultrasound result does not in itself guarantee that a breast lump is benign, since these tests miss more than 10 percent of breast cancers.

vaccine A form of biological therapy that would encourage a BREAST CANCER patient's immune system to recognize and destroy cancer cells. The immune system is constantly scanning the body for foreign invaders, but because cancer cells originate in the body, they are usually not detected by the immune system.

In cancer vaccine technology, tumor cells would be removed, marked as "foreign" by adding a special gene, and then injected beneath the skin along with an immunostimulant (such as interleukin-2). This technique would stimulate the immune system to "think" it had been newly infected with cancer, so that it would destroy this "new" antigen. Scientists hope such a vaccine would help the body recognize cancer, rejecting tumors and preventing cancer recurrence.

Unlike vaccines against infectious diseases, cancer vaccines are designed to be injected after the disease is diagnosed rather than before it develops. Cancer vaccines given when a tumor is small may be able to eradicate the cancer.

Early cancer vaccine studies primarily involved patients with melanoma, but scientists today are testing the vaccines for many other types of cancer, including breast cancer.

Scientists in California and Germany have successfully used an oral vaccine to stop cancerous tumor growth in animals by choking off the tumor's blood supply. Researchers first targeted a protein produced in new blood vessels (VEGF receptor 2), one of several substances that trigger new blood-vessel growth (a process called angiogenesis). New blood vessel growth is critical for cancerous tumor growth and spread. When researchers administered genetically engineered bacteria that contained a gene to express the VEGF receptor-2 protein, it triggered the animal's immune system to fight off the mild infection from the bacteria—and, in the process, killed the protein that spurs new blood vessel growth to the tumors.

Someday these exciting studies may prove useful in the treatment of cancer.

valley view Also called a cleavage view, a MAMMOGRAM image of the most central portions of the breasts that are in the "valley" between the two breasts. A valley view may be performed when there is a questionable density on the edge of the mammogram film and the radiologist needs to see more of this density. A valley view also may be performed if the radiologist sees something suspicious in one angle but cannot find the area on a different angle. In the procedure, the mammogram technologist places both breasts on the plate at the same time.

vegetarian diets Current studies of women who have a Western-style vegetarian diet have not shown that they have a lower risk of breast cancer than that of women whose diet includes meat. A recent study combining the data of five cohort studies examining vegetarians in the United States, Germany, and England found that the death rate of breast cancer in women on vegetarian diets was no different from that of women in the general population. The women in these studies were selected only because they did not eat meat. There was no evidence that they ate more fruits and vegetables, which may be associated with lower breast cancer risk. The major health difference noted between vegetarians and non-vegetarians was a lower death rate of heart disease among the vegetarians.

vesicant An intravenous CHEMOTHERAPY drug capable of damaging tissue and causing pain and swelling if it leaks into the skin. Many chemotherapy drugs cause local tissue damage if they leak out of the vein. These include the following:

- Anthracyclines (daunorubicin, doxorubicin [Adriamycin], epirubicin, idarubicin)

- Antibiotics (bleomycin, mitomycin, actinomycin)
- Mustards (mustine)
- Vinca alkaloids (vincristine, vinblastine, vindesine)
- Other (etoposide, tenoposide, amsacrine, mitoxantrone)

Wellness Community   A national nonprofit organization dedicated to providing free emotional support, education, and hope for patients with BREAST CANCER and their loved ones. Through participation in professionally led support groups, educational workshops, and mind–body programs that utilize the Patient Active Concept, people affected by cancer can learn vital skills to regain control, reduce feelings of isolation, and restore hope—regardless of their stage of disease.

With 21 facilities nationwide, the Virtual Wellness Community on the Internet, and international centers in Tel Aviv and Tokyo, the Wellness Community provides a free, homelike setting for people who are living with cancer and their loved ones to connect with and learn from each other. Services include counseling, support groups, networking groups, educational information, nutritional information, volunteer services, and survivor concerns.

The Wellness Community was founded by Dr. Harold Benjamin in Santa Monica, California, in 1982 as a result of his experience with his wife's breast cancer. After subsequent years of study of the psychological and social impacts of cancer, Dr. Benjamin formulated the Patient Active Concept, which was recognized years later, at the Walt Disney World EPCOT Metropolitan Life exhibit, as one of the most significant developments in the evolution of modern health care.

According to the Patient Active Concept, people who actively fight for recovery from cancer by adopting a particular series of actions and attitudes improve the quality of their life and may enhance their possibility of recovery. These patients consider themselves part of a team, fighting for recovery along with their physicians and other health-care providers.

From Dr. Benjamin's first program in a little yellow house in Santa Monica, The Wellness Community has grown to 22 facilities throughout the country with four additional facilities currently in development. A significant factor in expansion of facilities in the early 1990s was due to actress Gilda Radner, a participant at The Wellness Community until her death from ovarian cancer in 1989. For contact information, see Appendix I.

whole grains and breast cancer   The results of epidemiological studies suggest that eating whole grains may be associated with a small decrease in the risk of BREAST CANCER. Whole grains also have been associated with a decrease in the risk of other cancers and health problems, including heart disease.

Whole grains are the high-fiber unrefined products of various cereal plants including wheat, oats, rye, corn, rice, millet, sorghum, and barley; they contain the grain's starchy endosperm, the bran, and the germ. (Refined grains and flour include only the starchy endosperm of the grain.)

Although most studies have indicated a small decrease in breast cancer risk associated with eating whole grains, several studies have shown no association of whole grains with breast cancer risk. The lack of agreement among the studies could result from eating of a wide variety of foods; separating out the effect of single groups of food, such as grains, is difficult.

It does appear that fruit and vegetable fiber decreases breast cancer risk. Fiber may do this by decreasing the levels of estrogens in the body by binding estrogen in bile. Five studies have reported lower levels of estrogens in the blood of premenopausal women who ate a high-fiber diet. Fiber also can decrease the type of bacteria in the intestine that lead to reabsorption of estrogens from the bile into the body.

These studies present encouraging evidence that diets high in fiber may lower circulating estrogen levels in humans. More studies are needed in this area.

wine and cancer   There are many biologically active plant-based chemicals in wine. Some scientists believe that particular compounds called polyphenols found in red wine (such as catechins and resveratrol) may have antioxidant or anticancer properties.

Polyphenols are antioxidant compounds found in the skin and seeds of grapes, which are dissolved by alcohol produced by the fermentation process. Red wine contains more polyphenols than white wine because when white wine is made, the skins are removed after the grapes are crushed. The phenols in red wine include catechin, gallic acid, and epicatechin.

Polyphenols have been found to have antioxidant properties; that means they can protect cells from damage caused by molecules known as FREE RADICALS. These free radicals can damage important parts of cells (including proteins, membranes, and deoxyribonucleic acid [DNA]), and that damage may lead to cancer. Research on the antioxidants found in red wine has shown that they may help inhibit the development of certain cancers.

Resveratrol is a type of polyphenol that is produced as part of a plant's defense system in response to an invading fungus, stress, injury, infection, or ultraviolet irradiation. Red wine contains high levels of the antioxidant resveratrol, as do grapes, raspberries, peanuts, and other plants. Resveratrol has been shown to reduce tumor incidence in animals by affecting one or more stages of cancer development and has been shown to inhibit growth of many types of cancer cells in culture. It also appears to reduce inflammation and activation of a protein produced by the body's immune system when it is under attack. This protein affects cancer-cell growth and metastasis.

However, it is still too early to draw conclusions about the association between red wine consumption and cancer in humans. Although consumption of large amounts of alcoholic beverages may increase the risk of some cancers, there is growing evidence that the health benefits of red wine are related to its nonalcoholic components.

Women's Health and Cancer Rights Act (WHCRA)
A 1998 law that contains important protections for patients with breast cancer who choose breast reconstruction with a mastectomy. The law mandates that insurers cover mastectomy-related services, including prostheses, reconstruction and surgery to achieve symmetry between the breasts, and complications resulting from a mastectomy (including LYMPHEDEMA).

Several states also have their own laws requiring health plans that cover mastectomies to provide coverage for reconstructive surgery after mastectomy.

Because not all health plans are subject to state law, the new federal law covers those plans not currently covered by state law and sets a minimal standard securing this service for all women in all states—those with weaker state laws and those with no laws.

Although the law went into effect on October 21, 1998, it is a somewhat complicated and complex measure. The new law sets a federal floor so that all women will benefit from breast reconstruction after mastectomy, even if they live in states with no current mandates. Under the Women's Health Act, group health plans, insurance companies, and HMOs offering mastectomy coverage must also provide coverage for reconstructive surgery as determined by consultation between the attending physician and the patient. All group health plans, along with their insurance companies or HMOs that provide coverage for medical and surgical benefits with respect to a mastectomy, are subject to the requirements of the Women's Health Act. Deductibles and co-insurance may be charged, but only if they are consistent with those established for other benefits under the plan or coverage.

Both health plans and health insurance issuers are required to provide notice of WHCRA benefits at enrollment, and annually thereafter. WHCRA does not prevent a plan or health insurance issuer from negotiating the level and type of payment with attending providers. However, the law prohibits plans and issuers from penalizing providers or providing incentives that would cause a provider to give care that is inconsistent with WHCRA.

Y-ME National Breast Cancer Organization

National nonprofit breast cancer organization founded in 1978 by two patients with breast cancer dedicated to providing information, empowerment, and peer support, so that no one would face breast cancer alone.

The group operates a 24-hour breast cancer hotline (800-221-2141), the only hotline in the United States staffed by trained peer counselors who are breast cancer survivors. It is a convenient, anonymous resource for breast cancer and breast health information, as well as support for anyone touched by or concerned about this disease. Callers can be matched with a survivor, a patient, and/or a supporter who has had a similar experience with breast cancer. The group also offers a monthly one-hour teleconference featuring a breast cancer–related presentation by a medical professional, followed by a question-and-answer session. Participants are divided into small groups for discussion; groups are moderated by volunteers who match the profiles of the participants.

Publications include a national quarterly newsletter providing the latest information on breast cancer issues, research, and concerns surrounding breast cancer, and *Latina News,* a bilingual quarterly newsletter distributed nationwide to address breast cancer issues, research, and concerns specific to the Hispanic community. The organization also offers a program for men, to provide support and education while they are supporting a wife, mother, daughter, or friend through breast cancer.

The group's Web site (www.y-me.org) offers breast cancer information, resources, and support for patients, survivors, families, friends, caregivers, and medical professionals; guests can submit questions concerning breast health and/or breast cancer, which are answered by breast cancer survivors within 48 hours. The site is available in both English and Spanish.

The organization also offers free wigs and prostheses to women who have limited resources; monitors federal breast cancer–related legislation and regulations; and works with several patient-advocacy groups to impact breast cancer policy as it develops. For contact information, see Appendix I.

APPENDIXES

APPENDIX I
ASSOCIATIONS

APPEARANCE

American Board of Plastic and Reconstructive Surgeons
(800) 635-0635

Professional organization that provides a list of board-certified physicians in any area of the country

Look Good . . . Feel Better
CTFA Foundation
1101 17th Street, NW
Washington, DC 20036
(800) 395-5665
(202) 331-1770
http://www.lookgoodfeelbetter.org

BONE MARROW TRANSPLANT

National Bone Marrow Transplant Link
20411 West 12 Mile Road
Suite 108
Southfield, MI 48076
(800) LINK-BMT or (800) 546-5268
http://www.comnet.org

National Marrow Donor Program
3001 Broadway Street, NE
Suite 500
Minneapolis, MN 55413
(800) MARROW2 or (800) 627-7692
(888) 999-6743 (Office of Patient Advocacy)
http://www.marrow-donor.org

BRACHYTHERAPY

American Brachytherapy Society
11250 Roger Bacon Drive
Suite 8
Reston, VA 20190
(703) 234-4078
http://www.americanbrachytherapy.org

BRAIN TUMORS

American Brain Tumor Association
2720 River Road
Des Plaines, IL 60018
(847) 827-9910 (patient line)
(800) 886-2282
http://www.abta.org

Brain Tumor Society
124 Watertown Street
Suite 3-H
Watertown, MA 02472
(800) 770-8287
(617) 924-9998
http://www.tbts.org

Dana Alliance for Brain Initiatives, The
745 Fifth Avenue
Suite 700
New York, NY 10151
http://www.nsf.gov

The Dana Alliance, a nonprofit organization of 150 neuroscientists, was formed to help provide information about the personal and public benefits of brain research.

National Brain Tumor Foundation
785 Market Street
Suite 1600
San Francisco, CA 94103
(415) 284-0208
(800) 934-2873
http://www.braintumor.org

Foundation that offers resources and support, plus research. Affected patients can receive referrals to a network of support groups.

BREAST CANCER

ENCOREplus
YWCA of the USA
726 Broadway
New York, NY 10003
(212) 614-2827
http://www.ywca.org/html/B4d1.asp

National Alliance of Breast Cancer Associations
9 East 37th Street
New York, NY 10016
(888) 80-NABCO
(212) 719-0154
(212) 889-0606

National Breast Cancer Coalition
1707 L Street, NW
Suite 1060
Washington, DC 20036
(202) 296-7477
http://www.natlbcc.org

National Lymphedema Network
1611 Telegraph Avenue
Latham Square
Suite 1111
Oakland, CA 94612
(800) 541-3259
(510) 208-3200
http://www.lymphnet.org

Susan G. Komen Breast Cancer Foundation
P.O. Box 650309
Dallas, TX 75265
(800) 462-9273
http://www.komen.org

Women's Information Network (WIN) Against Breast Cancer
536 South Second Avenue
Suite K
Covina, California 91723
(866) 294-6222 (toll-free)
(626) 332-2255
http://www.winabc.org

Y-Me
212 West Van Buren
Suite 500
Chicago, IL 60607
(312) 986-8338
http://www.y-me.org

CANCER

American Cancer Society (ACS)
1599 Clifton Road, NE
Atlanta, GA 30329-4251
(800) 227-2345
http://www.cancer.org

A variety of breast cancer services, including Special Touch, a breast health program teaching breast self-examination, and Reach to Recovery, a support program for women initially diagnosed with breast cancer. Look Good . . . Feel Better is a program designed to help women with their appearance.

Cancer Care
1180 Avenue of the Americas
New York, NY 10036
(212) 221-3300
(800) 813-HOPE or (800) 813-4673
http://www.cancercare.org

Cancer Hope Network
Two North Road
Chester, NJ 07930
(877) 467-3638 or (877) HOPENET
http://www.cancerhopenetwork.org

Cancer Information and Counseling Line
1600 Pierce Street
Denver, CO 80214
(800) 525-3777
http://www.amc.org

Cancer Information Service
Building 31, Room 10A16
9000 Rockville Pike
Bethesda, MD 20892
(800) 4 CANCER
(301) 402-5874
http://www.icic.nci.nih.gov

Cancer Net
Building 31, Room 10A03
31 Center Drive
MSC 2580
Bethesda, MD 20892
(301) 435-3848
http://www.cancernet.nci.nih.gov/index.html

Cancer Research Institute
681 Fifth Avenue
New York, NY 10022
(212) 688-7515
http://www.cancerresearch.org

Cancer Survivors Network
American Cancer Society (ACS)
1599 Clifton Road, NE
Atlanta, GA 30329
(877) 333-4673
http://www.cancer.org

CanSurmount
(800) ACS-2345
http://www.bc.cancer.ca/ccs

I Can Cope
American Cancer Society (ACS)
1599 Clifton Road, NE
Atlanta, GA 30329
(800) 227-2345
http://www.cancer.org

International Union against Cancer
3 rue du Conseil General
1205 Geneva
Switzerland
http://www.uicc.org

CHEMOTHERAPY

CHEMOcare
231 North Avenue
Westfield, NJ 07090
(800) 552-4366
(908) 233-1103
http://www.chemocare.com

Chemotherapy Foundation
183 Madison Avenue
Suite 302
New York, NY 10016
(212) 213-9292
http://www.neoplastics.mssm.edu/sympbrochure.html

DEATH AND DYING

See also HOSPICE.

Choice in Dying
200 Varick Street
New York, NY 10014
(212) 366-5540
(800) 989-9455
http://www.choices.org

FINANCIAL AID

Corporate Angel Network
Westchester County Airport

Building 1
White Plains, NY 10604
(914) 328-1313
http://www.corpangelneetwork.org

Hill-Burton Free Hospital Care
5600 Fishers Lane
Rockville, MD 20857
(800) 638-0742
(301) 443-5656
www.discountrxmart.com

National Association of Hospital Hospitality
4915 Auburn Avenue
Bethesda, MD 20814
(800) 542-9730
http://www.comnet.org

National Patient Air Transport Hotline
http://www.vhl.org

GENETICS INFORMATION

Hereditary Cancer Institute
Creighton University School of Medicine
California at 24th
Omaha, NE 68178
(800) 648-8133
(402) 280-2942
http://www.medicine.Creighton.edu/medschool/
    prevmd/hc.jtml

GOVERNMENT AGENCIES

Centers for Disease Control and Prevention
1600 Clifton Road, NE
Atlanta, GA 30333
(404) 639-3534
(800) 311-3435
http://www.cdc.gov

National Cancer Institute
Building 31, Room 10A03
31 Center Drive, MSC 2580
Bethesda, MD 20892
(301) 435-3848
(800) 422-6237
http://www.nci.nih.gov

**National Center for Complementary and
    Alternative Medicine**
NCCAM Clearinghouse
P.O. Box 7923
Gaithersburg, MD 20898

(888) 644-6226 (toll-free)
(301) 519-3153 (international)
(866) 464-3615 (for hearing impaired)
E-mail: info@nccam.nih.gov
http://www.nccam.nih.gov

HOSPICE

Hospice Education Institute
3 Unity Square
P.O. Box 98
Machiasport, ME 04655
(207) 255-8800
http://www.hospiceworld.org

HospiceLink
Hospice Education Institute
190 Westbrook Road
Essex, CT 06426
(800) 331-1620
(203) 767-1620

National Hospice and Palliative Care Organization
1700 Diagonal Road
Suite 625
Alexandria, VA 22314
(703) 837-1500
http://www.nhpco.org

National Hospice Foundation
1700 Diagonal Road
Suite 625
Alexandria, VA 22314
(703) 516-4928
http://www.nhpco.org

LEGAL ISSUES

Cancer Legal Resource Center
919 South Albany Street
Los Angeles, CA 90019
(213) 736-1455
http://www.lls.edu/community/clrc.htm

LESBIAN/GAY GROUPS

Mary-Helen Mautner Project for Lesbians with Cancer
1707 I Street, NW
Washington, DC 20036
(202) 332-5536
http://www.mautnerproject.org

LYMPHEDEMA

National Lymphedema Network
2211 Post Street
Suite 404
San Francisco, CA 94115
(800) 541-3259
http://www.lymphnet.org

PROFESSIONAL GROUPS

American Society of Clinical Oncology
1900 Duke Street
Suite 200
Alexandria, VA 22314
(703) 299-0150
http://www.asco.org

Association of Community Cancer Centers
11600 Nebel Street
Suite 201
Rockville, MD 20852
(301) 984-9496 (ext. 200)
http://www.accc-cancer.org

Society of Gynecologic Oncologists
401 North Michigan Avenue
Chicago, IL 60611
(312) 644-6610
E-mail: sgo@sba.com
http://www.sgo.org

RADIATION THERAPY

American College of Radiology
(800) 227-5463
http://www.acr.org

Organization can provide a list of accredited facilities for mammography in any area in the country.

RESEARCH

American Institute for Cancer Research (AICR)
1759 R Street, NW
Washington, DC 20009
(202) 328-7744
(800) 843-8114
http://www.aicr.org

Breast Cancer Fund
2107 O'Farrell Street
San Francisco, CA 94115
(415) 346-8223

(800) 487-0492
http://www.breastcancerfund.org

Cancer Research Foundation of America
1600 Duke Street
Suite 110
Alexandria, VA 22314
(703) 836-4412
(800) 227-2732 or (800) 227-CRFA
http://www.preventcancer.org

Cancer Research Institute
681 Fifth Avenue
New York, NY 10022
(212) 688-7515
http://www.cancerresearch.org

European Organisation for Research and Treatment of Cancer
http://www.eortc.be/

SUPPORT GROUPS (GENERAL)

Gilda's Club Worldwide
322 Eighth Avenue
Suite 1402
New York, NY 10001

(800) GILDA-4-U
http://www.gildasclub.org

Make Today Count
2055 South Frem
Springfield, MO 65804
(800) 432-3373
http://www.members.tripod.com

WOMEN'S ISSUES

National Asian Women's Health Organization
250 Montgomery Street
Suite 900
San Francisco, CA 94104
(415) 989-9747
http://www.nawho.org

National Women's Health Information Center (NWHIC)
8550 Arlington Boulevard
Suite 300
Fairfax, VA 22031
(800) 994-9662
http://www.4woman.org

APPENDIX II
CANCER CENTERS

ALABAMA

University of Alabama at Birmingham Comprehensive Cancer Center*
1824 Sixth Avenue South
Birmingham, AL 35294
(205) 975-8222
(800) 822-0933 or (800) UAB-0933
http://www.ccc.uab.edu/

ARIZONA

Arizona Cancer Center*
The University of Arizona
1515 North Campbell Avenue
P.O. Box 245024
Tucson, AZ 85724
(520) 626-2900 (new patient registration line)
(800) 622-2673 or (800) 622-COPE
http://www.azcc.arizona.edu/

CALIFORNIA

Burnham Institute
10010 North Torrey Pines Road
La Jolla, California 92037
(858) 646-3400

Chao Family Comprehensive Cancer Center*
University of California at Irvine
Building 23
Route 81
101 The City Drive
Orange, CA 92868
(714) 456-8200
http://www.ucihs.uci.edu/cancer/

City of Hope*
1500 East Duarte Road
Cancer Center and Beckman Research Institute

Duarte, CA 91010
(626) 359-8111
(800) 826-4673 or (800) 826-HOPE
E-mail: becomingapatient@coh.org
http://www.cityofhope.org/

Jonsson Comprehensive Cancer Center at UCLA*
8-684 Factor Building
UCLA Box 951781
Los Angeles, CA 90095
(310) 825-5268
E-mail: jcccinfo@mednet.ucla.edu
http://www.cancer.mednet.ucla.edu/

Salk Institute
10010 North Torrey Pines Road
La Jolla, California 92037
(858) 453-4100 (ext.1386)

UC Davis Cancer Center**
University of California, Davis
4501 X Street
Suite 3003
Sacramento, California 95817
(916) 734-5800

University of California, San Diego Cancer Center*
9500 Gilman Drive
La Jolla, CA 92093
(858) 534-7600
http://www.cancer.ucsd.edu

University of California, San Francisco Comprehensive Cancer Center*
Box 0128, UCSF
2340 Sutter Street
San Francisco, CA 94143
(415) 476-2201 (general information)
(800) 888-8664 (cancer referral line)

*Comprehensive cancer centers
**Clinical cancer centers

E-mail: cceditor@cc.ucsf.edu
http://www.cc.ucsf.edu/

USC/Norris Comprehensive Cancer Center and Hospital*

1441 Eastlake Avenue
Los Angeles, CA 90033
(323) 865-3000
(800) 872-2273 or (800) USC-CARE
E-mail: cainfo@ccnt.hsc.usc.edu (for general information)
http://www.ccnt.hsc.usc.edu/

COLORADO

University of Colorado Cancer Center*

Box F-704
1665 North Ursula Street
Aurora, CO 80010
(720) 848-0300
(800) 473-2288 (cancer referral line)
http://www.uch.uchsc.edu/uccc/

CONNECTICUT

Yale Cancer Center*

Yale University School of Medicine
333 Cedar Street
P.O. Box 208028
New Haven, CT 06520
(203) 785-4095 (administrative offices)
http://www.info.med.yale.edu/ycc/

DISTRICT OF COLUMBIA

Lombardi Cancer Center*

Georgetown University Medical Center
3800 Reservoir Road, NW
Washington, DC 20007
(202) 784-4000
http://www.lombardi.georgetown.edu/

FLORIDA

H. Lee Moffitt Cancer Center & Research Institute at The University of South Florida*

12902 Magnolia Drive
Tampa, FL 33612
(813) 972-4673 or (813) 972-HOPE
http://www.moffitt.usf.edu/

HAWAII

Cancer Research Center of Hawaii**

1236 Lauhala Street
Honolulu, HI 96813
(808) 586-3010
http://www.hawaii.edu/crch/

ILLINOIS

Robert H. Lurie Comprehensive Cancer Center*

Northwestern University
Olson Pavilion 8250
710 North Fairbanks Court
Chicago, IL 60611
(312) 908-5250
E-mail: s-markman@northwestern.edu
http://www.lurie.nwu.edu/

University of Chicago Cancer Research Center*

Mail Code 9015
5758 South Maryland Avenue
Chicago, IL 60637
(773) 702-9200
(888) 824-0200 (new patients)
E-mail: aholub@mcis.bsd.uchicago.edu
http://www.-uccrc.uchicago.edu/

INDIANA

Indiana University Cancer Center**

535 Barnhill Drive
Indianapolis, IN 46202
(317) 278-4822
(888) 600-4822
http://www.iucc.iu.edu

Purdue University Cancer Center

Hansen Life Sciences Research Building
South University Street
West Lafayette, Indiana 47907
(765) 494-9129

IOWA

Holden Comprehensive Cancer Center at The University of Iowa*

5970-Z JPP
200 Hawkins Drive
Iowa City, IA 52242
(800) 777-8442 (patient referral)
(800) 237-1225 (general information)

E-mail: Cancer-Center@uiowa.edu
http://www.uihealthcare.com/DeptsClinicalServices/
   CancerCenter

MAINE

Jackson Laboratory
600 Main Street
Bar Harbor, Maine 04609
(207) 288-6041

MARYLAND

Johns Hopkins Oncology Center*
Weinberg Building
401 North Broadway
Baltimore, MD 21231
(410) 502-1033
http://www.hopkinskimmelcancercenter.org

**Sidney Kimmel Comprehensive Cancer Center
   at Johns Hopkins***
Room I57
North Wolfe Street
Baltimore, Maryland 21287
(410) 955-8822

MASSACHUSETTS

Center for Cancer Research
Massachusetts Institute of Technology
Room E17-110
77 Massachusetts Avenue
Cambridge, Massachusetts 02139
(617) 253-8511

Dana-Farber Cancer Institute*
44 Binney Street
Boston, MA 02115
(617) 632-3000 (ask for patient information)
http://www.dana-farber.org/

MICHIGAN

Barbara Ann Karmanos Cancer Institute*
Operating the Meyer L. Prentis Comprehensive
   Cancer Center of Metropolitan Detroit
Wertz Clinical Center
4100 John R. Street
Detroit, MI 48201
(800) 527-6266 or (800) KARMANOS
E-mail: info@karmanos.org
http://www.karmanos.org/

**University of Michigan Comprehensive
   Cancer Center***
1500 East Medical Center Drive
Ann Arbor, MI 48109
(800) 865-1125
http://www.cancer.med.umich.edu/

MINNESOTA

Mayo Clinic Cancer Center*
200 First Street, SW
Rochester, MN 55905
(507) 284-2111
http://www.mayo.edu/cancercenter/

University of Minnesota Cancer Center*
Box 806 Mayo
420 Delaware Street, SE
Minneapolis, MN 55455
(612) 624-8484
http://www.cancer.umn.edu/

MISSOURI

Siteman Cancer Center**
Barnes-Jewish Hospital and
Washington University School of Medicine
Box 8100
660 South Euclid
Street Louis, MO 63110
(314) 747-7222
(800) 600-3606
E-mail: info@ccadmin.wustl.edu
http://www.siteman.wustl.edu/

NEBRASKA

UNMC Eppley Cancer Center**
University of Nebraska Medical Center
986805 Nebraska Medical Center
Omaha, NE 68198
(402) 559-4238
http://www.unmc.edu/cancercenter/

NEW HAMPSHIRE

Norris Cotton Cancer Center*
Dartmouth-Hitchcock Medical Center
One Medical Center Drive
Lebanon, NH 03756
(603) 650-6300 (administration)

(800) 639-6918 (cancer help line)
E-mail: cancerhelp@dartmouth.edu
http://www.dartmouth.edu/dms/nccc

NEW JERSEY

Cancer Institute of New Jersey**
Robert Wood Johnson Medical School
195 Little Albany Street
New Brunswick, NJ 08901
(732) 235-2465
(732) 235-CINJ
http://www.cinj.umdnj.edu

NEW YORK

Albert Einstein Comprehensive Cancer Center*
Albert Einstein College of Medicine
1300 Morris Park Avenue
Bronx, NY 10461
(718) 430-2302
E-mail: aeccc@aecom.yu.edu
http://www.aecom.yu.edu/cancer

Herbert Irving Comprehensive Cancer Center*
Columbia Presbyterian Center
New York-Presbyterian Hospital
PH 18, Room 200
622 West 168th Street
New York, NY 10032
(212) 305-9327
http://www.ccc.columbia.edu/

Kaplan Comprehensive Cancer Center*
New York University School of Medicine
550 First Avenue
New York, NY 10016
(212) 263-6485
http://www.nyucancerinstitute.org/

Memorial Sloan-Kettering Cancer Center*
1275 York Avenue
New York, NY 10021
(800) 525-2225
http://www.mskcc.org/

Roswell Park Cancer Institute*
Elm and Carlton Streets
Buffalo, NY 14263
(800) 767-9355 or (800) ROSWELL
http://www.roswellpark.org/

NORTH CAROLINA

Comprehensive Cancer Center of Wake Forest University*
Wake Forest University Baptist Medical Center
Medical Center Boulevard
Winston-Salem, NC 27157
(336) 716-4464
http://www.bgsm.edu/cancer/

Duke Comprehensive Cancer Center*
Duke University Medical Center
Box 3843
301 MSRB
Durham, NC 27710
(919) 684-3377
http://www.cancer.duke.edu

UNC Lineberger Comprehensive Cancer Center*
School of Medicine
University of North Carolina at Chapel Hill
Campus Box 7295
Chapel Hill, NC 27599
(919) 966-3036
E-mail: dgs@med.unc.edu
http://www.cancer.med.unc.edu/

OHIO

Ireland Cancer Center*
University Hospitals of Cleveland
11100 Euclid Avenue
Cleveland, OH 44106
(216) 844-5432
(800) 641-2422
E-mail: info@irelandcancercenter.org
http://www.irelandcancercenter.org

Ohio State University Comprehensive Cancer Center*
The Arthur G. James Cancer Hospital and Richard J. Solove Research Institute
Suite 519
300 West 10th Avenue
Columbus, OH 43210
(800) 293-5066
E-mail: cancerinfo@jamesline.com
http://www.jamesline.com

OREGON

Oregon Cancer Center**
Oregon Health Sciences University
CR145

3181 Southwest Sam Jackson Park Road
Portland, OR 97201
(503) 494-1617
http://www.ohsu.edu/oci/

PENNSYLVANIA

Fox Chase Cancer Center*
7701 Burholme Avenue
Philadelphia, PA 19111
(215) 728-2570 (to schedule an appointment)
(888) 369-2427 or (888) FOX CHASE
E-mail: info@fccc.edu
http://www.fccc.edu/

Kimmel Cancer Center**
Thomas Jefferson University
Bluemle Life Sciences Building
233 South 10th Street
Philadelphia, PA 19107
(215) 503-4500
(800) 533-3669 or (800) JEFF-NOW (Jefferson
    Cancer Network)
(800) 654-5984 (TDD)
http://www.kcc.tju.edu/

University of Pennsylvania Cancer Center*
15th Floor, Penn Tower
3400 Spruce Street
Philadelphia, PA 19104
(215) 662-4000 (main)
(800) 789-7366 or (800) 789-PENN (referral/to
    schedule an appointment)
http://www.oncolink.upenn.edu/

University of Pittsburgh Cancer Institute*
Iroquois Building
3600 Forbes Avenue
Suite 206
Pittsburgh, PA 15213
(800) 237-4724 or (800) 237-4PCI
E-mail: PCI-INFO@msx.upmc.edu
http://www.upci.upmc.edu/

Wistar Institute
3601 Spruce Street
Philadelphia, Pennsylvania 19104
(215) 898-3926

TENNESSEE

Saint Jude Children's Research Hospital**
332 North Lauderdale Street
Memphis, TN 38105

(901) 495-3300
http://www.2.stjude.org

Vanderbilt-Ingram Cancer Center*
Vanderbilt University
649 The Preston Building
Nashville, TN 37232
(615) 936-1782
(615) 936-5847
(800) 811-8480 (clinical trial or treatment option
    information)
(888) 488-4089 (all other calls)
http://www.vicc.org/

TEXAS

San Antonio Cancer Institute*
8122 Datapoint Drive
San Antonio, TX 78229
(210) 616-5590
http://www.ccc.saci.org/

**University of Texas M. D. Anderson Cancer
    Center***
1515 Holcombe Boulevard
Houston, TX 77030
(713) 792-6161
(800) 392-1611
http://www.mdanderson.org/

UTAH

Huntsman Cancer Institute**
University of Utah
2000 Circle of Hope
Salt Lake City, UT 84112
(801) 585-0303
(877) 585-0303
http://www.hci.utah.edu/

VERMONT

Vermont Cancer Center*
University of Vermont
Medical Alumni Building
Burlington, VT 05401
(802) 656-4414
E-mail: vcc@uvm.edu
http://www.vermontcancer.org

VIRGINIA

Cancer Center at the University of Virginia**
University of Virginia Health System
Box 800334

Charlottesville, VA 22908
(804) 924-9333
(800) 223-9173
http://www.med.virginia.edu/medcntr/cancer/
   home.html

Massey Cancer Center**
Virginia Commonwealth University
P.O. Box 980037
401 College Street
Richmond, VA 23298
(804) 828-0450
http://www.vcu.edu/mcc/

WASHINGTON

Fred Hutchinson Cancer Research Center*
LA-205
P.O. Box 19024
1100 Fairview Avenue North

Seattle, WA 98109
(206) 288-1024
(800) 804-8824 (appointments and medical
   referral—Seattle Cancer Care Alliance)
E-mail: hutchdoc@seattlecca.org (patient
   information)
http://www.fhcrc.org/

WISCONSIN

**University of Wisconsin Comprehensive Cancer
   Center***
600 Highland Avenue, K5/601
Madison, WI 53792
(608) 263-8600
(608) 262-5223 (Cancer Connect)
(800) 622-8922 (Cancer Connect)
E-mail: uwccc@uwcc.wisc.edu/
http://www.cancer.wisc.edu

APPENDIX III
ONGOING CLINICAL TRIALS

More detailed information about the ongoing clinical trials assessing treatments for breast cancer is available from the National Cancer Institute (NCI) cancer.gov Web site at http://www.cancer.gov/clinical_trials/.

COMPARATIVE GENETIC STUDY OF SUSCEPTIBILITY GENOTYPES AND PROTEIN EXPRESSION IN HEALTHY WOMEN, WOMEN AT HIGH RISK FOR BREAST CANCER, AND WOMEN WITH BREAST CANCER

This is a genetic study to compare genes in healthy women, women at high risk for breast cancer, and women who have breast cancer. Participants will donate blood, tissue, and nipple fluid samples for genetic testing. They will also complete a questionnaire regarding diet and family history. Participants will not receive the results of genetic testing, and the results will not be kept in their medical records.

CORRELATION OF MENSTRUAL CYCLE PHASE AT THE TIME OF SURGERY WITH DISEASE-FREE SURVIVAL IN PREMENOPAUSAL WOMEN WITH STAGE I OR II BREAST CANCER

This clinical trial will determine whether timing of primary surgery in relation to menstrual cycle is associated with disease-free survival five years after surgery in women who have stage I or stage II breast cancer. Hormone levels and menstrual history will be obtained before patients undergo surgery. Patients will complete a questionnaire at six months and one year after surgery and be evaluated once a year for 10 years.

DIAGNOSTIC STUDY OF CONTRAST-ENHANCED BREAST MAGNETIC RESONANCE IMAGING FOR WOMEN WITH STAGE III

BREAST CANCER WHO ARE RECEIVING NEOADJUVANT CHEMOTHERAPY

This is a diagnostic trial to study the effectiveness of magnetic resonance imaging (MRI) in monitoring tumor response in women who are receiving chemotherapy for stage III breast cancer. Patients will undergo MRI before, during, and after chemotherapy. Patients will also undergo mammography, ultrasound, and biopsy at different times during treatment and will be evaluated every six months for up to ten years.

DIAGNOSTIC STUDY OF CONTRAST-ENHANCED MAGNETIC RESONANCE IMAGING AND CORRELATIVE MOLECULAR STUDIES IN WOMEN WITH LOCALLY ADVANCED BREAST CANCER WHO ARE RECEIVING NEOADJUVANT CHEMOTHERAPY

This is a diagnostic trial to study magnetic resonance imaging (MRI) and biomarkers in women who are receiving chemotherapy before surgery for locally advanced breast cancer. Patients will undergo MRI of the breast, biopsy, and blood collections before, during, and after chemotherapy. They will also undergo the same procedures, plus mammography with or without ultrasound, before surgery to remove the tumor. Patients will then be evaluated every six months for five years and once a year for the following 10 years.

GENETIC MAPPING OF INTERACTIVE SUSCEPTIBILITY LOCI IN PATIENTS AND SIBLINGS WITH BREAST, COLON, LUNG, OR PROSTATE CANCER

This is a clinical trial to identify genes that may be associated with cancer that certain cancer patients and their siblings may have in common. A questionnaire will be completed about the incidence of cancer in the family. Blood samples will be taken from the patient, the sibling, and their parents (if possible) and laboratory tests will be performed using those samples. Patients will receive a follow-up evaluation once a year. Patients will not receive the results of the genetic testing and the results will not influence the type and duration of treatment.

GENETIC, CLINICAL, AND EPIDEMIOLOGICAL STUDY OF INDIVIDUALS AND FAMILIES AT HIGH RISK OF CANCER

This is a study to identify genetic and environmental factors related to cancer risk in individuals and families at high risk of cancer. Individuals and families will undergo a physical evaluation and have blood samples drawn for testing. Some patients may undergo additional diagnostic studies and examinations. A family participating in the study may undergo genetic testing and genetic counseling if they were previously identified as having a gene that increases their risk for cancer. Families will receive follow-up evaluations at least once a year.

PHASE I PILOT STUDY OF HER2/NEU INTRACELLULAR DOMAIN PROTEIN PULSED AUTOLOGOUS DENDRITIC CELLS IN PATIENTS WITH HER2/NEU EXPRESSING ADVANCED MALIGNANCIES SHOWING NO EVIDENCE OF DISEASE AFTER STANDARD TREATMENT

This is a Phase I trial to study the effectiveness of biological therapy in treating patients who have advanced cancer that shows no signs of disease following treatment. White blood cells will be collected and treated in the laboratory. Patients will receive injections of the treated cells once every three weeks for up to four courses and will receive follow-up evaluations every three months for one year.

PHASE I PILOT STUDY OF VACCINATION WITH A HEPTAVALENT ANTIGEN-KEYHOLE LIMPET HEMOCYANIN CONJUGATE PLUS QS21 IN PATIENTS AT HIGH RISK FOR BREAST CANCER RECURRENCE

This is a Phase II trial to study the effectiveness of vaccine therapy in treating patients who are at high risk for breast cancer recurrence. Patients will receive injections of the vaccine once a week in weeks 1, 2, 3, 7, and 19. Patients will be evaluated every three months.

PHASE I STUDY OF BMS-247550 AND CAPECITABINE IN PATIENTS WITH METASTATIC BREAST CANCER PREVIOUSLY TREATED WITH A TAXANE AND AN ANTHRACYCLINE

This is a Phase I trial to study the effectiveness of combining BMS-247550 with capecitabine in treating patients who have metastatic breast cancer that has not responded to previous chemotherapy. Patients will be assigned to one of two groups. Patients in group one will receive a three-hour infusion of BMS-247550 on day 1, plus capecitabine by mouth twice a day for two weeks. Patients in group two will receive a one-hour infusion of BMS-247550 on days 1 to 3, and capecitabine as in group one. Treatment in both groups may be repeated every three weeks for up to 18 courses, and patients will be evaluated periodically for one month and every three months thereafter.

PHASE I STUDY OF BMS-247550 IN PATIENTS WITH ADVANCED OR RECURRENT SOLID TUMORS, OVARIAN CANCER, OR BREAST CANCER

This is a Phase I trial to study the effectiveness of BMS-247550 in treating patients who have metastatic, recurrent, or locally advanced ovarian cancer, breast cancer, or metastatic or unresectable solid tumors. Patients will receive an infusion of BMS-247550 once every three weeks, and treatment will continue for as long as benefit is shown.

PHASE I STUDY OF CAPECITABINE AND CISPLATIN IN PATIENTS WITH LOCALLY ADVANCED OR METASTATIC CANCER OF THE UPPER GASTROINTESTINAL TRACT, HEAD AND NECK, LUNG, BREAST, OR CARCINOMA OF UNKNOWN PRIMARY

This is a Phase I trial to study the effectiveness of capecitabine combined with cisplatin in treating patients who have locally advanced or metastatic solid tumors. Patients will receive capecitabine by mouth twice a day for five, 10, or 14 days, and will also receive an infusion of cisplatin on the first day of each treatment course. Treatment may be repeated every three weeks for as long as benefit is shown. Patients will receive follow-up evaluations every three months for six months and every six months thereafter.

PHASE I STUDY OF CRYOSURGERY IN WOMEN WITH HIGHLY SUSPICIOUS BREAST LESIONS

This is a Phase I trial to study the effectiveness of cryosurgery in treating women who have breast lesions. In this study, patients will undergo cryosurgery and within three to 21 days will undergo surgery to remove either the lesion or the entire breast. Patients will be evaluated at one week and then once a month for three months.

PHASE I STUDY OF INDOLE-3-CARBINOL FOR THE PREVENTION OF BREAST CANCER IN NONSMOKING WOMEN AT HIGH RISK FOR BREAST CANCER

This is a Phase I trial to study the effectiveness of indole-3-carbinol in preventing breast cancer in nonsmoking women who are at high risk for breast cancer. Participants will receive indole-3-carbinol or a placebo by mouth twice a day for 12 to 16 weeks. Quality of life will be assessed at the beginning of the study and every four weeks during the study.

PHASE I STUDY OF INTERLEUKIN-12, PACLITAXEL, AND TRASTUZUMAB (HERCEPTIN) IN PATIENTS WITH HER2/ NEU-OVEREXPRESSING MALIGNANCIES

This is a Phase I trial to study the effectiveness of interleukin-12, paclitaxel, and trastuzumab in treating patients who have solid tumors. Interleukin-12 may kill tumor cells by stopping blood flow to the tumor and by stimulating a person's white blood cells to kill cancer cells. Monoclonal antibodies such as trastuzumab can locate tumor cells and either kill them or deliver tumor-killing substances to them without harming normal cells. Combining interleukin-12, chemotherapy, and monoclonal antibody therapy may kill more tumor cells.

Patients will receive an infusion of trastuzumab once a week for three weeks and an infusion of paclitaxel on day 1 of week 1. Beginning with course two, patients will receive trastuzumab and paclitaxel as in course one and infusions of interleukin-12 twice a week for up to one year. Patients will be evaluated every three months for one year and every six months thereafter.

PHASE I STUDY OF INTRAVENOUS INTERLEUKIN-4 PE38KDEL CYTOTOXIN IN PATIENTS WITH RECURRENT OR UNRESP ONSIVE METASTATIC RENAL CELL,

NON-SMALL CELL LUNG, OR BREAST CANCER THAT OVEREXPRESSES INTERLEUKIN-4 RECEPTORS

This is a Phase I trial to study the effectiveness of intravenous interleukin-4 PE38KDEL cytotoxin in treating patients who have recurrent or metastatic kidney cancer, non-small cell lung cancer, or breast cancer that has not responded to previous treatment. Interleukin-4 PE38KDEL cytotoxin may be able to deliver cancer-killing substances directly to solid tumor cells.

Patients will receive an infusion of interleukin-4 PE38KDEL cytotoxin once a day for five days. Treatment may be repeated every four weeks for as long as benefit is shown.

PHASE I STUDY OF LMB-9 IMMUNOTOXIN IN PATIENTS WITH ADVANCED COLON, BREAST, NON-SMALL CELL LUNG, BLADDER, PANCREAS, OR OVARIAN CANCER

This is a Phase I trial to study the effectiveness of LMB-9 immunotoxin in treating patients who have advanced colon, breast, non-small cell lung, bladder, pancreatic, or ovarian cancer. The LMB-9 immunotoxin can locate tumor cells and kill them without harming normal cells.

Patients will receive a 10-day continuous infusion of LMB-9 immunotoxin; treatment may be repeated every 30 days for as long as benefit is shown. Patients will be evaluated at three weeks and then every two months thereafter.

PHASE I STUDY OF PERILLYL ALCOHOL IN WOMEN AT RISK FOR RECURRENT BREAST CANCER

This is a Phase I trial to study the effectiveness of perillyl alcohol in preventing the recurrence of breast cancer in women who have been treated with surgery with or without adjuvant therapy. The use of perillyl alcohol may be effective in preventing the recurrence of breast cancer. Patients will receive perillyl alcohol by mouth once a day for 12 weeks, and will then be evaluated once a week.

PHASE I STUDY OF SU5416 AND DOXORUBICIN IN PATIENTS WITH STAGE IIIB OR IV INFLAMMATORY BREAST CANCER

This is a Phase I trial to study the effectiveness of SU5416 and doxorubicin in treating patients who have stage IIIB or stage IV inflammatory breast cancer. SU5416 may stop the growth of breast cancer by stopping blood flow to the tumor. Drugs used in chemotherapy use different ways to stop tumor cells from dividing so they stop growing or die; combining SU5416 with chemotherapy may kill more cancer cells.

Patients will receive an infusion of SU5416 twice a week beginning in week 1 and an infusion of doxorubicin every three weeks beginning in week 2. Treatment may be repeated every three weeks for five courses. Following chemotherapy, all patients will undergo a modified radical mastectomy plus radiation therapy to the chest and nearby lymph nodes. Some patients will receive tamoxifen by mouth for five years after radiation therapy. Patients will be evaluated every three months.

PHASE I STUDY OF TRASTUZUMAB (HERCEPTIN) AND FLAVOPIRIDOL IN PATIENTS WITH HER2-POSITIVE METASTATIC BREAST CANCER

This is a Phase I trial to study the effectiveness of combining trastuzumab with flavopiridol in treating patients who have metastatic breast cancer. Monoclonal antibodies such as trastuzumab can locate tumor cells and either kill them or deliver tumor-killing substances to them without harming normal cells. Combining trastuzumab with flavopiridol may kill more tumor cells.

Patients will receive a 30- to 90-minute infusion of trastuzumab on days 1, 8, and 15 followed by a 24-hour continuous infusion of flavopiridol on days 1 and 8. Treatment may be repeated every three weeks for as long as benefit is shown.

PHASE I STUDY OF YTTRIUM Y 90 LABELED, HUMANIZED MONOCLONAL ANTIBODY BRE-3 AND INDIUM IN 111 LABELED, HUMANIZED MONOCLONAL ANTIBODY BRE-3 FOLLOWED BY AUTOLOGOUS BONE MARROW OR PERIPHERAL BLOOD STEM CELL TRANSPLANTATION IN PATIENTS WITH METASTATIC BREAST CANCER

This is a Phase I trial to study the effectiveness of radiolabeled monoclonal antibody therapy followed by bone marrow or peripheral stem cell transplantation in treating patients who have metastatic breast cancer. Radiolabeled monoclonal antibodies can locate tumor cells and either kill them or deliver tumor-killing substances to them. Peripheral stem cell transplantation or bone marrow transplantation may be able to replace immune cells that were destroyed by monoclonal antibody therapy used to kill tumor cells.

Before beginning treatment, peripheral stem cells or bone marrow will be collected from patients. Patients will receive infusions of two radiolabeled monoclonal antibodies on day 1. Peripheral stem cells or bone marrow will be infused on day 15. Patients will then receive infusions of filgrastim until blood counts return to normal. Patients will receive follow-up evaluations every three to four months for a year, and at least once a year thereafter.

PHASE I STUDY OF YTTRIUM Y 90 MONOCLONAL ANTIBODY B3 FOLLOWED BY AUTOLOGOUS OR SYNGENEIC PERIPHERAL BLOOD STEM CELL TRANSPLANTATION IN PATIENTS WITH RELAPSED OR METASTATIC BREAST CANCER

This is a Phase I trial to study the effectiveness of monoclonal antibody therapy followed by peripheral stem cell transplantation in treating patients with recurrent or metastatic breast cancer. Monoclonal antibodies can locate tumor cells and either kill them or deliver tumor-killing substances to them without harming normal cells. Peripheral stem cell transplantation may allow the doctor to give higher doses of monoclonal antibody therapy and kill more cancer cells.

Patients will receive injections of filgrastim once a day beginning four days before stem cell collection and continuing until stem cells have been collected. Two to three weeks after collecting of stem cells, patients will receive an infusion of the monoclonal antibody twice over eight days. Peripheral stem cells will be reinfused on day 7. Beginning one week later, patients will receive injections of filgrastim until blood counts return to normal. Patients will be evaluated at one month and every two months thereafter.

PHASE I STUDY OF YTTRIUM Y 90 MONOCLONAL ANTIBODY M170, CYCLOSPORINE AND PACLITAXEL IN PATIENTS WITH RECURRENT OR REFRACTORY METASTATIC BREAST CANCER

This is a Phase I trial to study the effectiveness of radiolabeled monoclonal antibody therapy, cyclosporine, and paclitaxel in treating patients who have recurrent or refractory metastatic breast cancer. Combining monoclonal antibody therapy with cyclosporine and paclitaxel may be an effective treatment for metastatic breast cancer.

Patients will receive injections of filgrastim once a day for four days. Peripheral stem cells will then be collected for up to five days. Patients will receive cyclosporine by mouth every 12 hours on days 1–29. Patients will receive infusions of unlabeled and radiolabeled monoclonal antibodies on days 4 and 11. Some patients may receive infusions of paclitaxel on day 13. Some patients may undergo peripheral stem cell transplantation on day 21, followed by injections of filgrastim once a day until blood counts return to normal. Patients will be evaluated once a month for three months, every three months for one year, and then every six months for one year.

PHASE I/II PILOT STUDY OF HERBA SCUTELLARIA BARBATAE (CHINESE HERBAL EXTRACT) IN WOMEN WITH METASTATIC BREAST CANCER

This is a Phase I/II trial to study the effectiveness of the Chinese herb *Scutellaria barbatae* in treating women who have metastatic breast cancer. *Scutellaria barbatae* contains ingredients that may slow the growth of cancer cells and may be an effective treatment for metastatic breast cancer. Patients will receive *Scutellaria barbatae* by mouth twice a day for up to one year. Quality of life will be assessed periodically.

PHASE I/II PILOT STUDY OF STEM CELL MOBILIZATION WITH PACLITAXEL AND CYCLOPHOSPHAMIDE FOLLOWED BY HIGH DOSE MELPHALAN AND ETOPOSIDE WITH AUTOLOGOUS PERIPHERAL BLOOD STEM CELL RESCUE IN PATIENTS WITH METASTATIC OR HIGH RISK BREAST CANCER

This is a Phase I/II trial to study the effectiveness of combination chemotherapy plus peripheral stem cell transplantation in treating patients who have stage III or stage IV recurrent or metastatic breast cancer. Combining chemotherapy with peripheral stem cell transplantation may allow the doctor to give higher doses of chemotherapy drugs and kill more tumor cells.

Patients will receive infusions of cyclophosphamide and 24-hour continuous infusions of paclitaxel for three days. They will also receive injections of filgrastim beginning on day 5 and continuing until peripheral stem cells have been collected. Treatment will be repeated every four weeks for up

to seven courses. Some patients may also receive infusions of doxorubicin and cyclophosphamide every three weeks for up to four courses. Patients will receive infusions of high-dose melphalan and etoposide for three days followed by reinfusion of the stem cells four days later. Some patients may receive pamidronate, radiation therapy, or hormone therapy. Patients will receive follow-up evaluations every six months for two years.

PHASE I/II RANDOMIZED STUDY OF ADJUVANT DOXORUBICIN AND CYCLOPHOSPHAMIDE WITH OR WITHOUT CHINESE HERBAL THERAPY FOR SYMPTOM MANAGEMENT IN WOMEN WITH STAGE I, II, OR EARLY STAGE III BREAST CANCER

This is a randomized Phase I/II trial to study the effectiveness of herbs used in traditional Chinese medicine in decreasing the side effects of chemotherapy after surgery in women who have stage I, stage II, or early stage III breast cancer.

Patients will be randomly assigned to one of two groups. Patients in both groups will receive infusions of doxorubicin and cyclophosphamide every three weeks for four doses. Beginning 10 days before chemotherapy, patients will receive either Chinese herbs or a placebo by mouth three times a day for 15 weeks. Quality of life will be assessed periodically, and patients will be evaluated at the completion of herbal therapy.

PHASE I/II STUDY OF ACTIVE IMMUNOTHERAPY WITH CARCINOEMBRYONIC ANTIGEN (CEA) RNA PULSED AUTOLOGOUS DENDRITIC CELLS IN PATIENTS WITH METASTATIC BREAST CANCER WHO ACHIEVE A COMPLETE RESPONSE AFTER HIGH DOSE CHEMOTHERAPY AND STEM CELL SUPPORT

This is a Phase I/II trial to study the effectiveness of immunotherapy with CEA-treated white blood cells in treating patients with metastatic breast cancer who have achieved a partial or complete response after chemotherapy and peripheral stem cell transplantation. Immunotherapy using CEA-treated white blood cells may help a person's body build an immune response to and kill tumor cells.

Prior to entry on this study, patients will undergo peripheral stem cell transplantation during which white blood cells will be removed. Approximately two to three months later, patients will receive immunotherapy with CEA-treated white blood cells every three weeks for four doses. Patients will then have more white blood cells removed. Patients will receive follow-up evaluations every three months for the first year and once a year thereafter.

PHASE I/II STUDY OF CPG 7909 AND TRASTUZUMAB (HERCEPTIN) IN WOMEN WITH METASTATIC BREAST CANCER REFRACTORY TO TRASTUZUMAB AND CHEMOTHERAPY

This is a Phase I/II trial to study the effectiveness of combining trastuzumab with CpG 7909 in treating women who have metastatic breast cancer that has not responded to previous treatment with trastuzumab and chemotherapy. Monoclonal antibodies such as trastuzumab can locate tumor cells and either kill them or deliver tumor-killing substances to them without harming normal cells. CpG 7909 may help trastuzumab kill more cancer cells by making tumor cells more sensitive to the drug.

Patients will receive a 30- to 90-minute infusion of trastuzumab followed by a two-hour infusion of CpG 7909 once a week for eight to 24 weeks. Patients will be evaluated within two weeks and every three months thereafter.

PHASE I/II STUDY OF DOCETAXEL AND FLAVOPIRIDOL IN PATIENTS WITH PREVIOUSLY TREATED LOCALLY ADVANCED OR METASTATIC BREAST CANCER

This is a Phase I/II trial to study the effectiveness of combination chemotherapy in treating patients who have locally advanced or metastatic breast cancer. Drugs used in chemotherapy use different ways to stop tumor cells from dividing so they stop growing or die. Combining more than one drug may kill more tumor cells.

Patients will receive a one-hour infusion of docetaxel on day 1. They will also receive either a one-hour infusion of flavopiridol or a three-day continuous infusion of flavopiridol beginning on day 2. Treatment may be repeated every three weeks for as long as benefit is shown. Quality of life will be assessed periodically.

PHASE I/II STUDY OF DOXORUBICIN HCI LIPOSOME AND TRASTUZUMAB (HERCEPTIN) IN WOMEN WITH ADVANCED HER-2/ NEU-OVEREXPRESSING BREAST CANCER

This is a Phase I/II trial to study the effectiveness of liposomal doxorubicin and trastuzumab in treating women who have advanced breast cancer. Monoclonal antibodies such as trastuzumab can locate tumor cells and either kill them or deliver tumor-killing substances to them without harming normal cells. Combining chemotherapy with monoclonal antibody therapy may kill more tumor cells.

Patients will receive an infusion of liposomal doxorubicin on day 1. They will also receive infusions of trastuzumab on days 1, 8, and 15. Treatment may be repeated every three weeks for as long as benefit is shown. Patients will be evaluated every three months.

PHASE I/II STUDY OF DOXORUBICIN HCI LIPOSOME AND TRASTUZUMAB (HERCEPTIN) IN WOMEN WITH LOCALLY ADVANCED, INFLAMMATORY, OR METASTATIC BREAST CANCER

This is a Phase I/II trial to study the effectiveness of liposomal doxorubicin and trastuzumab in treating women who have locally advanced, inflammatory, or metastatic breast cancer. Monoclonal antibodies such as trastuzumab can locate tumor cells and either kill them or deliver tumor-killing substances to them without harming normal cells. Patients will receive an infusion of liposomal doxorubicin on day 1 and an infusion of trastuzumab on days 1, 8, and 15. Treatment may be repeated every three weeks for as long as benefit is shown, and patients will be evaluated for at least three months.

PHASE I/II STUDY OF HIGH-DOSE CHEMOTHERAPY FOLLOWED BY AUTOLO-GOUS PERIPHERAL BLOOD STEM CELL TRANSPLANTATION AND IMMUNOTHERAPY WITH ACTIVATED T CELLS, INTERLEUKIN-2, AND SARGRAMOSTIM (GM-CSF) IN PATIENTS WITH STAGE IIIB OR IV BREAST CANCER OR OTHER SOLID TUMORS

This is a Phase I/II trial to study the effectiveness of chemotherapy followed by peripheral stem cell transplantation plus biological therapy in treating patients who have stage IIIB or stage IV breast cancer or other solid tumors. Combining chemotherapy with peripheral stem cell transplantation plus biological therapy may allow the doctor to give higher doses of chemotherapy drugs and kill more tumor cells.

Patients will receive an injection of filgrastim once a day for five days followed by collection of white blood cells. The white blood cells will then be treated in the laboratory with monoclonal antibody and interleukin-2. Patients will receive combination chemotherapy followed by stem cell collection. They will then receive one of two different combination chemotherapy regimens for six days, followed two or three days later by reinfusion of their stem cells. Beginning two weeks later, patients will receive an infusion of the treated white blood cells twice a week for eight weeks. They will also receive injections of interleukin-2 once a day and sargramostim twice a week for nine weeks. Patients will be evaluated at three months, six months, and once a year thereafter.

PHASE I/II STUDY OF IMMUNOTHERAPY WITH ARMED ACTIVATED T CELLS, INTERLEUKIN-2, AND SARGRAMOSTIM (GM-CSF) IN WOMEN WITH STAGE IV BREAST CANCER

This is a Phase I/II trial to study the effectiveness of combining different biological therapies in treating women who have stage IV breast cancer. Biological therapies use different ways to stimulate the immune system and stop cancer cells from growing. Combining different types of biological therapies may kill more tumor cells.

Patients' white blood cells will be collected and treated in the laboratory. Beginning two weeks later, patients will receive infusions of their treated white blood cells twice a week for four weeks. Patients will receive injections of interleukin-2 once a day and injections of sargramostim twice a week beginning one day before the first infusion of white blood cells and continuing until seven days after the last infusion. Patients will be evaluated at one, two, and five months and every six months thereafter.

PHASE I/II STUDY OF SEQUENTIAL PACLITAXEL, DOXORUBICIN, AND CYCLOPHOSPHAMIDE FOLLOWED BY IMMUNOTHERAPY WITH ACTIVATED T CELLS, INTERLEUKIN-2, AND SARGRAMOSTIM (GM-CSF) IN WOMEN WITH HIGH-RISK STAGE II OR III BREAST CANCER

This is a Phase I/II trial to study the effectiveness of combining chemotherapy with biological therapy in treating patients who have stage II or stage III breast cancer. Drugs used in chemotherapy use different ways to stop tumor cells from dividing so they stop growing or die. Biological therapies use different ways to stimulate the immune system and stop

tumor cells from growing. Combining chemotherapy with biological therapy may kill more tumor cells.

Patients will receive infusions of chemotherapy every other week for up to 18 weeks. They will also receive injections of filgrastim for eight days following each chemotherapy infusion. After chemotherapy is completed, patients' peripheral stem cells will be collected and treated in the laboratory. Within three to four weeks, patients will receive a reinfusion of stem cells once a week for eight weeks. Beginning three days before the stem cells are reinfused, patients will also receive injections of interleukin-2 once a day and sargramostim twice a week for nine weeks. Patients will be evaluated every three months for one year and once a year thereafter.

PHASE I/II STUDY OF TRASTUZUMAB (HERCEPTIN) AND ERLOTINIB AS FIRST-LINE THERAPY IN WOMEN WITH METASTATIC BREAST CANCER ASSOCIATED WITH HER-2/NEU OVEREXPRESSION

This is a Phase I/II trial to study the effectiveness of combining trastuzumab with erlotinib in treating women who have metastatic breast cancer. Monoclonal antibodies such as trastuzumab can locate tumor cells and either kill them or deliver tumor-killing substances to them without harming normal cells. Biological therapies such as erlotinib may interfere with the growth of tumor cells and slow the growth of the tumor. Combining trastuzumab with erlotinib may kill more tumor cells.

Patients will receive a 30- to 90-minute infusion of trastuzumab once a week beginning on day 1. Beginning on day 2, they will also receive erlotinib by mouth once a day. Treatment may continue for as long as benefit is shown. Patients will be evaluated every two months.

PHASE II NEOADJUVANT STUDY OF FOCUSED MICROWAVE THERMOTHERAPY IN WOMEN WITH STAGE I OR II INVASIVE BREAST CANCER IN AN INTACT BREAST

This is a Phase II trial to study the effectiveness of microwave thermotherapy in treating women who have stage I or stage II breast cancer. Microwave thermotherapy kills tumor cells by heating them to several degrees above body temperature. Patients will undergo a procedure to have sensors placed in and around the breast and will then undergo microwave thermotherapy for up to two hours. Some patients may receive a second treatment.

Within two months, patients will undergo surgery to remove the tumor. Some patients may then undergo radiation therapy and/or receive tamoxifen. Patients will be evaluated every six months for three years and once a year for two years.

PHASE II PILOT STUDY OF ADJUVANT PACLITAXEL, CYCLOPHOSPHAMIDE, FILGRASTIM (G-CSF), AND DOXORUBICIN FOLLOWED BY RADIOTHERAPY IN PATIENTS WITH STAGE II OR IIIA BREAST CANCER

This is a Phase II trial to study the effectiveness of combination chemotherapy and filgrastim followed by radiation therapy in treating patients who have stage II or stage IIIA breast cancer. Colony-stimulating factors such as filgrastim may increase the number of immune cells found in bone marrow or peripheral blood and may help a person's immune system recover from the side effects of chemotherapy. Radiation therapy uses high-energy X-rays to damage tumor cells.

Patients will receive a three-day continuous infusion of paclitaxel and infusions of cyclophosphamide once a day on the same three days. Patients will receive injections of filgrastim beginning on day 5 and continuing until blood counts return to normal. Treatment will be repeated every three weeks for three courses. Patients will then receive infusions of doxorubicin on day 1 and injections of filgrastim on days 2 through 11. Treatment will be repeated every three weeks for four courses. Some patients will also receive tamoxifen by mouth once a day for five years. Beginning three to six weeks after completing chemotherapy, patients will receive radiation therapy five days a week for up to seven weeks. Quality of life will be assessed periodically, and patients will receive follow-up evaluations every three months for two years and every six months thereafter.

PHASE II PILOT STUDY OF BEVACIZUMAB, DOCETAXEL, DOXORUBICIN, AND FILGRASTIM (G-CSF) IN PATIENTS WITH PREVIOUSLY UNTREATED STAGE IIIB OR IV INFLAMMATORY BREAST CANCER

This is a Phase II trial to study the effectiveness of bevacizumab plus chemotherapy and filgrastim in treating patients who have stage IIIB or stage IV inflammatory breast cancer that has not been previously treated with chemotherapy and/or radiation therapy. Monoclonal antibodies such as bevacizumab can locate tumor cells and either kill them or deliver tumor-killing substances to them without harming normal cells. Colony-stimulating factors such as filgrastim may increase the number of immune cells found in bone marrow or peripheral blood and may help a person's immune system recover from the side effects of chemotherapy. Combining monoclonal antibody therapy with chemotherapy and filgrastim may kill more tumor cells.

Patients will receive a 30- to 90-minute infusion of bevacizumab every three weeks for up to seven courses, and they will also receive one-hour infusions of doxorubicin and docetaxel every three weeks for six courses. On day 2 of courses two through seven, patients will receive injections of filgrastim once a day for 10 days. After completing course seven, patients may undergo surgery followed by an infusion of bevacizumab every three weeks for up to eight courses. Some patients may then receive tamoxifen by mouth once a day for up to five years. Patients will be evaluated every three months for one year and every three to six months for two years.

PHASE II RANDOMIZED STUDY OF DOXORUBICIN, CYCLOPHOSPHAMIDE, AND PACLITAXEL (ACT) VERSUS CYCLOPHOSPHAMIDE, THIOTEPA, AND CARBOPLATIN (STAMP V) IN PATIENTS WITH HIGH-RISK PRIMARY BREAST CANCER

This is a randomized Phase II trial to study the effectiveness of two regimens of combination chemotherapy in treating patients who have high-risk primary stage II or stage III breast cancer.

Patients will receive filgrastim twice a day until white blood cells are collected, and they will receive infusions of chemotherapy every three weeks for four doses. Patients will then be randomly assigned to receive one of two different chemotherapy regimens during an eight-day period. All patients will then undergo peripheral stem cell transplantation and will receive filgrastim until blood counts return to normal. Within four to six weeks after transplantation, some patients will begin receiving tamoxifen by mouth twice a day for five years, while some patients will receive infusions of pamidronate every four weeks for two years. Quality of life will be assessed periodically. Patients will receive follow-up evaluations every three months for one year and then every six months for at least 10 years.

PHASE II RANDOMIZED STUDY OF EXEMESTANE AND RALOXIFENE IN POSTMENOPAUSAL WOMEN WITH A HISTORY OF STAGE 0 (DUCTAL CARCINOMA IN SITU), I, II, OR III BREAST CANCER WHO HAVE NO CLINICAL EVIDENCE OF DISEASE

This is a randomized Phase II trial to evaluate the effectiveness of exemestane and raloxifene in treating postmenopausal women who have a history of ductal carcinoma in situ, stage I, stage II, or stage III breast cancer. Estrogen can stimulate the growth of breast cancer cells. Hormone therapy using exemestane may fight breast cancer by blocking the use of estrogen by the tumor cells. Raloxifene may be effective in preventing the recurrence of breast cancer.

Patients will be randomly assigned to receive either exemestane or raloxifene by mouth once a day for two weeks. After two weeks, all patients will receive a combination of raloxifene and exemestane once a day for one year. Patients may then continue to receive raloxifene alone or raloxifene plus exemestane for up to five years. Quality of life will be assessed before and periodically during treatment. Patients will be evaluated every three months for one year and then every six months through year 5.

PHASE II RANDOMIZED STUDY OF METHOTREXATE WITH OR WITHOUT ANTINEOPLASTON A10 CAPSULES IN WOMEN WITH ADVANCED BREAST CANCER

This is a randomized Phase II trial to study the effectiveness of methotrexate with or without antineoplaston therapy in treating postmenopausal women with advanced refractory breast cancer. Antineoplastons are naturally occurring substances found in urine that may inhibit the growth of cancer cells. It is not yet known whether giving antineoplastons with chemotherapy is more effective than chemotherapy alone in treating women with refractory breast cancer.

Patients will be randomized to one of two groups. Patients in group one will receive antineoplaston capsules by mouth seven times a day, followed by methotrexate capsules two to three times a day for five days, and repeated every 11 days. Patients in group two will receive methotrexate alone as in group one. Treatment may be repeated for as long as benefit is shown. Patients will be evaluated every four months for two years, every six months for two years, and then once a year for two years.

PHASE II RANDOMIZED STUDY OF PACLITAXEL, CARBOPLATIN, AND TRASTUZUMAB (HERCEPTIN) AS FIRST-LINE CHEMOTHERAPY IN WOMEN WITH OVEREXPRESSED HER-2, METASTATIC BREAST CANCER

This is a randomized Phase II trial to study the effectiveness of paclitaxel, carboplatin, and trastuzumab in treating women who have metastatic breast cancer that overexpresses *HER-2*. Monoclonal antibodies such as trastuzumab can locate tumor cells and either kill them or deliver tumor-killing substances to them without harming normal cells.

Patients will be randomly assigned to one of two groups. Patients in group one will receive a three-hour infusion of paclitaxel and an infusion of carboplatin every three weeks for up to eight courses. Patients in group two will receive a one-hour infusion of paclitaxel and an infusion of carboplatin once a week for three weeks. Treatment may be repeated every four weeks for up to six courses. Patients in both groups will receive a 90-minute infusion of trastuzumab on day 1 of course one and then a 30-minute infusion of trastuzumab once a week for as long as benefit is shown. Patients will be evaluated every three months for two years and every six months thereafter.

PHASE II RANDOMIZED STUDY OF SOY ISOFLAVONE IN PATIENTS WITH BREAST CANCER

This is a randomized Phase II trial to study the effectiveness of soy isoflavone compared with no treatment before surgery in treating patients who have breast cancer. Soy isoflavone may stop the growth of cancer by stopping blood flow to the tumor, but it is not yet known if isoflavone is more effective than no treatment before surgery for breast cancer.

Patients will be randomly assigned to one of two groups. Patients in group one will receive soy isoflavone by mouth once a day for two weeks followed by surgery to remove all or part of the breast. Patients in group two will receive no therapy before surgery.

PHASE II RANDOMIZED STUDY OF SOY PROTEIN IN POSTMENOPAUSAL WOMEN WITH BREAST CANCER TAKING TAMOXIFEN AND EXPERIENCING HOT FLASHES

This is a randomized Phase II trial to determine the effectiveness of soy protein supplements in reducing hot flashes in postmenopausal women who are receiving tamoxifen for breast cancer. Soy protein supplements may be effective in reducing hot flashes in postmenopausal women who are receiving tamoxifen for this purpose.

All patients will keep a daily record of hot flashes and receive a placebo by mouth once a day for one week. Patients will then be randomly assigned to one of two groups. Patients in group one will receive a soy supplement by mouth once a day. Patients in group two will receive a placebo by mouth once a day. Treatment may continue for up to three months. All patients will continue to keep a daily record of hot flashes. Quality of life will be assessed periodically, and patients will be evaluated every three months.

PHASE I/II STUDY OF TIPIFARNIB, DOXORUBICIN, AND CYCLOPHOSPHAMIDE IN WOMEN WITH LOCALLY ADVANCED OR METASTATIC BREAST CANCER

This is a Phase I/II trial to study the effectiveness of combining tipifarnib with doxorubicin and cyclophosphamide in treating women who have locally advanced or metastatic breast cancer. Tipifarnib may stop the growth of tumor cells by blocking the enzymes necessary for tumor cell growth. Combining tipifarnib with doxorubicin and cyclophosphamide may kill more tumor cells.

Patients will receive tipifarnib by mouth twice a day for two weeks, and will also receive infusions of doxorubicin and cyclophosphamide on day 1. Treatment may be repeated every three weeks for up to four courses. Some patients may then undergo surgery to completely remove the tumor. Patients will be evaluated every three to four months for three years, every six months for two years, and once a year thereafter.

PHASE II PILOT STUDY OF BEVACIZUMAB, DOCETAXEL, DOXORUBICIN, AND FILGRASTIM (G-CSF) IN PATIENTS WITH PREVIOUSLY UNTREATED STAGE IIIB OR IV INFLAMMATORY BREAST CANCER

This is a Phase II trial to study the effectiveness of bevacizumab plus chemotherapy and filgrastim in treating patients who have stage IIIB or stage IV inflammatory breast cancer that has not been previously treated with chemotherapy and/or radiation therapy. Monoclonal antibodies such as beva-

cizumab can locate tumor cells and either kill them or deliver tumor-killing substances to them without harming normal cells. Colony-stimulating factors such as filgrastim may increase the number of immune cells found in bone marrow or peripheral blood and may help a person's immune system recover from the side effects of chemotherapy. Combining monoclonal antibody therapy with chemotherapy and filgrastim may kill more tumor cells.

Patients will receive a 30- to 90-minute infusion of bevacizumab every three weeks for up to seven courses, and they will also receive one-hour infusions of doxorubicin and docetaxel every three weeks for six courses. On day 2 of courses two through seven, patients will receive injections of filgrastim once a day for 10 days. After completing course seven, patients may undergo surgery followed by an infusion of bevacizumab every three weeks for up to eight courses. Some patients may then receive tamoxifen by mouth once a day for up to five years. Patients will be evaluated every three months for one year and every three to six months for two years.

PHASE II PILOT STUDY OF CDNA MICROARRAY AS A MEASURE OF TUMOR RESPONSE TO NEOADJUVANT DOCETAXEL AND CAPECITABINE FOLLOWED BY SURGERY AND ADJUVANT DOXORUBICIN AND CYCLOPHOSPHAMIDE IN PATIENTS WITH STAGE II OR III BREAST CANCER

This is a Phase II trial to study the effectiveness of combination chemotherapy and surgery in treating patients who have stage II or stage III breast cancer. Radiation therapy uses high-energy X-rays to damage tumor cells; combining chemotherapy with radiation therapy may kill more tumor cells.

Patients will receive an infusion of docetaxel on day 1 and capecitabine by mouth twice a day on days 2 through 15 every three weeks for four courses. Patients will then undergo surgery to remove the tumor and axillary lymph nodes, followed by infusions of doxorubicin and cyclophosphamide every three weeks for four courses. Patients may receive radiation therapy after completing chemotherapy. Some patients will receive tamoxifen by mouth daily for five years. Tumor tissue will be collected periodically and evaluated, and patients will receive follow-up evaluations every six months.

PHASE II PILOT STUDY OF ERLOTINIB IN PATIENTS WITH LOCALLY ADVANCED OR METASTATIC BREAST CANCER

This is a Phase II trial to study the effectiveness of erlotinib in treating patients who have locally advanced or metastatic breast cancer. Biological therapies such as erlotinib may interfere with the growth of tumor cells and slow the growth of the tumor. Patients will receive erlotinib by mouth once a day for as long as benefit is shown, and will be evaluated within four weeks.

PHASE II PILOT STUDY OF MRI-GUIDED FOCUSED ULTRASOUND ABLATION IN WOMEN WITH STAGE I–IIIA BREAST CANCER

This is a Phase II trial to study the effectiveness of magnetic resonance imaging (MRI)–guided ultrasound energy in treating women who have stage I, stage II, or stage IIIA breast cancer. Imaging procedures, such as MRI, may allow the doctor to better detect the tumor. Highly focused ultrasound energy may be able to kill tumor cells by heating the breast-tumor cells without affecting the surrounding tissue.

Patients will receive MRI-guided ultrasound energy to the breast tumor. Within three days, patients will undergo MRI to evaluate tumor changes. Seven to ten days after MRI-guided ultrasound energy, patients will undergo an ultrasound exam in which guide wires will be used to mark the tumor area to be removed. Within 10 to 21 days later, patients will undergo surgery to remove the tumor or breast. Patients will receive follow-up evaluations five to 10 days after surgery.

PHASE II PILOT STUDY OF TRASTUZUMAB (HERCEPTIN) PLUS DOCETAXEL AND VINORELBINE WITH FILGRASTIM (G-CSF) SUPPORT IN WOMEN WITH HER2-POSITIVE STAGE IV BREAST CANCER

This is a Phase II trial to study the effectiveness of trastuzumab combined with docetaxel, vinorelbine, and filgrastim in treating women who have stage IV breast cancer. Monoclonal antibodies such as trastuzumab can locate tumor cells and either kill them or deliver tumor-killing substances to them without harming normal cells. Colony-stimulating factors such as filgrastim may help a person's immune system recover from the side effects of chemotherapy.

Patients will receive a one-hour infusion of docetaxel on day 1, an injection of filgrastim on days 2 through 21, an infusion of vinorelbine on days 8 and 15, and an infusion of trastuzumab on days 1, 8, and 15. Treatment may be repeated every three weeks for as long as benefit is shown. Patients will be evaluated every six months for three years.

PHASE II RANDOMIZED CHEMOPREVENTION STUDY OF LY353381 HYDROCHLORIDE IN WOMEN WITH FINE NEEDLE ASPIRATION CYTOLOGIC EVIDENCE OF HYPERPLASIA AND AT HIGH RISK FOR BREAST CANCER

This is a randomized Phase II trial to study the effectiveness of LY353381 in preventing breast cancer in women who have hyperplasia.

Patients will be randomly assigned to one of two groups: patients in group one will receive LY353381 by mouth once a day for six months. Patients in group two will receive a placebo by mouth once a day for six months. Patients in both groups will then receive LY353381 by mouth once a day for an additional six months. Quality of life will be assessed periodically. Patients will receive follow-up evaluations at two weeks and then once a year for five years.

PHASE II RANDOMIZED NEOADJUVANT STUDY OF CYTOREDUCTIVE DOXORUBICIN AND CYCLOPHOSPHAMIDE WITH OR WITHOUT FOCUSED MICROWAVE THERMOTHERAPY IN WOMEN WITH LOCALLY ADVANCED BREAST CANCER IN AN INTACT BREAST

This is a randomized Phase II trial to compare the effectiveness of combination chemotherapy with or without microwave therapy before surgery in treating women who have locally advanced breast cancer. Microwave therapy kills tumor cells by heating them to several degrees above body temperature. Combining chemotherapy with microwave therapy before surgery may shrink the tumor so that it can be removed during surgery.

Patients will be randomly assigned to one of two groups. Patients in group one will have sensors placed in and around the breast, and they will then undergo microwave therapy for up to one hour. Beginning on day 1 of the first course of therapy, patients will also receive infusions of cyclophosphamide and doxorubicin. Treatment with therapy and chemotherapy may be repeated every three weeks for up to three courses. Patients will receive a fourth course of chemotherapy alone.

Patients in group two will receive chemotherapy alone as in group one. After completion of chemotherapy, patients in both groups will undergo partial or total mastectomy. Some patients may then undergo radiation therapy and/or receive tamoxifen by mouth twice a day for up to five years. Patients will be evaluated every six months for three years and once a year for two years.

PHASE II RANDOMIZED PILOT STUDY OF CAPECITABINE IN WOMEN WITH ADVANCED OR METASTATIC BREAST CANCER

This is a randomized Phase II trial to compare the effectiveness of two different doses of capecitabine in treating women who have advanced or metastatic breast cancer. Patients will be randomly assigned to one of two groups to receive one of two different doses of capecitabine by mouth twice a day for two weeks. Treatment may be repeated in both groups every three weeks for as long as benefit is shown. Quality of life will be assessed periodically.

PHASE II RANDOMIZED PILOT STUDY OF P53 VACCINE IN PATIENTS WITH STAGE IV, RECURRENT, OR PROGRESSIVE ADENOCARCINOMA OF THE BREAST

This is a randomized Phase II trial to study the effectiveness of vaccine therapy in treating patients who have stage IV, recurrent, or progressive breast cancer. Vaccines may make the body build an immune response to kill tumor cells.

Patients will be randomly assigned to one of two groups. All patients will have peripheral stem cells collected and treated in the laboratory with sargramostim, interleukin-4, and the vaccine. Patients in group one will receive injections of the vaccine and interleukin-2. Patients in group two will receive an infusion of the vaccine and an injection of interleukin-2. Treatment for both groups will be repeated every three weeks for four doses. During course three, all patients will receive an injection of interleukin-2 on days 4 to 8 and 11 to 15. Treatment may continue for up to two years. Patients will be evaluated at one month.

PHASE II RANDOMIZED STUDY OF CELECOXIB IN WOMEN WITH METASTATIC OR RECURRENT BREAST CANCER

This is a randomized Phase II trial to study the effectiveness of celecoxib in treating women who have metastatic or recurrent breast cancer. Celecoxib may stop the growth of tumor cells by blocking the enzymes necessary for tumor cell growth. Patients will be randomly assigned to one of two groups. Patients in group one will receive high-dose celecoxib by mouth twice a day, whereas patients in group two will receive low-dose celecoxib by mouth twice a day. Treatment may continue for as long as benefit is shown. If the cancer progresses, patients may continue treatment in the same group or opposite group for up to one year. Patients will be evaluated for up to five years.

PHASE II RANDOMIZED STUDY OF CYCLOPHOSPHAMIDE, METHOTREXATE, AND FLUOROURACIL WITH OR WITHOUT TRASTUZUMAB (HERCEPTIN) IN WOMEN WITH C-ERBB2-POSITIVE METASTATIC BREAST CANCER

This is a randomized Phase II trial to compare the effectiveness of combination chemotherapy with or without trastuzumab in treating women who have metastatic breast cancer. Monoclonal antibodies, such as trastuzumab, can locate tumor cells and either kill them or deliver tumor-killing substances to them without harming normal cells. Combining chemotherapy with trastuzumab may kill more tumor cells. Patients will be randomly assigned to one of two groups. Patients in group one will receive cyclophosphamide by mouth on days 1 through 14, or by infusion on days 1 and 8. They will also receive infusions of methotrexate and fluorouracil on days 1 and 8. Treatment may be repeated every four weeks for up to eight courses. Patients in group two will receive chemotherapy as in group one plus a 30- to 90-minute infusion of trastuzumab once during each week of chemotherapy. Patients will then receive trastuzumab alone once every three weeks for as long as benefit is shown. Patients will be evaluated every eight to 12 weeks.

PHASE II RANDOMIZED STUDY OF DOCETAXEL WITH OR WITHOUT BEVACIZUMAB, FOLLOWED BY SURGERY, RADIOTHERAPY, AND DOXORUBICIN AND CYCLOPHOSPHAMIDE IN PATIENTS WITH LOCALLY ADVANCED BREAST CANCER

This is a randomized Phase II trial to study the effectiveness of docetaxel with or without bevacizumab followed by surgery, radiation therapy, and combination chemotherapy in treating patients who have stage III breast cancer. Monoclonal antibodies such as bevacizumab can locate tumor cells and either kill them or deliver tumor-killing substances to them without harming normal cells.

Patients will be randomly assigned to one of two groups. Patients in group one will receive an infusion of docetaxel once a week in weeks 1 through 6 and an infusion of bevacizumab once every two weeks during weeks 1 through 8. Patients in group two will receive docetaxel alone as in group one. Treatment in both groups may be repeated every eight weeks for up to three courses. Some patients may then undergo surgery to remove the tumor, followed within three to six weeks by radiation therapy given five days a week for seven weeks. Approximately four weeks after completing radiation therapy, these patients will receive infusions of doxorubicin and cyclophosphamide every three weeks for up to four courses. Some patients may also receive tamoxifen by mouth once a day for five years. Patients will be evaluated at three, six and 12 months, every six months for four years, and once a year thereafter.

PHASE II RANDOMIZED STUDY OF DOXORUBICIN, CYCLOPHOSPHAMIDE, AND PACLITAXEL (ACT) VERSUS CYCLOPHOSPHAMIDE, THIOTEPA, AND CARBOPLATIN (STAMP V) IN PATIENTS WITH HIGH-RISK PRIMARY BREAST CANCER

This is a randomized Phase II trial to study the effectiveness of two regimens of combination chemotherapy in treating patients who have high-risk primary stage II or stage III breast cancer.

Patients will receive filgrastim twice a day until white blood cells are collected, and will receive infusions of chemotherapy every three weeks for four doses. Patients will then be randomly assigned to receive one of two different chemotherapy regimens during an eight-day period. All patients will then undergo peripheral stem cell transplantation and will receive filgrastim until blood counts return to normal. Within four to six weeks after transplantation, some patients will begin receiving tamoxifen by mouth twice a day for five years. Some patients will receive infusions of pamidronate every four weeks for two years. Quality of life will be assessed periodically. Patients will receive follow-up evaluations every three months for one year and then every six months for at least 10 years.

PHASE II RANDOMIZED STUDY OF EXEMESTANE AND RALOXIFENE IN POSTMENOPAUSAL WOMEN WITH A

HISTORY OF STAGE 0 (DUCTAL CARCINOMA IN SITU), I, II, OR III BREAST CANCER WHO HAVE NO CLINICAL EVIDENCE OF DISEASE

This is a randomized Phase II trial to evaluate the effectiveness of exemestane and raloxifene in treating postmenopausal women who have a history of ductal carcinoma in situ, stage I, stage II, or stage III breast cancer.

Estrogen can stimulate the growth of breast cancer cells, and hormone therapy using exemestane may fight breast cancer by blocking the use of estrogen by the tumor cells. Raloxifene may be effective in preventing the recurrence of breast cancer.

Patients will be randomly assigned to receive either exemestane or raloxifene by mouth once a day for two weeks. After two weeks, all patients will receive a combination of raloxifene and exemestane once a day for one year. Patients may then continue to receive raloxifene alone or raloxifene plus exemestane for up to five years. Quality of life will be assessed before and periodically during treatment. Patients will be evaluated every three months for one year and then every six months through year 5.

PHASE II RANDOMIZED STUDY OF METHOTREXATE WITH OR WITHOUT ANTINEOPLASTON A10 CAPSULES IN WOMEN WITH ADVANCED BREAST CANCER

This is a randomized Phase II trial to study the effectiveness of methotrexate with or without antineoplaston therapy in treating postmenopausal women with advanced refractory breast cancer. Antineoplastons are naturally occurring substances found in urine that may inhibit the growth of cancer cells. It is not yet known whether giving antineoplastons with chemotherapy is more effective than chemotherapy alone in treating women with refractory breast cancer.

Patients will be randomized to one of two groups. Patients in group one will receive antineoplaston capsules seven times a day. Methotrexate capsules will be given by mouth two to three times a day for five days, and repeated every 11 days. Patients in group two will receive methotrexate alone. Treatment may be repeated for as long as benefit is shown. Patients will be evaluated every four months for two years, every six months for two years, and then once a year for two years.

PHASE II RANDOMIZED STUDY OF TWO DIFFERENT DOSE SCHEDULES OF

DOXORUBICIN HCl LIPOSOME IN WOMEN WITH METASTATIC BREAST CANCER

This is a randomized Phase II trial to compare the effectiveness of two regimens of liposomal doxorubicin in treating women who have metastatic breast cancer. It is not yet known which regimen of liposomal doxorubicin is more effective for metastatic breast cancer.

Patients will be randomly assigned to one of two groups. Patients in group one will receive an infusion of liposomal doxorubicin every six weeks, and patients in group two will receive an infusion of liposomal doxorubicin every four weeks. Treatment may be repeated for at least 36 weeks. Patients will be evaluated every three months.

PHASE II RANDOMIZED STUDY OF TWO DIFFERENT SCHEDULES OF DOCETAXEL OR PACLITAXEL IN WOMEN WITH UNRESECTABLE LOCALLY ADVANCED OR METASTATIC BREAST CANCER

This is a randomized Phase II trial to compare the effectiveness of two different regimens of docetaxel or paclitaxel in treating women who have unresectable locally advanced or metastatic breast cancer.

Patients will be randomly assigned to one of four groups. Patients in group one will receive an infusion of docetaxel every three weeks, and those in group two will receive an infusion of paclitaxel every three weeks. Patients in group three will receive an infusion of docetaxel once a week for six weeks, and patients in group four will receive an infusion of paclitaxel once a week for six weeks. Treatment may be repeated every three weeks or every eight weeks for as long as benefit is shown. Quality of life will be assessed before treatment and then every eight weeks.

PHASE II RANDOMIZED STUDY OF VINORELBINE/EPIRUBICIN VERSUS VINORELBINE/MITOXANTRONE VERSUS CYCLOPHOSPHAMIDE/DOXORUBICIN AS PREOPERATIVE CHEMOTHERAPY IN WOMEN WITH EARLY STAGE BREAST CANCER

This is a randomized Phase II trial to compare the effectiveness of three regimens of combination chemotherapy in treating women who have stage I or stage II breast cancer.

Patients will be randomly assigned to one of three groups. Patients in group one will receive an infusion of vinorelbine on days 1 and 8 and an infusion of epirubicin on day 1. Patients in group two will receive an infusion of vinorelbine on days 1 and 8 and an infusion of mitoxantrone on day 1. Patients in group three will receive infusions of doxorubicin and cyclophosphamide on day 1. Treatment may be repeated every three weeks for six courses. Some patients will also receive tamoxifen by mouth once a day. Patients may undergo surgery or radiation therapy. Patients will receive follow-up evaluations every three months for two years, every six months for three years, and once a year thereafter.

PHASE II STUDY OF ANASTROZOLE AND ZD 1839 IN POST-MENOPAUSAL WOMEN WITH ESTROGEN RECEPTOR–POSITIVE, HORMONE REFRACTORY, METASTATIC BREAST CANCER

This is a Phase II trial to study the effectiveness of combining anastrozole with ZD 1839 in treating postmenopausal women who have metastatic breast cancer that has not responded to hormone therapy. Estrogen can stimulate the growth of breast cancer cells, and anastrozole may fight breast cancer by blocking the production of estrogen by the tumor cells. Biological therapies such as ZD 1839 may interfere with the growth of the tumor cells and slow the growth of advanced solid tumors. Scientists suspect that combining anastrozole with ZD 1839 may be effective in treating postmenopausal women who have metastatic breast cancer.

Patients will receive anastrozole alone by mouth once a day for two weeks. Beginning in week 3, they will receive both anastrozole and ZD 1839 by mouth once a day. Treatment may continue for as long as benefit is shown. Patients will be evaluated once a month.

PHASE II STUDY OF ANTINEOPLASTONS A10 AND AS2-1 IN PATIENTS WITH STAGE IV BREAST CARCINOMA

This is a Phase II trial to study the effectiveness of antineoplaston therapy in treating women with stage IV breast cancer. Patients will receive infusions of antineoplastons six times a day; treatment may be repeated for as long as benefit is shown. Patients will be evaluated every two months for the first year and every three months for the second year.

PHASE II STUDY OF AUTOLOGOUS HEAT SHOCK PROTEIN 70 VACCINE IN PATIENTS WITH HIGH-RISK BREAST CANCER

This is a Phase II trial to study the effectiveness of vaccine therapy in treating women who have high-risk breast cancer. Vaccines made from a person's tumor cells may make the body build an immune response to kill more tumor cells and may be an effective treatment for breast cancer.

The vaccine will be made in the laboratory using tumor cells collected from the patient during previous surgery. Patients will receive an injection of the vaccine once a week for six weeks. They will be evaluated at week 8, every three months for two years, and every six months thereafter.

PHASE II STUDY OF BMS-247550 IN PATIENTS WITH INCURABLE, LOCALLY ADVANCED OR METASTATIC BREAST CANCER

This is a Phase II trial to study the effectiveness of BMS-247550 in treating patients who have locally advanced or metastatic breast cancer. Patients will receive a one-hour infusion of BMS-247550 on days 1 through 5. Treatment may be repeated every three weeks for as long as benefit is shown.

PHASE II STUDY OF BRYOSTATIN 1 FOR THE TREATMENT OF STAGE IV BREAST CANCER

This is a Phase II trial to study the effectiveness of bryostatin 1 in treating patients with stage IV breast cancer. Patients will receive a 24-hour continuous infusion of bryostatin 1 once a week for as long as benefit is shown. All patients will receive evaluations every four to eight weeks.

PHASE II STUDY OF CELECOXIB AND TRASTUZUMAB (HERCEPTIN) IN WOMEN WITH HER2/NEU-OVEREXPRESSING METASTATIC BREAST CANCER THAT IS REFRACTORY TO PRIOR TRASTUZUMAB

This is a Phase II trial to study the effectiveness of combining celecoxib and trastuzumab in treating women who have metastatic breast cancer that has not responded to previous trastuzumab. Celecoxib may be effective in preventing the further development of cancer. Monoclonal antibodies such as trastuzumab can locate tumor cells and either kill them or deliver tumor-killing substances to them without harming normal cells.

Combining trastuzumab with celecoxib may kill more tumor cells.

At least three weeks after the last dose of chemotherapy, patients will receive celecoxib by mouth two times a day plus infusions of trastuzumab once a week or once every three weeks for as long as benefit is shown.

PHASE II STUDY OF CI-1040 IN PATIENTS WITH ADVANCED NON-SMALL CELL LUNG, BREAST, COLON, OR PANCREATIC CANCER

This is a Phase II trial to study the effectiveness of CI-1040 in treating patients who have metastatic or unresectable breast, colon, pancreatic, or non-small cell lung cancer. CI-1040 may stop the growth of tumors by blocking the enzymes necessary for cancer cell growth and by stopping blood flow to the tumor. Patients will receive CI-1040 by mouth twice a day for three weeks; treatment may be repeated every four weeks for as long as benefit is shown. Quality of life will be assessed periodically, and patients will be evaluated every two months.

PHASE II STUDY OF CONCURRENT BEVACIZUMAB AND VINORELBINE IN PATIENTS WITH STAGE IV BREAST CANCER

This is a Phase II trial to study the effectiveness of bevacizumab combined with vinorelbine in treating patients who have stage IV breast cancer. Monoclonal antibodies such as bevacizumab can locate tumor cells and either kill them or deliver tumor-killing substances to them without harming normal cells.

Patients will receive an infusion of vinorelbine once a week and an infusion of bevacizumab every other week. Treatment may be repeated every eight weeks for four courses. Some patients may continue to receive bevacizumab and vinorelbine either once every other week or as scheduled during the first four courses.

PHASE II STUDY OF CONCURRENT PACLITAXEL AND RADIOTHERAPY FOLLOWING ADJUVANT DOXORUBICIN AND CYCLOPHOSPHAMIDE IN WOMEN WITH STAGE II OR III BREAST CANCER

This is a Phase II trial to study the effectiveness of paclitaxel and radiation therapy in treating women who have stage II or stage III breast cancer. Radiation therapy uses high-energy X-rays to damage tumor cells. Combining paclitaxel with radiation therapy may kill more tumor cells.

Patients will receive an infusion of paclitaxel every three weeks for four courses plus radiation therapy five days a week for six to seven weeks. Patients will be evaluated at one month, every three months for one year, every six months for five years, and once a year thereafter.

PHASE II STUDY OF DOCETAXEL AND IFOS-FAMIDE AS FIRST-LINE CHEMOTHERAPY IN WOMEN WITH METASTATIC BREAST CANCER

This is a Phase II trial to study the effectiveness of docetaxel and ifosfamide in treating women who have metastatic breast cancer. Patients will receive an infusion of docetaxel on day 1 followed by an infusion of ifosfamide on days 1 through 3. Treatment may continue every four weeks for as long as benefit is shown. Quality of life will be assessed periodically. Patients will be evaluated every three months.

PHASE II STUDY OF DOCETAXEL IN ELDERLY WOMEN WITH METASTATIC BREAST CANCER

This is a Phase II trial to study the effectiveness of docetaxel in treating older women who have metastatic breast cancer. Patients will receive an infusion of docetaxel once every three weeks for as long as benefit is shown, and will be evaluated every three months for three years.

PHASE II STUDY OF DOCETAXEL, DOXORU-BICIN, AND AD5CMV-P53 GENE THERAPY (INGN 201) IN PATIENTS WITH LOCALLY ADVANCED BREAST CANCER

This is a Phase II trial to study the effectiveness of combining chemotherapy with gene therapy in treating patients who have stage III or stage IV breast cancer. Inserting the *p53* gene into the tumor may increase the effectiveness of a chemotherapy drug by making tumor cells more sensitive to the drug. Combining chemotherapy with gene therapy may kill more tumor cells.

Patients will receive an injection of *p53* gene into the tumor on days 1 and 2, and infusions of doxorubicin and docetaxel on day 1. Treatment may be repeated every three weeks for up to six courses. Some patients will then undergo surgery.

PHASE II STUDY OF DOCETAXEL, VINORELBINE, AND FILGRASTIM (G-CSF)

IN WOMEN WITH HER-2-NEGATIVE STAGE IV BREAST CANCER

This is a Phase II trial to study the effectiveness of combining docetaxel, vinorelbine, and filgrastim in treating women who have stage IV breast cancer. Colony-stimulating factors such as filgrastim may increase the number of immune cells found in bone marrow or peripheral blood and may help a person's immune system recover from the side effects of chemotherapy.

Patients will receive an infusion of docetaxel on day 1 and an infusion of vinorelbine on days 8 and 15. Patients also will receive an injection of filgrastim on days 2 through 21. Treatment may be repeated every three weeks for as long as benefit is shown. Patients will be evaluated every six months for three years.

PHASE II STUDY OF DOSE-INTENSIVE CHEMOTHERAPY AND STEM CELL RESCUE IN PATIENTS WITH INFLAMMATORY STAGE IIIB BREAST CANCER

This is a Phase II trial to study the effectiveness of chemotherapy and stem cell transplantation in treating patients with stage IIIB breast cancer. Combining chemotherapy with peripheral stem cell transplantation may allow the doctor to give higher doses of chemotherapy drugs and kill more tumor cells.

Patients will be assigned to one of two groups. Patients in group one will receive infusions of doxorubicin and paclitaxel plus filgrastim, followed by a modified radical mastectomy. Patients in group two will receive no treatment at this time. All patients will then receive paclitaxel and cyclophosphamide plus filgrastim, followed by removal of their stem cells. All patients will receive two courses of high-dose chemotherapy followed by filgrastim and reinfusion of stem cells. Radiation therapy will then be given. Some patients will receive tamoxifen within two weeks of discharge. All patients will be given follow-up evaluations every three months for two years and then once a year for the next three years.

PHASE II STUDY OF DOXORUBICIN HCI LIPOSOME AND DOCETAXEL WITH OR WITHOUT TRASTUZUMAB (HERCEPTIN) IN WOMEN WITH METASTATIC BREAST CANCER

This is a Phase II trial to study the effectiveness of combination chemotherapy with or without trastuzumab in treating women who have metastatic breast cancer. Patients will be assigned to one of two treatment groups. Patients in group one will receive infusions of liposomal doxorubicin and docetaxel every three weeks for eight courses, followed by infusions of docetaxel alone either weekly or every three weeks for as long as benefit is shown. Patients in group two will receive an infusion of trastuzumab once a week, plus infusions of liposomal doxorubicin and docetaxel as in group one. They may then receive trastuzumab once a week, followed by docetaxel either once a week or every three weeks for as long as benefit is shown. Patients will be evaluated every three months for two years, every six months for three years, and once a year thereafter.

PHASE II STUDY OF DOXORUBICIN HCl LIPOSOME AND GEMCITABINE IN WOMEN WITH METASTATIC BREAST CANCER

This is a Phase II trial to study the effectiveness of combining doxorubicin with gemcitabine in treating women who have metastatic breast cancer.

Patients will receive an infusion of doxorubicin on day 1 and infusions of gemcitabine on days 1 and 8. Treatment may be repeated every four weeks for as long as benefit is shown. Quality of life will be assessed periodically, and patients will be evaluated at four weeks and then every three months for five years.

PHASE II STUDY OF DOXORUBICIN-MONOCLONAL ANTIBODY BR96 IMMUNOCONJUGATE (SGN-15) AND DOCETAXEL IN WOMEN WITH METASTATIC OR RECURRENT BREAST CANCER

This is a Phase II trial to study the effectiveness of combining docetaxel and monoclonal antibody therapy in treating women who have metastatic or recurrent breast cancer. Patients will receive an infusion of monoclonal antibody followed by an infusion of docetaxel once a week for six weeks. Treatment may be repeated every eight weeks for up to six courses, and patients will be evaluated at one month.

PHASE II STUDY OF ETOPOSIDE, IFOSFAMIDE, MESNA, AND CISPLATIN IN PATIENTS WITH METASTATIC BREAST CANCER

This is a Phase II trial to study the effectiveness of combination chemotherapy consisting of etoposide, ifosfamide, mesna, and cisplatin in treating patients

who have metastatic breast cancer. Drugs such as mesna may be effective in preventing some of the side effects of chemotherapy.

Patients will receive infusions of etoposide, cisplatin, and ifosfamide on days 1 to 3. Mesna will be given by infusion before and after ifosfamide. Eight hours after the infusion of ifosfamide, patients will receive mesna by mouth. Treatment may be repeated every four weeks for as long as benefit is shown, and patients will be evaluated every three months.

PHASE II STUDY OF FULVESTRANT (ICI 182780) IN WOMEN WITH METASTATIC BREAST CANCER WHO HAVE FAILED AROMATASE INHIBITOR THERAPY

This is a Phase II trial to study the effectiveness of ICI 182780 in treating patients who have metastatic breast cancer that has not responded to previous hormone therapy. Hormone therapy using ICI 182780 may fight breast cancer by blocking the activity of estrogen in the tumor cells.

Patients will receive an injection of ICI 182780 every four weeks for as long as benefit is shown. Patients will be evaluated every three months for five years.

PHASE II STUDY OF HIGH-DOSE COMBINATION CHEMOTHERAPY AND AUTOLOGOUS OR SYNGENEIC PERIPHERAL BLOOD STEM CELL RESCUE FOLLOWED BY IMMUNOTHERAPY WITH INTERLEUKIN-2 AND SARGRAMOSTIM (GM-CSF) IN PATIENTS WITH INFLAMMATORY STAGE IIIB AND RESPONSIVE METASTATIC STAGE IV BREAST CANCER

This is a Phase II trial to study the effectiveness of combination chemotherapy and peripheral stem cell transplantation followed by interleukin-2 and sargramostim in treating patients who have inflammatory stage IIIB or metastatic stage IV breast cancer. Combining chemotherapy with peripheral stem cell transplantation may allow doctors to give higher doses of chemotherapy drugs and kill more tumor cells. Interleukin-2 and colony-stimulating factors such as sargramostim may help a person's immune system kill more tumor cells.

Following treatment with cyclophosphamide, paclitaxel, and filgrastim, peripheral stem cells will be collected. Patients will receive busulfan by mouth every six hours for three days, followed by infusions of melphalan and thiotepa. Peripheral stem cells will be infused beginning 36 to 48 hours after the last dose of thiotepa. All patients will receive tamoxifen by mouth once a day for up to five years. Some patients will receive injections of interleukin-2 once a day plus sargramostim three days a week for 12 weeks beginning five to 15 weeks after transplantation. Some patients will also receive radiation therapy. Patients will receive follow-up evaluations every three months for two years, and every six months thereafter.

PHASE II STUDY OF IMATINIB MESYLATE IN PATIENTS WITH METASTATIC BREAST CANCER

This is a Phase II trial to study the effectiveness of imatinib mesylate in treating patients who have metastatic breast cancer. Imatinib mesylate may stop the growth of cancer by blocking the enzymes necessary for tumor cell growth. Patients will receive imatinib mesylate by mouth twice a day for up to eight weeks.

PHASE II STUDY OF IROFULVEN IN PATIENTS WITH METASTATIC BREAST CANCER

This is a Phase II trial to study the effectiveness of irofulven in treating patients who have metastatic breast cancer. Patients will receive an infusion of irofulven once a week for two weeks; treatment may be repeated every four weeks for as long as benefit is shown.

PHASE II STUDY OF LY231514 AND GEMCITABINE IN WOMEN WITH METASTATIC BREAST CANCER

This is a Phase II trial to study the effectiveness of combining LY231514 plus gemcitabine in treating women who have metastatic breast cancer. Patients will receive an infusion of gemcitabine on days 1 and 8 and an infusion of LY231514 on day 8. Treatment may be repeated every three weeks for as long as benefit is shown. Patients will receive follow-up evaluations every three months for five years.

PHASE II STUDY OF MITOXANTRONE, LEUCOVORIN CALCIUM, AND FLUOROURACIL IN ELDERLY WOMEN WITH METASTATIC BREAST CANCER

This is a Phase II trial to study the effectiveness of combination chemotherapy in treating older women who have metastatic breast cancer. Patients will receive infusions of mitoxantrone and leucovorin followed by a two-day continuous infusion of fluorouracil. Treatment may be repeated every three weeks for up to eight courses. Quality of life will be assessed periodically, and patients will receive follow-up evaluations every three months.

PHASE II STUDY OF NEOADJUVANT DOXORUBICIN, CYCLOPHOSPHAMIDE, AND PACLITAXEL WITH OR WITHOUT TRASTUZUMAB (HERCEPTIN) FOLLOWED BY LOCAL SURGERY WITH OR WITHOUT ADJUVANT TRASTUZUMAB OR ADJUVANT DOXORUBICIN, CYCLOPHOSPHAMIDE, PACLITAXEL, AND TRASTUZUMAB IN WOMEN WITH STAGE IIB, IIIA, IIIB, OR IV BREAST CANCER

This is a Phase II trial to study the effectiveness of combination chemotherapy, monoclonal antibody therapy, and surgery in treating women who have stage II, stage III, or stage IV breast cancer. Combining chemotherapy, monoclonal antibody therapy, and surgery may be a more effective treatment for breast cancer.

Patients will be assigned to one of three groups. Patients in group one will receive infusions of doxorubicin, cyclophosphamide, and paclitaxel every three weeks for four courses. Patients will then undergo surgery with or without radiation therapy and/or tamoxifen. Patients in group two will receive doxorubicin and cyclophosphamide as in group one.

Following completion of course four, patients will receive infusions of paclitaxel and trastuzumab once a week during weeks 13 through 24. Patients will then undergo surgery with or without radiation therapy plus additional trastuzumab during weeks 29 through 69 or weeks 36 through 76. Patients in group three will receive doxorubicin and cyclophosphamide as in group one and paclitaxel and trastuzumab as in group two. They will then receive radiation therapy followed by trastuzumab in weeks 29 through 69 or 36 through 76. Patients will receive follow-up evaluations every three months for two years, every six months for three years, and then once a year for five years.

PHASE II STUDY OF ORAL ANTINEOPLASTONS A10 AND AS2-1 IN PATIENTS WITH ADVANCED BREAST CANCER

This is a Phase II trial of antineoplaston therapy in treating women who have stage IV breast cancer.

Antineoplastons are naturally-occurring substances found in urine. Antineoplastons may inhibit the growth of cancer cells. Patients will receive antineoplaston therapy by mouth six to seven times a day for as long as benefit is shown, and will receive follow-up evaluations.

PHASE II STUDY OF ORAL VINORELBINE IN ELDERLY WOMEN WITH STAGE IV BREAST CANCER

This is a Phase II trial to study the effectiveness of vinorelbine in treating older women who have stage IV breast cancer. Patients will receive vinorelbine by mouth once a week for as long as benefit is shown. Quality of life will be assessed periodically, and patients will be evaluated every three months for five years.

PHASE II STUDY OF PS-341 IN WOMEN WITH METASTATIC BREAST CANCER

This is a Phase II trial to study the effectiveness of PS-341 in treating women who have metastatic breast cancer. PS-341 may stop the growth of tumor cells by blocking the enzymes necessary for cancer cell growth.

Patients will receive an infusion of PS-341 twice a week for two weeks. Treatment may be repeated every three weeks for as long as benefit is shown.

PHASE II STUDY OF R101933 IN COMBINATION WITH PACLITAXEL OR DOCETAXEL IN PATIENTS WITH TAXANE-REFRACTORY METASTATIC BREAST CANCER

This is a Phase II trial to study the effectiveness of combining R101933 with either paclitaxel or docetaxel in treating patients who have metastatic breast cancer that has not responded to previous chemotherapy. Combining R101933 with paclitaxel or docetaxel may reduce resistance to the drug and allow the tumor cells to be killed. Patients will receive an infusion of R101933 followed immediately by an infusion of either paclitaxel or docetaxel. Treatment may be repeated every three weeks for seven or more courses, and patients will be evaluated every six weeks.

PHASE II STUDY OF REBECCAMYCIN ANALOGUE IN PATIENTS WITH STAGE IIIB OR IV BREAST CANCER

This is a randomized Phase II trial to compare the effectiveness of two regimens of rebeccamycin analogue in treating patients who have stage IIIB or stage IV breast cancer. The best way to give rebeccamycin analogue in patients with breast cancer is not yet known.

Patients will be randomly assigned to one of two groups. Patients in group one will receive one infusion of rebeccamycin analogue. Patients in group two will receive infusions of rebeccamycin analogue for five days. Treatment may be repeated every three weeks for as long as benefit is shown.

PHASE II STUDY OF SENTINEL NODE BIOPSY TO ASSESS AXILLARY NODAL STATUS IN PATIENTS WITH RESECTABLE STAGE I OR II BREAST CANCER

This is a Phase II trial to study the effectiveness of sentinel-node biopsy to assess axillary lymph nodes in women who have stage I or stage II breast cancer. Diagnostic procedures such as sentinel-node biopsy may improve the ability to detect breast cancer and determine the extent of disease.

Patients will receive injections of a radioactive substance and/or a blue dye that will enable the sentinel lymph node and other affected lymph nodes to be identified. These lymph nodes will be removed during surgery to remove the tumor.

PHASE II STUDY OF SULINDAC AND DOCETAXEL IN WOMEN WITH METASTATIC OR RECURRENT ADENOCARCINOMA OF THE BREAST

This is a Phase II trial to study the effectiveness of combining sulindac with docetaxel in treating women who have metastatic or recurrent breast cancer.

Patients will receive sulindac by mouth twice a day, and a one-hour infusion of docetaxel every three weeks. Treatment may continue for as long as benefit is shown. Patients will be evaluated within three to four weeks.

PHASE II STUDY OF T-CELL DEPLETED ALLOGENEIC PERIPHERAL BLOOD STEM CELL TRANSPLANTATION IN PATIENTS WITH METASTATIC BREAST CANCER

This is a Phase II trial to study the effectiveness of peripheral stem cell transplantation in treating patients who have stage IV breast cancer. Peripheral stem cell transplantation may be able to replace immune cells that were destroyed by chemotherapy used to kill tumor cells.

Patients will receive daily injections of filgrastim. Five days later, specific blood cells will be collected and treated in the laboratory. Patients will then receive infusions of fludarabine and cyclophosphamide for four days followed by daily injections of filgrastim beginning on day 5 and continuing until blood counts return to normal. Treatment may be repeated three weeks later. Patients will then receive infusions of fludarabine and cyclophosphamide for four days followed by an infusion of peripheral stem cells and injections of filgrastim. Patients will receive cyclosporine given by infusion every 12 hours for 16 days and then by mouth until day 40. Some patients will also receive donor white blood cells in weeks 6, 10, and 14. Patients will be evaluated twice a week until week 15 and then at six, nine, 12, 18, and 24 months.

PHASE II STUDY OF TRASTUZUMAB (HERCEPTIN) AND PACLITAXEL IN PATIENTS WITH HER2-OVEREXPRESSING METASTATIC BREAST CANCER

This is a Phase II trial to study the effectiveness of trastuzumab plus paclitaxel in treating patients who have metastatic breast cancer that overexpresses *HER-2*. Monoclonal antibodies such as trastuzumab can locate tumor cells and deliver tumor-killing substances to them without harming normal cells. Combining monoclonal antibody therapy with chemotherapy may kill more tumor cells.

Patients will receive infusions of trastuzumab once a week for four weeks, and will then receive infusions of trastuzumab and paclitaxel once a week. Treatment may be repeated every four weeks for as long as benefit is shown.

PHASE II STUDY OF TRASTUZUMAB (HERCEPTIN) AND ZD 1839 IN PATIENTS WITH METASTATIC BREAST CANCER THAT OVEREXPRESSES HER2-NEU

This is a Phase I/II trial to study the effectiveness of combining trastuzumab and ZD 1839 in treating patients who have *HER-2*-positive breast cancer. The monoclonal antibody trastuzumab can locate breast cancer cells that have *HER-2* on their surface and either kill them or deliver tumor-killing substances to them without harming normal cells. Bio-

logical therapies such as ZD 1839 may also interfere with the growth of the tumor cells, and may enhance the effects of trastuzumab. Combining trastuzumab and ZD 1839 may be an effective treatment for metastatic breast cancers with high amounts of *HER-2*.

Patients will receive ZD 1839 by mouth once a day for as long as benefit is shown. They will also receive an infusion of trastuzumab once a week for approximately six months followed by trastuzumab once every three weeks for as long as benefit is shown. Patients will be evaluated every three months for two years, every six months for three years, and once a year thereafter.

PHASE II STUDY OF TRASTUZUMAB (HERCEPTIN) PLUS INTERLEUKIN-2 IN PATIENTS WITH HER2-POSITIVE METASTATIC BREAST CANCER WHO HAVE FAILED PRIOR TRASTUZUMAB THERAPY

This is a Phase II trial to study the effectiveness of trastuzumab plus interleukin-2 in treating patients who have metastatic breast cancer that has not responded to previous trastuzumab therapy. Monoclonal antibodies such as trastuzumab can locate tumor cells and either kill them or deliver tumor-killing substances to them without harming normal cells. Interleukin-2 may stimulate a person's white blood cells to kill breast cancer cells.

Patients will receive an infusion of trastuzumab on days 1 and 8 and injections of interleukin-2 on days 2 through 7 and 9 through 21. Beginning on day 22, patients will receive an infusion of trastuzumab every two weeks, plus injections of interleukin-2 daily for two weeks. Treatment may continue for up to one year, and patients will be evaluated for at least 30 days.

PHASE II STUDY OF WHOLE BODY HYPER-THERMIA COMBINED WITH DOXORUBICIN HCI LIPOSOME AND FLUOROURACIL IN PATIENTS WITH METASTATIC BREAST, OVARIAN, ENDOMETRIAL, OR CERVICAL CANCER

This is a Phase II trial to study the effectiveness of fluorouracil and liposomal doxorubicin combined with systemic hyperthermia in treating patients with metastatic breast, ovarian, endometrial, or cervical cancer. Hyperthermia therapy kills tumor cells by heating them to several degrees above body temperature. Combining chemotherapy with hyperthermia may kill more tumor cells than either treatment alone.

Patients will receive a 24-hour continuous infusion of fluorouracil on days 1 through 5 followed by an infusion of liposomal doxorubicin on day 6. One day later, patients will receive up to four six-hour hyperthermia treatments. Treatment may be repeated every four to five weeks for four courses. Some patients may receive further chemotherapy without hyperthermia. Patients will be evaluated at four weeks and every six months for one year.

PHASE II/III RANDOMIZED STUDY OF ANASTROZOLE WITH OR WITHOUT TRASTUZUMAB (HERCEPTIN) IN POSTMENOPAUSAL WOMEN WITH HORMONE-RECEPTOR POSITIVE HER2-OVEREXPRESSING METASTATIC BREAST CANCER

This is a randomized Phase II/III trial to compare the effectiveness of anastrozole plus trastuzumab with that of anastrozole alone in treating postmenopausal women who have metastatic breast cancer. Anastrozole may fight breast cancer by blocking the production of estrogen by the tumor cells. Monoclonal antibodies such as trastuzumab can locate tumor cells and either kill them or deliver tumor-killing substances to them without harming normal cells. It is not yet known whether anastrozole is more effective with or without trastuzumab in treating metastatic breast cancer.

Patients will be randomly assigned to one of two groups. Patients in group one will receive anastrozole by mouth once a day and an infusion of trastuzumab once a week. Patients in group two will receive anastrozole alone as in group one. Treatment will continue in both groups for at least two years. Patients will be evaluated at four weeks.

PHASE II/III RANDOMIZED STUDY OF CAPECITABINE VERSUS VINORELBINE IN WOMEN WITH METASTATIC BREAST CANCER PREVIOUSLY TREATED WITH TAXANES WITH OR WITHOUT ANTHRACYCLINES

This is a randomized Phase II/III trial to compare the effectiveness of capecitabine with that of vinorelbine in treating women who have metastatic breast cancer that has been previously treated with chemotherapy. It is not yet known if capecitabine is more effective than vinorelbine in treating metastatic breast cancer.

Patients will be randomly assigned to one of two groups. Patients in group one will receive an infusion of vinorelbine once a week for two weeks. Patients in group two will receive capecitabine by mouth twice a day for two weeks. Treatment in both groups may be repeated every three weeks for as long as benefit is shown. Patients and their quality of life will be assessed periodically.

PHASE II/III RANDOMIZED STUDY OF FIRST-LINE HORMONAL THERAPY WITH EXEMESTANE VERSUS TAMOXIFEN IN POSTMENOPAUSAL WOMEN WITH LOCALLY RECURRENT OR METASTATIC BREAST CANCER

This is a randomized Phase II/III trial to compare the effectiveness of exemestane with that of tamoxifen in treating postmenopausal women who have locally recurrent or metastatic breast cancer. Hormone therapy using exemestane or tamoxifen may fight cancer by blocking the uptake of estrogen.

Patients will be randomly assigned to one of two groups. Patients in group one will receive exemestane by mouth once a day. Patients in group two will receive tamoxifen by mouth once a day. Treatment may continue for as long as benefit is shown. Patients will be evaluated every three months for 18 months and at least every six months thereafter.

PHASE III PROGNOSTIC STUDY OF SENTINEL NODE AND BONE MARROW MICROMETASTASES IN WOMEN WITH STAGE I OR IIA BREAST CANCER

This is a Phase III prognostic study of sentinel lymph node metastases and bone marrow metastases in women who have stage I or stage IIA breast cancer. Biopsy of sentinel lymph nodes and bone marrow may improve the ability to detect and determine the extent of cancer.

Patients will undergo segmental mastectomy and surgery to remove sentinel lymph nodes, and may have bone marrow removed from the hip and tested for the presence of tumor cells. Some patients may have additional lymph nodes removed from the armpit. All patients will receive radiation therapy five days a week for up to eight weeks. Patients will be evaluated at 30 days, every six months for 36 months, and once a year thereafter.

PHASE III RANDOMIZED ADJUVANT STUDY OF FLUOROURACIL, EPIRUBICIN, AND

CYCLOPHOSPHAMIDE (FEC) OR EPIRUBICIN FOLLOWED BY CYCLOPHOSPHAMIDE, METHOTREXATE, AND FLUOROURACIL (EPI-CMF) VERSUS FEC FOLLOWED BY SEQUENTIAL DOCETAXEL IN WOMEN WITH RESECTED STAGE I OR II BREAST CANCER

This is randomized Phase III trial to compare the effectiveness of different combination chemotherapy regimens in treating women who have resected stage I or stage II breast cancer. Patients will be randomly assigned to one of two groups. Patients in group one will receive one of two combination chemotherapy regimens every three to four weeks for up to eight courses. Patients in group two will receive four courses of one of the chemotherapy regimens as in group one followed by infusions of docetaxel once every three weeks for four courses. Within four weeks after completing chemotherapy, some patients will receive radiation therapy five days a week for three to five weeks and/or tamoxifen by mouth once a day for at least five years. Quality of life will be assessed periodically. Patients will be evaluated every three months for two years and every six months thereafter.

PHASE III RANDOMIZED ADJUVANT STUDY OF TAMOXIFEN IN WOMEN WITH EARLY BREAST CANCER

This is a randomized Phase III trial to compare the effectiveness of at least two years of tamoxifen with that of five additional years of tamoxifen in treating women who have breast cancer that has been surgically removed. Patients will be randomly assigned to one of two groups. Patients in group one will stop taking tamoxifen after two years. Patients in group two will continue to receive tamoxifen for five additional years. Patients will be evaluated once a year.

PHASE III RANDOMIZED NEOADJUVANT STUDY OF ICI 182780 IN WOMEN WITH STAGE I OR II PRIMARY BREAST CANCER

This is a randomized Phase III trial to study the effectiveness of ICI 182780 given before surgery in treating women who have stage I or stage II primary breast cancer. Hormone therapy using ICI 182780 before surgery may block the uptake of estrogen by the tumor cells and prevent metastases. It is not yet known if ICI 182780 is effective in preventing breast cancer metastases.

Patients will be randomly assigned to receive one injection of either ICI 182780 or a placebo. Patients

will undergo surgery within two to four weeks after the injection. Patients will receive follow-up evaluations every three months for two years, every six months for three years, and once a year thereafter.

PHASE III RANDOMIZED STUDY OF ACUPRESSURE FOR CHEMOTHERAPY-INDUCED NAUSEA IN WOMEN WITH BREAST CANCER RECEIVING DOXORUBICIN AND CYCLOPHOSPHAMIDE WITH OR WITHOUT FLUOROURACIL

This is a randomized Phase III trial to determine the effectiveness of acupressure in treating nausea in women who are receiving combination chemotherapy for breast cancer. Acupressure may help to reduce or prevent nausea in patients treated with chemotherapy. It is not yet known if acupressure plus standard nausea care is more effective than standard nausea care alone in women who are receiving chemotherapy for breast cancer.

Patients will be randomly assigned to one of three groups. Patients in group one will receive acupressure applied to a specific site each morning, and whenever nausea is experienced, for three to six minutes, plus standard nausea care during the second or third course of chemotherapy. Patients in group two will receive placebo acupressure applied to a nonspecific site plus the standard nausea care as in group one. Patients in group three will receive standard nausea care alone during the second or third course of chemotherapy. Patients in all groups will complete a daily log. Quality of life will be assessed periodically.

PHASE III RANDOMIZED STUDY OF ADJUVANT BREAST RADIOTHERAPY WITH OR WITHOUT REGIONAL RADIOTHERAPY IN WOMEN WITH RESECTED, EARLY STAGE, INVASIVE BREAST CANCER

This is a randomized Phase III trial to compare the effectiveness of radiation therapy to the breast alone following surgery with that of radiation therapy to the breast plus surrounding tissue in treating women who have early-stage invasive breast cancer. It is not yet known if radiation therapy to the breast alone after surgery is more effective than radiation therapy to the breast plus surrounding tissue for invasive breast cancer.

Patients will be randomly assigned to one of two groups. Patients in group one will undergo radiation therapy to the breast alone five days a week for up to five weeks. Patients in group two will undergo radiation therapy to the breast and surrounding tissue five days a week for up to five weeks. Quality of life will be assessed periodically. Patients will be evaluated at three and nine months, every six months for two years, and once a year thereafter.

PHASE III RANDOMIZED STUDY OF ADJUVANT CHEMOTHERAPY COMPRISING STANDARD CYCLOPHOSPHAMIDE, METHOTREXATE, AND FLUOROURACIL (CMF) OR DOXORUBICIN AND CYCLOPHOSPHAMIDE (AC) VERSUS ORAL CAPECITABINE IN ELDERLY WOMEN WITH OPERABLE ADENOCARCINOMA OF THE BREAST

This is a randomized Phase III trial to compare the effectiveness of different chemotherapy regimens in treating older women who have undergone surgery for breast cancer. It is not yet known which chemotherapy regimen is more effective in treating older women with breast cancer.

Patients will be randomly assigned to one of two groups. Patients in group one will receive one of two different combination chemotherapy regimens by infusion and/or by mouth every three to four weeks for up to six courses. Patients in group two will receive capecitabine by mouth twice a day for two weeks. Treatment for these patients may be repeated every three weeks for up to six courses. Within four to six weeks after treatment, some patients from both groups will undergo radiation therapy. Within 12 weeks after treatment, some patients from both groups may receive tamoxifen by mouth once a day for up to five years. Quality of life will be assessed periodically. All patients will be evaluated every six months for two years and then once a year for 15 years.

PHASE III RANDOMIZED STUDY OF ADJUVANT CLODRONATE WITH OR WITHOUT SYSTEMIC CHEMOTHERAPY AND/OR TAMOXIFEN IN WOMEN WITH EARLY-STAGE BREAST CANCER

This is a randomized Phase III trial to determine the effectiveness of clodronate in preventing metastases in women who have stage I or stage II breast cancer. Clodronate may be effective in preventing the spread of cancer to the bones and other parts of the body. It is not yet known if clodronate is more effective alone or combined with chemotherapy in preventing metastatic breast cancer.

Patients will be randomly assigned to one of two groups. Patients in group one will receive clodronate by mouth once a day for up to three years. Patients in group two will receive a placebo by mouth once a day for up to three years. Some patients may also receive chemotherapy and/or tamoxifen. Patients will be evaluated every six months for five years and once a year thereafter.

PHASE III RANDOMIZED STUDY OF ADJUVANT CYCLOPHOSPHAMIDE AND DOXORUBICIN VERSUS PACLITAXEL IN WOMEN WITH HIGH-RISK NODE-NEGATIVE BREAST CANCER

This is a randomized Phase III trial to compare the effectiveness of cyclophosphamide and doxorubicin to that of paclitaxel in treating women who have breast cancer. Patients will be randomly assigned to one of four groups. Patients in groups one and two will receive infusions of cyclophosphamide and doxorubicin once every three weeks for four and six courses, respectively. Patients in groups three and four will receive a one-hour infusion of paclitaxel once a week for 12 and 18 weeks, respectively. All patients will be evaluated at four to six weeks, every six months for two years, and once a year for 15 years.

PHASE III RANDOMIZED STUDY OF ADJUVANT CYCLOPHOSPHAMIDE, EPIRUBICIN AND FLUOROURACIL VERSUS CYCLOPHOSPHAMIDE, EPIRUBICIN, FILGRASTIM (G-CSF), AND EPOETIN ALFA FOLLOWED BY PACLITAXEL VERSUS CYCLOPHOSPHAMIDE AND DOXORUBICIN FOLLOWED BY PACLITAXEL IN PRE-MENOPAUSAL OR EARLY POSTMENOPAUSAL WOMEN WITH PREVIOUSLY RESECTED NODE POSITIVE OR HIGH-RISK NODE NEGATIVE STAGE I–IIIA BREAST CANCER

This is a randomized Phase III trial to compare the effectiveness of combination chemotherapy given with or without epoetin alfa in treating women who have undergone surgery for stage I, stage II, or stage III breast cancer. Colony-stimulating factors such as epoetin alfa and filgrastim may decrease the side effects of chemotherapy. It is not yet known which treatment regimen is most effective for breast cancer.

Patients will be randomly assigned to one of three groups. Patients in group one will receive chemotherapy by infusion and by mouth for two weeks. Treatment may be repeated every four weeks for six courses. Patients in group two will receive infusions of chemotherapy on day 1 and an injection of filgrastim once a day on days 2 through 13. These patients will also receive an injection of epoetin alfa once a week. Treatment may continue every two to three weeks for up to 10 courses. Patients in group three will receive combination chemotherapy once every three weeks for up to eight courses. Quality of life will be assessed periodically and patients will receive follow-up evaluations.

PHASE III RANDOMIZED STUDY OF ADJUVANT CYCLOPHOSPHAMIDE, METHOTREXATE, AND FLUOROURACIL WITH OR WITHOUT EPIRUBICIN IN WOMEN WITH EARLY STAGE BREAST CANCER

This is a randomized Phase III trial to compare the effectiveness of combination chemotherapy with or without epirubicin in treating women who have early-stage breast cancer and who have undergone surgery to remove the tumor. It is not yet known whether combination chemotherapy plus epirubicin is more effective than combination chemotherapy alone for stage I or stage II breast cancer.

Patients will be randomly assigned to one of two groups. Patients in group one will receive cyclophosphamide by mouth for four days and an infusion of methotrexate and fluorouracil on days 1 and 8. Treatment may be repeated every four weeks for six courses. Patients in group two will receive an infusion of epirubicin every three weeks for four courses plus combination chemotherapy as in group one. Some patients may also receive radiation therapy during or after chemotherapy. Quality-of-life will be assessed periodically, and patients will receive follow-up evaluations once a year for 10 years.

PHASE III RANDOMIZED STUDY OF ADJUVANT DOXORUBICIN AND CYCLOPHOSPHAMIDE FOLLOWED BY DOCETAXEL VERSUS DOXORUBICIN AND DOCETAXEL VERSUS DOXORUBICIN, DOCETAXEL, AND CYCLOPHOSPHAMIDE IN WOMEN WITH BREAST CANCER AND POSITIVE AXILLARY LYMPH NODES

This is a randomized Phase III trial to compare the effectiveness of different regimens of combination chemotherapy in treating women who have stage I, stage II, or stage IIIA breast cancer and positive axil-

lary lymph nodes and who have previously undergone surgery for breast cancer. It is not yet known which regimen of combination chemotherapy is more effective for treating breast cancer with positive axillary lymph nodes.

Patients will be randomly assigned to one of three groups. Patients in group one will receive infusions of doxorubicin and cyclophosphamide every three weeks for four courses. Three weeks later these patients will receive an infusion of docetaxel every three weeks for four courses. Patients in group two will receive infusions of doxorubicin and docetaxel every three weeks for four courses. Patients in group three will receive infusions of doxorubicin, cyclophosphamide, and docetaxel every three weeks for four courses. Some patients may also receive tamoxifen by mouth once a day for five years. Radiation therapy may also be given. Quality of life will be assessed periodically. Patients will receive follow-up evaluations every six months for five years and once a year thereafter.

PHASE III RANDOMIZED STUDY OF ADJUVANT DOXORUBICIN, CYCLOPHOSPHAMIDE, AND DOCETAXEL WITH OR WITHOUT TRASTUZUMAB (HERCEPTIN) VERSUS TRASTUZUMAB, DOCETAXEL, AND EITHER CARBOPLATIN OR CISPLATIN IN WOMEN WITH HER2-NEU-EXPRESSING NODE-POSITIVE OR HIGH-RISK NODE-NEGATIVE OPERABLE BREAST CANCER

This is a randomized Phase III trial to compare the effectiveness of combination chemotherapy with or without trastuzumab in treating women who have undergone surgery for breast cancer.

Patients will be randomly assigned to one of three groups. Patients in each group will receive different regimens of combination chemotherapy with or without trastuzumab. Treatment may be repeated every three weeks for up to six courses. Patients may continue to receive trastuzumab for approximately one year. Beginning three to four weeks after completing chemotherapy, some patients will receive tamoxifen by mouth once a day for five years. Beginning three to eight weeks after completing chemotherapy, some patients may undergo radiation therapy. Quality of life will be assessed periodically. Patients will be evaluated at one month, every three months for two years, every six months for three years, and once a year for five years.

PHASE III RANDOMIZED STUDY OF ADJUVANT EXEMESTANE VERSUS ADJUVANT TAMOXIFEN IN POSTMENOPAUSAL WOMEN WITH EARLY BREAST CANCER

This is a randomized Phase III trial to compare the effectiveness of exemestane with that of tamoxifen in treating postmenopausal women who have undergone surgery to remove early-stage breast cancer. It is not yet known if exemestane is more effective than tamoxifen in preventing the recurrence of breast cancer.

Patients will be randomly assigned to one of two groups. Patients in group one will receive tamoxifen by mouth once a day for at least five years. Patients in group two will receive exemestane by mouth once a day for at least five years. Quality of life will be assessed periodically for one year. Patients will be evaluated at least once a year.

PHASE III RANDOMIZED STUDY OF ADJUVANT INDUCTION CHEMOTHERAPY WITH OR WITHOUT CYCLOPHOSPHAMIDE AND METHOTREXATE AS MAINTENANCE CHEMOTHERAPY IN PATIENTS WITH STAGE I, II, OR III BREAST CANCER

This is a randomized Phase III trial to compare different combination chemotherapy regimens in treating patients who have stage I, stage II, or stage III breast cancer.

Patients will be randomly assigned to one of two groups. Patients in group one will receive infusions of one of six combination chemotherapy regimens every three to four weeks for up to six courses. Patients in group two will receive the same treatment as in group one; beginning four weeks after the last course of chemotherapy, they will also receive chemotherapy by mouth one of two times a day twice a week for one year. Some patients will receive radiation therapy. Quality of life will be assessed periodically, and patients will be evaluated every six months for five years and once a year thereafter.

PHASE III RANDOMIZED STUDY OF ADJUVANT LETROZOLE VERSUS TAMOXIFEN IN POSTMENOPAUSAL WOMEN WITH OPERABLE, HORMONE RECEPTOR–POSITIVE BREAST CANCER

This is a randomized, double-blind phase III trial to compare the effectiveness of letrozole with that of tamoxifen in treating postmenopausal women who

have breast cancer that has been surgically removed. Hormone therapy using letrozole may fight breast cancer by reducing the production of estrogen. Hormone therapy using tamoxifen may fight breast cancer by blocking the uptake of estrogen by the tumor cells. It is not yet known which treatment regimen is most effective for breast cancer.

Patients will be randomly assigned to one of four groups. Patients in group one will receive tamoxifen by mouth once a day for five years. Patients in group two will receive letrozole by mouth once a day for five years. Patients in group three will receive tamoxifen by mouth once a day for two years followed by letrozole by mouth once a day for three years. Patients in group four will receive letrozole by mouth once a day for two years, followed by tamoxifen by mouth once a day for three years. Patients may receive radiation therapy. Some patients may also receive chemotherapy beginning within eight weeks following surgery and continuing for up to six months. Patients will receive follow-up evaluations once a year.

PHASE III RANDOMIZED STUDY OF ADJUVANT PACLITAXEL, EPIRUBICIN, AND CYCLOPHOSPHAMIDE WITH OR WITHOUT GEMCITABINE IN WOMEN WITH COMPLETELY RESECTED EARLY-STAGE BREAST CANCER

This is a randomized Phase III trial to compare the effectiveness of paclitaxel, epirubicin, and cyclophosphamide with or without gemcitabine in treating women who have undergone surgery for breast cancer. Patients will be randomly assigned to one of two groups. Patients in group one will receive a three-hour infusion of epirubicin, cyclophosphamide, and paclitaxel on day 1, and an infusion of gemcitabine on days 1 and 8. Patients in group two will receive an infusion of epirubicin, cyclophosphamide, and paclitaxel as in group one. Treatment may be repeated every three weeks for four courses. Patients will be evaluated every three months for six months, every six months for three years, and once a year for six years.

PHASE III RANDOMIZED STUDY OF AXILLARY LYMPH NODE DISSECTION IN WOMEN WITH STAGE I OR IIA BREAST CANCER WHO HAVE A POSITIVE SENTINEL NODE

This is a randomized Phase III trial to determine the effectiveness of removing lymph nodes in the armpit in treating women who have stage I or stage IIA breast cancer. Surgery to remove lymph nodes in the armpit may remove cancer cells that have spread from tumors in the breast.

Patients will be randomly assigned to one of two groups. Patients in group one will undergo surgery to remove lymph nodes in the armpit. They will then receive radiation therapy to the breast five days a week for up to seven weeks. Patients in group two will receive radiation therapy only. Some patients in both groups may receive chemotherapy. Patients will receive follow-up evaluations at 30 days and six months, then every six months for three years, and then once a year thereafter.

PHASE III RANDOMIZED STUDY OF BREAST-CONSERVING LOCAL THERAPY VERSUS MASTECTOMY FOLLOWED BY RADIOTHERAPY IN WOMEN WITH LOCALLY ADVANCED BREAST CANCER WHO HAVE RECEIVED PRIOR INDUCTION CHEMOTHERAPY

Randomized Phase III trial to compare the effectiveness of breast-conserving therapy versus mastectomy followed by radiation therapy in treating women who have locally advanced breast cancer that has been previously treated with chemotherapy. Breast-conserving treatments such as radiation therapy or limited surgery are less invasive than mastectomy and may improve the quality of life. It is not yet known if breast-conserving treatments are as effective as mastectomy followed by radiation therapy in treating locally advanced breast cancer.

Patients will be randomly assigned to one of two groups. Patients in group one will undergo a mastectomy followed by radiation therapy. Patients in group two will receive either radiation therapy alone, limited surgery followed by radiation therapy, or radiation therapy followed by limited surgery. Quality of life will be assessed periodically. Patients will be evaluated within one month, every three months for two years, every six months for three years, and once a year thereafter.

PHASE III RANDOMIZED STUDY OF CHEMOTHERAPY AND SURGERY COMPARING ADJUVANT DOXORUBICIN FOLLOWED BY CMF (CYCLOPHOSPHAMIDE, METHOTREXATE, AND FLUOROURACIL) VERSUS ADJUVANT DOXORUBICIN AND PACLITAXEL FOLLOWED BY CMF VERSUS PRIMARY DOXORUBICIN AND PACLITAXEL

FOLLOWED BY CMF IN WOMEN WITH OPERABLE BREAST CANCER AND TUMOR GREATER THAN TWO CENTIMETERS

This is a randomized Phase III trial to study the effectiveness of chemotherapy plus surgery in treating women who have breast cancer. Patients will be randomly assigned to one of three groups: Patients in groups one and two will undergo surgery to remove the tumor, followed three weeks later with one of two regimens of combination chemotherapy for 31 weeks. Patients in group three will receive combination chemotherapy followed by surgery. All patients will receive radiation therapy four weeks after other therapies and will receive tamoxifen for five years. Patients will receive follow-up evaluations at six, 12, 18, and 24 months, and once a year thereafter.

PHASE III RANDOMIZED STUDY OF COMPLETE AXILLARY LYMPH NODE DISSECTION VERSUS AXILLARY RADIOTHERAPY IN SENTINEL LYMPH NODE–POSITIVE WOMEN WITH OPERABLE INVASIVE BREAST CANCER

This is a randomized Phase III trial to compare the effectiveness of complete axillary lymph-node dissection with that of axillary radiation therapy in treating women who have invasive breast cancer. Radiation therapy uses high-energy X-rays to damage tumor cells and may be a less invasive treatment and cause fewer side effects than complete axillary lymph-node dissection. It is not yet known which treatment is more effective for invasive breast cancer.

All patients will undergo lymphoscintigraphy, and they will then have surgery to remove either the tumor or the entire breast. Within eight weeks after surgery, patients will be randomly assigned to one of two groups. Patients in group one will undergo complete axillary lymph node dissection, whereas patients in group two will undergo radiation therapy to the axillary lymph nodes five days a week for five weeks. Some patients in group one may also receive radiation therapy to the axillary lymph nodes. Quality of life will be assessed periodically, and patients will be evaluated once a year for five years.

PHASE III RANDOMIZED STUDY OF DOCETAXEL AND TRASTUZUMAB (HERCEPTIN) WITH OR WITHOUT CARBOPLATIN IN WOMEN WITH HER2-POSITIVE STAGE IIIB OR IV BREAST CANCER

This is a randomized Phase III trial to study the effectiveness of combining docetaxel and trastuzumab with or without carboplatin in treating women who have *HER-2*-positive stage IIIB or stage IV breast cancer. It is not yet known if docetaxel and trastuzumab is more effective with or without carboplatin in treating women who have *HER-2*-positive breast cancer.

Patients will be randomly assigned to one of two groups: Patients in group one will receive a 30- to 90-minute infusion of trastuzumab on days 1, 8, and 15, a one-hour infusion of docetaxel, and a 30- to 60-minute infusion of carboplatin on day 2 of course one and on day 1 for all other courses. Patients in group two will receive infusions of docetaxel and trastuzumab as in group one. Treatment in both groups may be repeated every three weeks for up to eight courses. All patients may then continue to receive infusions of trastuzumab once every three weeks for as long as benefit is shown. Patients will be evaluated every two months for three years.

PHASE III RANDOMIZED STUDY OF DOCETAXEL IN WOMEN WITH METASTATIC BREAST CANCER

This is a randomized Phase III trial to determine the effectiveness of docetaxel in treating patients who have metastatic breast cancer. Patients will be randomly assigned to one of two groups: Patients in group one will receive an infusion of docetaxel every three weeks for as long as benefit is shown. Patients in group two will receive an infusion of docetaxel once a week for three weeks. Treatment may be repeated every four weeks for as long as benefit is shown. Patients will be evaluated at three weeks, every three to four months for one year, and then once a year for four years.

PHASE III RANDOMIZED STUDY OF DOCETAXEL VERSUS PACLITAXEL IN WOMEN WITH METASTATIC OR LOCALLY ADVANCED, INOPERABLE ADENOCARCINOMA OF THE BREAST

This is a randomized Phase III trial to study the effectiveness of paclitaxel or docetaxel in treating women with stage IIIB or metastatic breast cancer. It is not yet known whether paclitaxel is more effective than docetaxel for breast cancer.

Patients will be randomly assigned to one of two groups. Patients in group one will receive an infusion of paclitaxel, and patients in group two will receive an infusion of docetaxel. Treatment for patients in both groups will be repeated every three

weeks for as long as benefit is shown. Quality of life will be assessed periodically, and patients will be evaluated every three months.

PHASE III RANDOMIZED STUDY OF DOXORUBICIN AND CYCLOPHOSPHAMIDE FOLLOWED BY PACLITAXEL WITH OR WITHOUT TRASTUZUMAB (HERCEPTIN) IN WOMEN WITH NODE-POSITIVE BREAST CANCER THAT OVEREXPRESSES HER2

This is a randomized Phase III trial to compare the effectiveness of combination chemotherapy with or without trastuzumab in treating women who have stage I, stage II, or stage IIIA breast cancer that has spread to lymph nodes in the armpit. Monoclonal antibodies such as trastuzumab can locate tumor cells and either kill them or deliver tumor-killing substances to them without harming normal cells. It is not yet known whether combination chemotherapy plus trastuzumab is more effective than combination chemotherapy alone for treating breast cancer.

Patients will be randomly assigned to one of two groups: Patients in group one will receive infusions of doxorubicin and cyclophosphamide every three weeks for four courses. About three weeks after the last course, these patients will receive an infusion of paclitaxel every three weeks for four courses. Patients in group two will receive chemotherapy as in group one, plus an infusion of trastuzumab on day 1 of the first course of paclitaxel. They will continue to receive an infusion of trastuzumab once a week for 51 weeks. Some patients will receive tamoxifen by mouth once a day for five years, and some patients may receive radiation therapy daily for five to six weeks. All patients will receive follow-up evaluations every six months for five years and once a year thereafter.

PHASE III RANDOMIZED STUDY OF DOXORUBICIN PLUS CYCLOPHOSPHAMIDE FOLLOWED BY PACLITAXEL WITH OR WITHOUT TRASTUZUMAB (HERCEPTIN) IN WOMEN WITH HER-2-OVEREXPRESSING NODE-POSITIVE BREAST CANCER

This is a randomized Phase III trial to compare the effectiveness of combination chemotherapy with or without trastuzumab in treating women who have breast cancer. Monoclonal antibodies such as trastuzumab can locate tumor cells and either kill them or deliver tumor-killing substances to them without harming normal cells. It is not yet known whether combination chemotherapy is more effective with or without trastuzumab in treating breast cancer.

Patients will be randomly assigned to one of three groups: Patients in group one will receive infusions of doxorubicin and cyclophosphamide every three weeks for four courses, plus infusions of paclitaxel beginning in week 13 and continuing once a week for 12 courses. Patients in group two will receive chemotherapy as in group one plus infusions of trastuzumab beginning in week 25 and continuing once a week for one year. Patients in group three will receive chemotherapy as in group one plus infusions of trastuzumab beginning in week 13 and continuing for 12 courses. Within five weeks of completing chemotherapy, patients may undergo radiation therapy, and some patients will receive tamoxifen by mouth once a day for five years. Patients will be evaluated every three months for one year, every six months for four years, and then once a year for 15 years.

PHASE III RANDOMIZED STUDY OF EXEMESTANE IN POSTMENOPAUSAL WOMEN WITH RESECTED STAGE I, II, OR IIIA BREAST CANCER WHO HAVE COMPLETED FIVE YEARS OF TAMOXIFEN

This is a randomized Phase III trial to study the effectiveness of exemestane in preventing cancer recurrence in postmenopausal women who have resected stage I, stage II, or stage IIIA breast cancer and have completed five years of tamoxifen. It is not yet known whether exemestane is effective in preventing the recurrence of breast cancer.

Patients will be randomly assigned to one of two groups: Patients in group one will receive exemestane by mouth once a day for two years, and patients in group two will receive a placebo by mouth once a day for two years. Quality of life will be assessed periodically, and patients will be evaluated every six months for one year and once a year thereafter.

PHASE III RANDOMIZED STUDY OF FIRST-LINE TRASTUZUMAB (HERCEPTIN) ALONE FOLLOWED BY COMBINATION TRASTUZUMAB AND PACLITAXEL VERSUS FIRST-LINE COMBINATION TRASTUZUMAB AND PACLITAXEL IN WOMEN WITH HER-2-OVEREXPRESSING METASTATIC BREAST CANCER

This is a randomized Phase III trial to compare the effectiveness of the monoclonal antibody trastuzumab with or without paclitaxel in treating women who have metastatic breast cancer that overexpresses HER-2. It is not yet known whether combining monoclonal antibody therapy with chemotherapy is more effective than antibody therapy alone in treating patients with metastatic breast cancer.

Patients will be randomly assigned to one of two groups: Patients in group one will receive an infusion of trastuzumab once a week. If the disease progresses, patients will receive treatment as in group two. Patients in group two will receive an infusion of trastuzumab once a week plus an infusion of paclitaxel once a week for three weeks followed by one week of rest. Treatment may continue for as long as benefit is shown. Quality of life will be assessed before treatment and periodically during treatment. Patients will be evaluated at one, three, and six months, and then every six months thereafter.

PHASE III RANDOMIZED STUDY OF FLUOROURACIL, EPIRUBICIN, AND CYCLOPHOSPHAMIDE VERSUS DOCETAXEL, EPIRUBICIN, AND CYCLOPHOSPHAMIDE IN WOMEN WITH PRIMARY BREAST CANCER

This is a randomized Phase III trial to compare the effectiveness of two different combination chemotherapy regimens in treating women who have primary breast cancer. Combining more than one drug and giving them after surgery may kill any remaining tumor cells following surgery, but it is not yet known which combination chemotherapy regimen is more effective in treating breast cancer.

Patients will be randomly assigned to one of two groups: Patients in group one will receive infusions of fluorouracil and epirubicin once in weeks 1 and 2, plus cyclophosphamide by mouth once a day for two weeks. Treatment may be repeated every four weeks for up to six courses. Patients in group two will receive an infusion of epirubicin and a one-hour infusion of cyclophosphamide in weeks 1, 3, 6, and 9, followed by a one-hour infusion of docetaxel in weeks 12, 14, 16, and 21.

Patients in both groups will undergo radiation therapy five days a week for five and one-half weeks, either during the last three courses of chemotherapy or within three weeks after completing chemotherapy. Some patients may receive tamoxifen by mouth once a day for up to five years, and some also may receive goserelin injections once every four weeks for up to two years. Quality of life will be assessed periodically. Patients will be evaluated every three months for three years, every six months for three years, and once a year thereafter.

PHASE III RANDOMIZED STUDY OF HIGH-DOSE CYCLOPHOSPHAMIDE, THIOTEPA, AND CARBOPLATIN AND AUTOLOGOUS BONE MARROW OR PERIPHERAL BLOOD STEM CELL TRANSPLANTATION IN CONJUNCTION WITH CYCLOSPORINE AND INTERFERON GAMMA VERSUS INTERLEUKIN-2 AS IMMUNOMODULATION IN WOMEN WITH HIGH-RISK STAGE II OR III BREAST CANCER

This is a randomized Phase III trial to compare the effectiveness of cyclosporine and interferon gamma to that of interleukin-2 following combination chemotherapy and bone marrow or peripheral stem cell transplantation in women who have stage II or stage III breast cancer. Combining chemotherapy with peripheral stem cell transplantation or bone marrow transplantation may allow the doctor to give higher doses of chemotherapy drugs and kill more tumor cells. Biological therapy may interfere with the growth of the cancer cells, but it is not yet known which post-transplant biological therapy regimen is more effective for breast cancer.

Patients will receive four-day continuous infusions of cyclophosphamide and thiotepa, plus an infusion of carboplatin once a day on days 1 through 4. Bone marrow or peripheral stem cells will be infused on day 7. Patients will be randomly assigned to one of two groups: Patients in group one will receive an infusion of cyclosporine twice a day beginning on day 7 and continuing until leaving the hospital, plus interferon gamma injections every two days on days 14 through 35. Patients in group two will receive injections of interleukin-2 once a day for four weeks. Treatment in both groups may be repeated for as long as benefit is shown. Patients will be evaluated every three months for one year and then once a year for five years.

PHASE III RANDOMIZED STUDY OF HORMONE REPLACEMENT THERAPY IN MENOPAUSAL OR PERIMENOPAUSAL WOMEN WITH PRIOR STAGE 0–II BREAST CANCER

This is a randomized Phase III trial to determine the risk of breast cancer recurrence in women with previous early-stage breast cancer who are receiving hormone replacement therapy for menopause symptoms. It is not yet known if hormone replacement therapy increases the risk of breast cancer recurrence in women previously treated for early-stage breast cancer.

Patients will be randomized to receive either daily hormone replacement therapy by mouth or non-hormonal therapy, such as drug therapy, counseling, exercise, or acupuncture. Treatment may continue for as long as benefit is shown. Quality of life will be assessed three times during the study and every two years thereafter. Patients will be evaluated at three and six months, every six months until year 3, and once a year thereafter.

PHASE III RANDOMIZED STUDY OF HYPERICUM PERFORATUM (ST. JOHN'S WORT) COMBINED WITH DOCETAXEL IN PATIENTS WITH UNRESECTABLE SOLID TUMORS

This is a randomized Phase III trial to compare the effectiveness of docetaxel with or without St. John's wort in treating patients who have solid tumors that cannot be removed by surgery. St. John's wort may interfere with the effectiveness of chemotherapy, but it is not yet known if chemotherapy is more effective with or without St. John's wort in treating solid tumors.

Patients who have not previously received St. John's wort will be randomly assigned to one of two groups. Patients in group one will receive a placebo by mouth three times a day for two weeks, followed by a one-hour infusion of docetaxel on day 15. Patients in group two will receive St. John's wort by mouth three times a day for two weeks followed by docetaxel as in group one. Patients who have previously received St. John's wort will receive their usual regimen for two weeks followed by docetaxel as in group one. Treatment in all groups may be repeated every three weeks for two courses. Patients will be evaluated periodically.

PHASE III RANDOMIZED STUDY OF INTERNAL MAMMARY AND MEDIAL SUPRACLAVICULAR LYMPH NODE CHAIN IRRADIATION VERSUS NO FURTHER THERAPY IN WOMEN WITH RESECTED STAGE I/II/III BREAST CANCER

This is a randomized Phase III trial to study the effectiveness of radiation therapy in treating women who have stage I, stage II, or stage III breast cancer that has been surgically removed. Patients will be randomly assigned to one of two groups: Patients in group one will receive no further therapy after surgery. Patients in group two will receive radiation therapy five days a week for five weeks to the lymph nodes located near the sides of the breastbone under the ribs and the medial supraclavicular lymph nodes. Patients will receive follow-up evaluations at least once a year for up to 20 years.

PHASE III RANDOMIZED STUDY OF LETROZOLE VERSUS PLACEBO IN POSTMENOPAUSAL WOMEN WITH PRIMARY BREAST CANCER WHO HAVE COMPLETED AT LEAST FIVE YEARS OF ADJUVANT TAMOXIFEN

This is a randomized Phase III trial to compare the effectiveness of letrozole with that of a placebo in treating women who have resected breast cancer after completing treatment with tamoxifen. Hormone therapy using letrozole may fight breast cancer by reducing the production of estrogen. Patients will be randomly assigned to receive letrozole or a placebo by mouth daily for five years. Quality of life will be assessed periodically, and patients will be evaluated once a year.

PHASE III RANDOMIZED STUDY OF MEDROXYPROGESTERONE ACETATE VERSUS OBSERVATION FOR PREVENTION OF ENDOMETRIAL PATHOLOGY IN POSTMENOPAUSAL WOMEN WITH BREAST CANCER TREATED WITH ADJUVANT TAMOXIFEN

This is a randomized Phase III trial to study the effectiveness of medroxyprogesterone in preventing endometrial disorder in postmenopausal women who have ductal carcinoma in situ, lobular carcinoma in situ, Paget's disease of the nipple, stage I breast cancer, or stage II breast cancer, and who are taking tamoxifen. It is not yet known whether medroxyprogesterone is effective in preventing endometrial disorder in patients with breast cancer who are taking tamoxifen.

Patients will be randomly assigned to one of two groups: Patients in group one will receive tamoxifen by mouth once a day for five years and will undergo observation. Patients in group two will receive tamoxifen by mouth once a day for five years, plus medroxyprogesterone by mouth once a day for two weeks; treatment may be repeated every three months for five years. Patients will be evaluated every six months for two years and once a year thereafter.

PHASE III RANDOMIZED STUDY OF MITOXANTRONE WITH OR WITHOUT DOCETAXEL AS FIRST-LINE CHEMOTHERAPY FOR WOMEN WITH POOR PROGNOSIS METASTATIC BREAST CANCER

This is a randomized Phase III trial to compare the effectiveness of mitoxantrone with or without docetaxel in treating women who have metastatic breast cancer with a poor prognosis. It is not yet known if mitoxantrone is more effective with or without docetaxel.

Patients will be randomly assigned to one of two groups. Patients in group one will receive an infusion of mitoxantrone every three weeks for as long as benefit is shown. Patients in group two will receive infusions of mitoxantrone plus docetaxel every three weeks for up to six courses. Quality of life will be assessed periodically.

PHASE III RANDOMIZED STUDY OF NEOADJUVANT DOXORUBICIN AND CYCLOPHOSPHAMIDE WITH OR WITHOUT FILGRASTIM (G-CSF) IN WOMEN WITH INFLAMMATORY OR ESTROGEN-RECEPTOR-NEGATIVE LOCALLY ADVANCED BREAST CANCER

This is a randomized Phase III trial to compare the effectiveness of combining doxorubicin and cyclophosphamide with or without filgrastim in treating women who have locally advanced breast cancer. It is not yet known whether combination chemotherapy is more effective with or without filgrastim in treating breast cancer.

Patients will be randomly assigned to one of two groups: Patients in group one will receive an infusion of doxorubicin and an infusion of cyclophosphamide every three weeks for up to five courses. Patients in group two will receive an infusion of doxorubicin on day 1, cyclophosphamide by mouth once a day on days 1 through 7, and an injection of filgrastim once a day on days 2 through 7. Treatment may be repeated once a week for up to 15 courses. Three to six weeks after completing chemotherapy, some patients will undergo surgery to remove the tumor and affected lymph nodes. Patients will be evaluated every six months for one year and once a year for four years.

PHASE III RANDOMIZED STUDY OF NEOADJUVANT FLUOROURACIL, DOXORUBICIN, AND CYCLOPHOSPHAMIDE (FAC) VERSUS CYCLOPHOSPHAMIDE, METHOTREXATE, AND FLUOROURACIL (CMF) IN PATIENTS WITH STAGE III BREAST CANCER

This is a randomized Phase III trial to compare cyclophosphamide, doxorubicin, and fluorouracil with cyclophosphamide, methotrexate, and fluorouracil in treating women with stage III breast cancer.

Patients will be randomly assigned to one of two groups: Patients in group one will receive infusions of cyclophosphamide, doxorubicin, and fluorouracil every three weeks for up to three courses. Patients in group two will receive infusions of cyclophosphamide, methotrexate, and fluorouracil every four weeks for up to three courses. Following chemotherapy, some patients from both groups may undergo surgery with or without additional chemotherapy and/or radiation therapy. Quality of life will be assessed periodically. Patients will be evaluated every three to four months for two years, every four to six months for three years, and once a year thereafter.

PHASE III RANDOMIZED STUDY OF NEOADJUVANT FLUOROURACIL, EPIRUBICIN, AND CYCLOPHOSPHAMIDE VERSUS NEOADJUVANT DOCETAXEL AND EPIRUBICIN FOLLOWED BY RADIOTHERAPY AND SURGERY IN WOMEN WITH LOCALLY ADVANCED, INFLAMMATORY, OR LARGE OPERABLE BREAST CANCER

This is a randomized Phase III trial to compare the effectiveness of different regimens of chemotherapy plus radiation therapy with or without surgery in treating women who have locally advanced or inflammatory breast cancer.

Patients will be randomly assigned to one of two groups: Patients in group one will receive one of three combination chemotherapy regimens every three or four weeks for up to six courses. Patients in group two will receive a different chemotherapy regimen in weeks 1, 4, 7, 10, 13, and 16. Following

chemotherapy, patients in both groups may undergo radiation therapy with or without surgery to remove part or all of the breast. Patients will be evaluated every three months for one year, every four months for two years, and every six months thereafter.

PHASE III RANDOMIZED STUDY OF PACLITAXEL VIA ONE HOUR INFUSION EVERY WEEK VERSUS THREE HOUR INFUSION EVERY THREE WEEKS WITH OR WITHOUT TRASTUZUMAB (HERCEPTIN) IN PATIENTS WITH INOPERABLE, RECURRENT, OR METASTATIC BREAST CANCER WITH OR WITHOUT OVEREXPRESSION OF HER2-NEU

This is a randomized Phase III trial to compare the effectiveness of two regimens of paclitaxel, with or without trastuzumab, in treating women who have breast cancer that is inoperable, recurrent, or metastatic, with or without overexpression of *HER-2/neu*. It is not yet known which of two regimens of paclitaxel, with or without trastuzumab, is more effective in treating women with inoperable, recurrent, or metastatic breast cancer.

Patients will be randomly assigned to receive one of the following: an infusion of paclitaxel on day 1; an infusion of paclitaxel once a week for three weeks; an infusion of paclitaxel on day 1 plus an infusion of trastuzumab once a week for three weeks; or infusions of paclitaxel and trastuzumab once a week for three weeks. Treatment may be repeated every three weeks for as long as benefit is shown. Quality of life will be assessed periodically. Patients will receive follow-up evaluations at six, 12, and 18 months, and then once a year for at least five years.

PHASE III RANDOMIZED STUDY OF PACLITAXEL WITH OR WITHOUT BEVACIZUMAB IN PATIENTS WITH LOCALLY RECURRENT OR METASTATIC BREAST CANCER

This is a randomized Phase III trial to determine the effectiveness of chemotherapy with or without bevacizumab in treating patients who have locally recurrent or metastatic breast cancer. Monoclonal antibodies such as bevacizumab can locate tumor cells and either kill them or deliver tumor-killing substances to them without harming normal cells. It is not yet known if chemotherapy is more effective with or without bevacizumab in treating breast cancer.

Patients will be randomly assigned to one of two groups: Patients in group one will receive an infusion of paclitaxel in weeks 1 through 3 and an infusion of bevacizumab in weeks 1 and 3. Patients in group two will receive paclitaxel alone as in group one. Treatment in both groups may be repeated every four weeks for up to 18 courses. Quality of life will be assessed periodically. Patients will be evaluated every three months for two years, every six months for three years, and once a year thereafter.

PHASE III RANDOMIZED STUDY OF PALLIATIVE THERAPY FOR BONE METASTASES FROM BREAST OR PROSTATE CANCER

This is a randomized Phase III trial to compare different radiation therapy regimens in treating patients who have bone metastases from breast or prostate cancer. It is not yet known which radiation therapy regimen is more effective for bone metastases.

Patients will be randomly assigned to one of two groups: Patients in group one will receive ten radiation treatments over two weeks. Patients in group two will receive a single dose of radiation therapy. Treatment may be repeated after four weeks. Patients will receive follow-up evaluations and quality-of-life assessments at two and four weeks; then at two, three, six, nine, and 12 months; every six months for three years; and once a year thereafter.

PHASE III RANDOMIZED STUDY OF PROLONGED VERSUS SHORTER ADJUVANT TAMOXIFEN IN PATIENTS WITH CURATIVELY TREATED BREAST CANCER

This is a randomized Phase III trial to compare the effectiveness of prolonged tamoxifen with that of shorter tamoxifen therapy in treating patients who have had a breast tumor removed. It is not yet known if prolonged tamoxifen is more effective than shorter tamoxifen therapy.

After approximately five years of treatment with tamoxifen, patients will be randomly assigned to stop tamoxifen therapy immediately or to continue to receive tamoxifen daily for at least five more years. Patients will receive follow-up evaluations once a year.

APPENDIX IV
DRUGS USED TO TREAT BREAST CANCER

5-FU (5-fluorouracil, fluorouracil, Adrucil) A standard intravenous (IV) chemotherapy agent that belongs to the family of drugs called antimetabolites. 5-FU is sometimes used to treat cancers of the breast, in addition to those of the colon, ovary, prostate, stomach, liver, and pancreas. It may also be administered by infusion over days or months or may be given as a cream for basal cell skin cancer. This drug is often combined with other chemotherapy agents.

Adriamycin See DOXORUBICIN.

Adrucil See 5-FU.

Alkeran See L-PHENYLALANINE MUSTARD.

amethopterin See METHOTREXATE.

aminoglutethimide (Cytadren) An oral chemotherapy agent that belongs to the family of drugs called nonsteroidal aromatase inhibitors and is used to treat breast cancer as well as prostate and adrenal cancers. Aminoglutethimide is used to decrease the production of sex hormones (estrogen or testosterone) and to suppress the growth of tumors that need sex hormones for growth. Because of its function, it may also be called a medical adrenalectomy.

amsacrine (*m*-acridinylamine methane-sulfon anisidide [AMSA]) An intravenous (IV) chemotherapy agent that belongs to the family of drugs called topoisomerase inhibitors. This agent is cur-

rently being studied for use in treating breast cancer and other cancers, including acute nonlymphocytic leukemia, lymphoma, melanoma, and colon cancer.

anastrozole (Arimidex) An oral chemotherapy drug used to treat breast cancer that has not responded to tamoxifen.

Anzemet See DOLASETRON.

Arimidex See ANASTROZOLE.

Aromasin See EXEMESTANE.

CAF A combination of the chemotherapy drugs cyclophosphamide (Cytoxan), doxorubicin (Adriamycin), and 5-fluorouracil (5-FU) that is sometimes used to treat breast cancer.

capecitabine (Xeloda) An oral chemotherapy agent that belongs to the family of drugs called antimetabolites; it is used to treat metastatic breast cancer that is resistant to paclitaxel (Taxol) and anthracyclines.

CFM A combination of the chemotherapy drugs cyclophosphamide (Cytoxan), 5-fluorouracil (5-FU), and methotrexate that may be used to treat breast cancer.

CFPT A combination of the chemotherapy drugs cyclophosphamide (Cytoxan), 5-fluorouracil (5-FU), prednisone, and methotrexate that may be used to treat breast cancer.

chlorambucil (Leukeran) A chemotherapy agent that belongs to the family of drugs called alkylating agents, sometimes used to treat breast cancer; it may also be used to treat cancers of the ovary and testis, chronic lymphocytic leukemia, lymphomas, and choriocarcinoma.

cisplatin (Platinol, formerly *cis*-platinum) A very common intravenous (IV) chemotherapy agent that belongs to the family of drugs called platinum compounds, which are sometimes used to treat breast cancer. It also may be used to treat lymphomas, myeloma, melanoma, and osteogenic sarcoma or cancers of the testes, head and neck, bladder, ovary, prostate, lung, esophagus, and cervix.

***cis*-platinum** See CISPLATIN.

clomiphene An experimental antiestrogen medication used to treat some patients with breast cancer.

CMF A combination of the chemotherapy drugs cyclophosphamide (Cytoxan), methotrexate, and 5-fluorouracil (5-FU) used to treat breast cancer. CMF was the first type of adjuvant therapy proved effective in this type of cancer.

CMFP A combination of the chemotherapy drugs cyclophosphamide (Cytoxan), methotrexate, 5-fluorouracil (5-FU), and prednisone sometimes used to treat breast cancer.

CMFVP A combination of the chemotherapy drugs cyclophosphamide (Cytoxan), methotrexate, 5-fluorouracil (5-FU), vincristine, and prednisone (also called the Cooper regimen) sometimes used to treat breast cancer.

Compazine See PROCHLORPERAZINE.

cyclophosphamide (Cytoxan) One of the most commonly used chemotherapy drugs, sometimes used to treat breast cancer and other malignancies, including lymphoma, leukemia, myeloma, neuroblastoma, Ewing's sarcoma, mycosis fungoides, rhabdomyosarcoma, and cancers of the ovary, lung, testis, and endometrium. It can be administered either intravenously or orally and belongs to the family of alkylating agents.

cyclosporin A drug used to help reduce the risk of rejection of organ and bone marrow transplants by the body. It is also used in clinical trials to make cancer cells more sensitive to chemotherapy drugs.

Cytadren See AMINOGLUTETHIMIDE.

Cytovene See GALLIUM NITRATE.

Cytoxan See CYCLOPHOSPHAMIDE.

Decadron (dexamethasone, Hexadrol) See DEXAMETHASONE.

2'-deoxycytidine A drug that protects healthy tissues from the toxic effects of anticancer drugs.

Demerol See MEPERIDINE.

Depo-Provera See MEDROXYPROGESTERONE.

Depo-Testosterone A long-acting male hormonal drug that is injected into the muscle and used to treat breast cancer.

dexamethasone (Decadron) An antinausea drug and synthetic adrenocorticoid prescribed to ease nausea and vomiting in chemotherapy patients. It is also used to reduce swelling of brain tissue in patients with brain cancer, and, sometimes, to treat leukemia and lymphoma.

dexrazoxane (Zinecard) A drug used to protect the heart from the toxic effects of anthracycline drugs such as doxorubicin. It belongs to the family of drugs called chemoprotective agents.

DHAD   See MITOXANTRONE.

DHA-paclitaxel   A combination of docosahexaenoic acid (DHA) (a natural fatty acid) and paclitaxel (an anticancer drug) that is being studied as a treatment for cancer.

Didronel   See ETIDRONATE.

docetaxel (Taxotere)   A chemotherapy drug used to treat metastatic or locally advanced breast cancer; its usefulness with other types of cancer is also being studied. Taxotere received approval in September of 2001 for treating patients with metastatic breast cancer whose cancer has progressed after treatment with an anthracycline-containing cancer therapy (such as doxorubicin [Adriamycin]). Taxotere received approval in May 1996 for the treatment of locally advanced or metastatic breast cancer that has progressed during anthracycline-based treatment or relapsed during anthracycline-based adjuvant therapy. Taxotere injection received additional approval in June of 1998 for the treatment of patients with locally advanced or metastatic breast cancer after failure of prior chemotherapy.

dolasetron (Anzemet)   An antiemetic drug that prevents or reduces nausea and vomiting that typically occur during chemotherapy. It can be given intravenously or orally.

doxorubicin (Adriamycin)   A major intravenous (IV) antibiotic chemotherapy drug used to treat cancer of the breast and many other cancers, including Wilms' tumor, neuroblastoma, rhabdomyosarcoma, Ewing's sarcoma, retinoblastoma, Kaposi's sarcoma, and cancers of the bladder, thyroid, lung, and ovary. This drug must be given carefully, since it can cause severe skin damage if it leaks out into the surrounding area. Patients who are taking this drug should drink plenty of fluids to prevent kidney or bladder problems. In addition to typical side effects common to many chemotherapy drugs, this drug can cause direct damage to the muscle cells of the heart (cardiomyopathy). This

damage is related to total accumulative lifetime dosage.

dronabinol (Marinol)   A synthetic pill form of delta-9-tetrahydrocannabinol, an active ingredient in marijuana that is used to treat nausea and vomiting associated with cancer chemotherapy.

Eldisine   See VINDESINE.

Ellence   See EPIRUBICIN.

endostatin   A drug that is being studied for its ability to prevent the growth of new blood vessels into a solid tumor. Endostatin belongs to the family of drugs called angiogenesis inhibitors.

epirubicin (Ellence)   An intravenous (IV) antibiotic chemotherapy drug sometimes used to treat breast cancer and other malignancies, including soft tissue sarcoma, non-Hodgkin's lymphoma, and cancers of the ovaries, stomach, colon or rectum, pancreas, head, or neck.

EPO   See ERYTHROPOIETIN.

epoetin alfa   See ERYTHROPOIETIN.

Epogen   See ERYTHROPOIETIN.

Eprex   See ERYTHROPOIETIN.

erythropoietin (EPO, Epogen, Procrit, epoetin alfa, Eprex)   A colony-stimulating factor that activates the production of red blood cells. It is sometimes used to treat anemia in patients with nonmyeloid cancer or in certain chemotherapy patients.

etanidazole   A drug that increases the effectiveness of radiation therapy.

etidronate (Didronel)   An oral and intravenous (IV) drug that belongs to the family of drugs called bisphosphonates and is used as treatment for breast cancer that has spread to the bone.

Evista See RALOXIFENE.

exemestane (Aromasin) An anticancer drug used to decrease estrogen production and suppress the growth of estrogen-dependent tumors.

FAC A combination of the chemotherapy drugs 5-fluorouracil (5-FU), doxorubicin (Adriamycin), and cyclophosphamide (Cytoxan) sometimes used to treat breast cancer.

Fareston See TOREMIFENE.

fentanyl citrate A narcotic opioid drug that is used in the treatment of pain and often administered in lollipop form.

flecainide A drug used to treat abnormal heart rhythms that also may relieve nerve pain—the burning, stabbing, or stinging pain that may arise from damage to nerves caused by breast cancer or its treatment.

Folex See METHOTREXATE.

gabapentin A substance being studied as a treatment for relieving hot flashes of women who have breast cancer. Gabapentin belongs to a family of drugs called anticonvulsants.

goserelin acetate (Zoladex) A drug that blocks the production of male hormones and is used as a palliative treatment for advanced breast cancer. It is administered monthly as a pellet injected under the skin of the abdomen, where it slowly releases the drug.

granisetron (Kytril) An antinausea drug given to chemotherapy patients with breast cancer to prevent or control nausea and vomiting. It can be given either as an IV or by mouth.

halofuginone hydrobromide A substance that is being studied for its ability to slow the growth of connective tissue and prevent the growth of new blood vessels to a solid tumor. It belongs to a family of drugs called quinazolinone alkaloids.

hematopoietin-1 See INTERLEUKIN-1.

Herceptin See TRASTUZUMAB.

Hexadrol See DEXAMETHASONE.

IMF A combination of the chemotherapy drug ifosfamide with mesna, methotrexate, and 5-fluorouracil (5-FU); sometimes used to treat breast cancer.

imiquimod A substance that improves the body's natural response to infection and disease. Imiquimod is currently being studied as a topical agent to prevent some types of cancer. It belongs to the family of drugs called biological response modifiers.

indomethacin A drug that belongs to the family of drugs called nonsteroidal anti-inflammatory drugs. It is used to reduce tumor-induced suppression of the immune system and to increase the effectiveness of anticancer drugs.

Kytril See GRANISETRON.

Leukeran See CHLORAMBUCIL.

Levo-Dromoran See LEVORPHANOL.

levorphanol (Levo-Dromoran) A narcotic injectable and oral drug used to control pain.

L-phenylalanine mustard (Alkeran) An oral alkylating chemotherapy drug sometimes used to treat breast cancer, ovarian cancer, or myeloma.

L-sarcolysin See L-PHENYLALANINE MUSTARD.

m-AMSA See AMSACRINE.

Marinol See DRONABINOL.

Medrol See METHYLPREDNISOLONE.

methylprednisolone (Medrol) An oral corticosteroid hormonal drug sometimes used to treat breast cancer and other malignancies, including lymphoma, Hodgkin's disease, acute leukemia, and myeloma.

medroxyprogesterone (Provera, Depo-Provera) A female sex hormone that has sometimes been used to treat breast cancer, kidney cancer, and endometrial cancer.

Megace See MEGESTROL.

MEG See MEGESTROL.

megestrol (Megace, MEG, Pallace) A hormonal type of oral chemotherapy sometimes used to treat cancers of the breast.

meperidine (Demerol) A strong narcotic used to treat pain for a short period of time (between two and three hours). For this reason, it is not given for patients with chronic pain, but instead for occasional episodes of pain after surgery.

mesna (Mesnex) A drug approved in March of 2002 to reduce the incidence of ifosfamide-induced hemorrhagic cystitis. Ifosfamide is a type of chemotherapy agent given as a treatment for breast cancer. After ifosfamide and the first dose of mesna are administered intravenously, subsequent doses of mesna may be given intravenously or orally. The most frequently reported adverse reactions were headache, injection site reactions, flushing, dizziness, nausea, vomiting, fatigue, diarrhea, anorexia, fever, sore throat, flulike symptoms, and coughing.

Mesna does not prevent hemorrhagic cystitis in all patients and does not decrease other chemotherapy-related side effects.

methotrexate (Mexate, Folex, amethopterin) An important antimetabolite chemotherapy drug sometimes used to treat cancers of the breast, and other malignancies, including an acute leukemia sarcoma, lymphoma, mycosis fungoides, and cancers of the cervix, head and neck, colon, lung, and testes. This drug can be given either intravenously or orally.

metoclopramide (Reglan) An antinausea drug that may be given to chemotherapy patients before treatment to prevent nausea and vomiting. It can be administered either intravenously or orally.

Mexate See METHOTREXATE.

mifepristone (RU486) A French abortion drug that is currently being studied as a possible chemotherapy drug to treat metastatic breast cancer, ovarian cancer, some brain tumors, and prostate cancer.

mitomycin (Mutamycin) An intravenous antibiotic chemotherapy drug sometimes used to treat cancers of the breast, stomach, cervix, colon, pancreas, or bladder. In addition to typical chemotherapy side effects, this drug may lead to the destruction of red blood cells (hemolysis), which can be fatal.

mitoxantrone (Novantrone, DHAD) An important intravenous chemotherapy drug sometimes used to treat breast cancer and other cancers, including leukemia, lymphoma, and prostate cancer. It is also used in combination with steroids to ease symptoms in patients with advanced prostate cancer. This drug was developed as an alternative to adriamycin, because it has a milder side effect profile.

MTX See METHOTREXATE.

Mutamycin See MITOMYCIN.

Navelbine   See VINORELBINE.

Nolvadex   See TAMOXIFEN.

Novantrone   See MITOXANTRONE.

Oncovin   See VINCRISTINE.

paclitaxel (Taxol)   A chemotherapy drug used to treat advanced metastatic breast cancer and other malignancies, including advanced ovarian cancer, Kaposi's sarcoma, and lung cancer. Originally produced from the bark of the Pacific yew tree, it is now manufactured in a semisynthetic process in much larger amounts. Research is ongoing to find other types of cancer that will respond to this drug. This drug received additional approval in October of 1999 for adjuvant treatment of node-positive breast cancer. In clinical trials, the drug improved overall survival rate of women who had receptor-positive and receptor-negative tumors. However, the improvement has been specifically demonstrated only in women who have estrogen- and progesterone-receptor-negative tumors.

Pallace   See MEGESTROL.

Platinol   See CISPLATIN.

prochlorperazine (Compazine)   An antinausea drug commonly prescribed for chemotherapy patients to control severe nausea and vomiting.

Procrit   See ERYTHROPOIETIN.

Provera   See MEDROXYPROGESTERONE.

raloxifene (Evista)   The first in a new class of drugs known as selective estrogen-receptor modulators. Raloxifene is being studied as a drug to prevent breast cancer. Like tamoxifen, it is a synthetic drug that blocks the action of estrogen, which encourages the growth of breast tumors. Some studies have suggested raloxifene can lower a woman's risk of having breast cancer and cause fewer side effects than tamoxifen, including fewer hot flashes and possibly a lower risk of uterine cancer. The two drugs are currently being compared as part of the study of tamoxifen and raloxifene, which began in 1999.

Reglan   See METOCLOPRAMIDE.

RU 486   See MIFEPRISTONE.

tamoxifen (Nolvadex)   A nonsteroidal antiestrogen drug used as adjuvant chemotherapy to prevent a recurrence of breast cancer and as a treatment for advanced breast cancer. Tamoxifen is far less toxic than most types of chemotherapy agents. Although it increases the risk of uterine cancer and potentially fatal blood clots, its benefits are considered to outweigh the risks.

Tamoxifen lowers the risk of invasive breast cancer by 49 percent in women at increased risk for development of the disease. However, few studies have been done to see whether tamoxifen is effective in women who have *BRCA1* or *BRCA2* mutations. One study did find that tamoxifen reduced the incidence of breast cancer by 62 percent in women who had alterations in *BRCA2*, but the results showed no reduction in breast cancer incidence with tamoxifen use among women who had *BRCA1* alterations. A prevention trial that is currently under way (the Study of Tamoxifen and Raloxifene) compares the effect of tamoxifen with that of raloxifene in reducing the incidence of breast cancer.

Taxol   See PACLITAXEL.

Taxotere   See DOCETAXEL.

teniposide (VM-26, Vunom)   An intravenously administered chemotherapy drug being studied for use against cancers of the breast, among others.

thiotEPA (triethylenethiophosphoramide [TSPA])   An injectable alkylating chemotherapy drug sometimes used to treat cancers of the breast.

toremifene (Fareston) An oral hormonal chemotherapy drug used to treat metastatic breast cancer of postmenopausal women who have estrogen-receptor-positive or receptor-unknown tumors.

trastuzumab (Herceptin) An intravenously administered monoclonal antibody genetically engineered to attack the protein generated by the *HER-2/neu* gene and used to treat metastatic patients with breast cancer who have this gene. It has been studied in combination with taxol to treat advanced breast or ovarian cancer. Herceptin works best in the 30 percent of patients with breast cancer and 20 percent of patients with ovarian cancer whose tumor shows high levels of this gene.

triethylenethiophosphoramide See THIOTEPA.

TSPA See THIOTEPA.

VATH A combination of the chemotherapy drugs vinblastine, doxorubicin (Adriamycin), and thiotepa sometimes used to treat breast cancer.

Velban See VINBLASTINE.

vinblastine (Velban) An important intravenously administered chemotherapy drug sometimes used to treat cancers of the head and neck, breast, kidney, or testes, or lymphoma or Kaposi's sarcoma.

vincristine (Oncovin) An intravenously administered chemotherapy drug sometimes used to treat cancers of the brain, breast, cervix, and testes, as well as lymphoma, acute leukemia, Wilms' tumor, neuroblastoma, and rhabdomyosarcoma. Vincristine is derived from the periwinkle plant.

vindesine (Eldisine, vinblastine amide sulfate) An investigational intravenously administered drug being studied as a possible treatment for breast cancer and other malignancies, including lymphoma, melanoma, leukemia, and cancers of the lung, colon, or testes.

vinorelbine (Navelbine) A chemotherapy drug used alone or in combination with cisplatin to treat breast cancer and unresectable, advanced non-small cell lung cancer. Vinorelbine is given either intravenously or orally.

VM-26 See TENIPOSIDE.

Vunom See TENIPOSIDE.

Xeloda See CAPECITABINE.

Zinecard See DEXRAZOXANE.

Zoladex See GOSERELIN ACETATE.

APPENDIX V
PRODUCTS FOR PATIENTS WITH BREAST CANCER*

Nearly You
http://www.nearlyyou.com

Breast prosthetics, mastectomy products, lingerie, and bras

A New Image Boutique
(319) 232-3219
(800) 359-2357
http://www.anewimageboutique.com

Breast forms, equalizer forms, mastectomy bras, camisoles, swimwear, hats, wigs, turbans, and compression therapy products

A New You, Mastectomy Boutique
(888) 737-2511
http://www.newyouboutique.com

Silicone breast forms, mastectomy bras, and other products

Breast Prosthesis and Post Surgery Fashions
http://www.cpmart.com

Silicone and foam breast prostheses, forms, fashions, adhesives, bras, and swimwear

Cancer Boutique
22941 Ventura Boulevard
Suite M
Woodland Hills, CA 91326
(818) 999-9719

2421 Tustin Avenue
Santa Ana, CA 92705
(714) 835-9656

Cancer Center of Santa Barbara
Santa Barbara, CA
(888) 848-7965
http://www.cancerboutique.com/index.html

Breast prostheses, bras, wigs, hats, enhancers, swimwear, activewear, and so on

Josephine's
9514 Kenwood Road
Cincinnati, OH 45242
(800) 442-8236
(513) 745-9501
http://www.josephinesshops.com

Postmastectomy shop

SOUBRA Breast Prosthesis Supports
O.M.T. Limited
61 Herring Cove Road
Halifax, Nova Scotia B3N 1P9
Canada
(902) 479-0419
(866) 476-8272 or (866) 4SOUBRA (toll-free in North America)
http://www.soubra.ca

Breast prostheses with adhesive-free attachments

Undie Box—Mastectomy Boutique
http://www.undiebox.com

Breast prostheses, attachable and nonattachable breast forms, contours, enhancers, and bras 32–54 AA–H cups

Woman's Personal Health Resource
(877) 463-1343 (toll-free)
(845) 369-0560
http://www.womanspersonalhealth.com/
postmastectomyproducts.htm

Breast forms, mastectomy bras, camisoles, and all mastectomy supplies and accessories

*Inclusion does not indicate endorsement; exclusion does not indicate disapproval.

ContourMed
2821 Kavanaugh Boulevard
Suite 2
Little Rock, AR 72205
(501) 907-0530
(888) 301-0520
http://www.contourmed.com

Custom and standard prostheses

Nicola Jane Mastectomy Wear Collection
http://www.nicolajane.com

Swimwear, bras, breast prostheses, and numerous accessories, designed for use after a partial or full mastectomy

Webb Prosthetics
http://www.webbprosthetics.net

Custom and prefabricated prosthetics and orthotics, including breast prostheses and bras

Maizy Grace Mastectomy and Lumpectomy Camisole
http://www.maizygrace.com

A camisole worn as a tank top

Ladies First, Inc.
(800) 497-8285
http://www.wvi.com/~ladies1

Silicone breast prostheses and other postmastectomy products designed for women after breast cancer or breast surgery

Dignity Mastectomy Products
1386-A Westgate Center Drive
Winston-Salem, NC 27103
(336) 760-4333
http://www.mastectomyboutique.com

Breast prostheses, forms, lingerie, bras, swimwear, and headcoverings.

Park Prosthetics
Park Mastectomy Supply
2222 Morgan Avenue
Suite 110
Corpus Christi, Texas 78405
(361) 385-1041
http://www.parkmastectomy.com

Wigs, mastectomy forms, bras, swimsuits, and similar products

GLOSSARY

adjuvant   A substance that speeds or improves the action of a medicine or therapy.

adrenal glands   A pair of small glands, one located on top of each kidney, that produce steroid hormones, adrenaline, and noradrenaline to help control heart rate, blood pressure, and other important body functions.

agonists   Drugs that trigger an action from a cell or another drug.

agranulocyte   A type of white blood cell that includes monocytes and lymphocytes.

allogeneic   Originating from another person.

anaplastic   A term used to describe cancer cells that divide rapidly and bear little or no resemblance to normal cells.

antibody   A protein in the blood that fights against an invading foreign agent (antigen). Each antibody bonds to a particular antigen.

apoptosis   Programmed cell death.

autologous   Originating from the same person.

axilla   The underarm or armpit.

B cell   White blood cell that makes antibodies and is an important part of the immune system. B cells are from bone marrow. Also called B lymphocyte.

biopsy   The surgical removal of a small piece of tissue for microscopic examination to determine whether cancer cells are present.

blood-brain barrier   A network of blood vessels with closely spaced cells that make it difficult for potentially toxic substances (such as chemotherapy drugs) to enter the brain.

B lymphocytes   See **B cell**.

cell   The basic structural unit of all life. All living matter is composed of cells.

cervix   The lower, narrow end of the uterus that forms a canal between the uterus and vagina.

chromosome   Part of a cell that contains genetic information. Except sperm and eggs, all human cells contain 46 chromosomes.

coenzyme   A substance needed for the proper functioning of an enzyme.

colony-stimulating factors   Biological products (including erythropoietin, granulocyte colony-stimulating factor [G-CSF], and granulocyte-macrophage colony-stimulating factor [GM-CSF]) that stimulate the growth of normal blood cells.

cyst   An abnormal, saclike structure that contains liquid or semisolid material. A cyst may be benign or malignant.

cytokines   A class of substances produced by immune system cells that affect the immune response. Cytokines can also be produced in the laboratory and administered to people to influence immune response.

cytopenia   A reduction in the number of blood cells.

cytotoxic   Cell-killing.

diploid   The characteristic of having two sets of chromosomes in a cell. This is normal for a breast cell.

diuretic   A drug that increases the volume of urine.

DNA   Deoxyribonucleic acid; one of two nucleic acids (the other is ribonucleic acid [RNA]) found in the nucleus of all cells. DNA contains genetic information for cell growth, division, and cell function.

endocrine glands   Glands that manufacture and secrete hormones into the blood. Endocrine glands include the pituitary, thyroid, parathyroid, and adrenal glands; ovary and testis; placenta; and part of the pancreas.

endometrium   The lining of the uterus.

enzyme   A protein that promotes essential functions involved in cell growth and metabolism.

eosinophil   Type of white blood cell.

genes   Located in the nucleus of the cell, these substances contain hereditary information that is transferred from cell to cell.

granulocyte   A type of white blood cell that fights bacterial infection. Neutrophils, eosinophils, and basophils are granulocytes.

hemoglobin   A protein in red blood cells that carries oxygen from the lungs to the body's tissues.

hypoxia   A lack of oxygen flow to the tissues of the body.

immunotherapy   Treatment that involves use of biological response modifiers to strengthen the body's immune system.

killer cells   White blood cells that attack tumor cells and body cells that have been invaded by foreign substances.

leukocytes   A white blood cell that does not contain hemoglobin. White blood cells include lymphocytes, neutrophils, eosinophils, macrophages, and mast cells, all of which are produced by bone marrow and help the body fight infection.

lobular   The part of the breast (the lobes) farthest from the nipple.

lymph   The clear fluid of the lymphatic system through which cells travel as they fight infection and disease.

lymphocyte   A type of white blood cell that helps produce antibodies and other substances that fight infection and diseases.

mastalgia   Pain in the breast.

mast cell   A type of white blood cell.

metastasis   Cancer that has spread from the site of origin to another part of the body, usually through the lymphatic system or the blood.

monocyte   A type of white blood cell.

monoclonal antibodies   Substances produced in the lab that can locate and bind to cancer cells wherever they are in the body. Many monoclonal antibodies are used in cancer diagnosis or treatment. Each recognizes a different protein on certain cancer cells. Monoclonal antibodies can be used alone, or they can be used to deliver drugs, toxins, or radioactive material directly to a tumor.

myeloid   Derived from or pertaining to bone marrow.

myometrium   The muscular outer layer of the uterus.

natural killer cells (NK cells)   White blood cells that can kill tumor cells.

necrosis   Tissue death.

neoplasm   A new growth of tissue that serves no physiological function.

neutrophil   A type of white blood cell.

nodule   A small, solid lump that can be detected by touch. This term usually refers to a lump that is malignant but can also refer to one that is benign.

oropharynx   The middle part of the throat. It includes the soft palate, the base of the tongue, and the tonsils.

parathyroid glands   Four pea-sized glands found on the thyroid that produce parathyroid hormone, which increases calcium level in the blood.

peptide   Any compound consisting of two or more amino acids, the building blocks of proteins.

plasma   The clear, yellowish fluid part of the blood that carries the blood cells.

platelets   Blood cells that help prevent bleeding by causing blood clot formation.

polyp   A growth that protrudes from a mucus membrane.

precancerous   Also called *premalignant,* abnormal change in cells that indicates the potential for development of cancer.

protein   A molecule made up of amino acid chains that the body needs for proper function. Proteins form the structure of skin, hair, enzymes, cytokines, and antibodies.

radiation sensitizer   Chemical that makes a cell more susceptible to the effects of radiation therapy.

radioisotope An unstable element that releases radiation as it breaks down. Radioisotopes can be used in imaging tests and in treatment for cancer.

receptor A molecule inside or on the surface of a cell that binds to a specific substance.

red blood cell A cell (also called an erythrocyte) that carries oxygen to all parts of the body.

regional involvement The spread of cancer from its original site to nearby areas.

serum The clear liquid part of the blood that remains after blood cells and clotting proteins have been removed.

stem cells Cells from which other types of cells can develop.

supraclavicular nodes The lymph nodes located above the collarbone in the area of the neck.

systemic Affecting the whole body.

T cell A type of white blood cell that attacks invaders such as cancer cells and produces substances that regulate immune response.

thyroid gland A gland located beneath the larynx that produces thyroid hormone and helps regulate growth and metabolism.

white blood cell A blood cell that does not contain hemoglobin, including lymphocytes, neutrophils, eosinophils, macrophages, and mast cells. These cells are made by bone marrow and help the body fight infection and other diseases.

BIBLIOGRAPHY

Abbott, D. W., M. L. Freeman, and J. T. Holt. "Double-strand Break Repair Deficiency and Radiation Sensitivity in *BRCA2* Mutant Cancer Cells." *Journal of the National Cancer Institute* 90, no. 13 (1998): 978–985.

Adami, H. O., et al. "Absence of Association between Reproductive Variables and the Risk of Breast Cancer in Young Women in Sweden and Norway." *British Journal of Cancer* 62 (1990): 122–126.

Adlercreutz, H. "Evolution, Nutrition, Intestinal Microflora, and Prevention of Cancer: A Hypothesis." *Proceedings of the Society for Experimental Biology and Medicine* 217 (1998): 241–246.

Albanes, D., A. Blair, and P. R. Taylor. "Physical Activity and Risk of Cancer in the NHANES I Population." *American Journal of Public Health* 79 (1989): 744–750.

Albertazzi, P., et al. "Dietary Soy Supplementation and Phytoestrogen Levels." *Obstetrics and Gynecology* 94 (1999): 229–231.

Ambrosone, C. B., et al. "Breast Cancer Risk, Meat Consumption, and N-acetyltransferase Genetic Polymorphisms." *International Journal of Cancer* 75 (1998): 30.

Anderson, J. J. B., and S. C. Garner. "Phytoestrogens and Human Function." *Nutrition Today* 32 (1997): 39.

Apter, D. "Hormonal Events during Female Puberty in Relation to Breast Cancer Risk." *European Journal of Cancer Prevention* 5 (1996): 476–482.

Ardies, C. M., and C. Dee. "Xenoestrogens Significantly Enhance Risk for Breast Cancer during Growth and Adolescence." *Medical Hypotheses* 50 (1998): 457–464.

Aulmann, S., et al. "CTCF Gene Mutations in Invasive Ductal Breast Cancer." *Breast Cancer Research and Treatment* 80, no. 3 (August 2003): 347–352.

Bal, D. G., and S. B. Forester. "Dietary Strategies for Cancer Prevention." *Cancer* 72 (1992): 1005–1010.

Barger-Lux, M. J., and R. P. Heaney. "The Role of Calcium Intake in Preventing Bone Fragility, Hypertension, and Certain Cancers." *Journal of Nutrition* 124 (1994): 1406S–1411S.

Beaty, O., et al. "Subsequent Malignancies in Children and Adolescents after Treatment for Hodgkin's Disease." *Journal of Clinical Oncology* 13 (1995): 603–609.

Beecher, C. W. W. "Cancer Preventive Properties of Varieties of *Brassica oleracea:* A Review." *American Journal of Clinical Nutrition* 59 (1994): 166S–1170S.

Bennicke, K., et al. "Cigarette Smoking and Breast Cancer." *British Medical Journal* 310 (1995): 1431–1433.

Bernstein, L., et al. "Physical Exercise and Reduced Risk of Breast Cancer in Young Women." *Journal of the National Cancer Institute* 86 (1994): 1403–1408.

Bhatia, S., et al. "Breast Cancer and Other Second Neoplasms after Childhood Hodgkin's Disease." *New England Journal of Medicine* 334 (1996): 745–751.

Biganzoli, E., et al. "Prognosis in Node-Negative Primary Breast Cancer: A Neural Network Analysis of Risk Profiles Using Routinely Assessed Factors." *Annals of Oncology* 14, no. 10 (October 2003): 1484–1493.

Bingham, S. A. "Meat or Wheat for the Next Millennium? High-Meat diets and Cancer Risk." *Proceedings of the Nutrition Society* 58 (1999): 243–248.

Bingham, S. A., et al. "Phyto-oestrogens: Where Are We Now?" *British Journal of Nutrition* 79 (1998): 393–406.

Blot, W., B. Henderson, and J. J. Boice. "Childhood Cancer in Relation to Cured Meat Intake: Review of the Epidemiological Evidence." *Nutrition and Cancer* 34 (1999): 111–118.

Bouker, K. B., and L. Hilakivi-Clarke. "Genistein: Does It Prevent or Promote Breast Cancer?" *Environmental Health Perspectives* 108 (2000): 701–708.

Bourne, T. H., et al. "Screening for Early Familial Ovarian Cancer with Transvaginal Ultrasonography and Colour Blood Flow Imaging." *British Medical Journal* 306 (1993): 1025–1029.

Bowlin, S. J., et al. "Breast Cancer Risk and Alcohol Consumption: Results from a Large Case-Control Study." *International Journal of Epidemiology* 26 (1997): 915–923.

Boyd, N. F., et al. "A Meta-analysis of Studies of Dietary Fat and Breast Cancer Risk." *British Journal of Cancer* 68 (1993): 627–636.

Bradlow, H. L., et al. "Indole-3-carbinol: A Novel Approach to Breast Cancer Prevention." *Annals of the New York Academy of Science* 768 (1995): 180–200.

Braga, C., et al. "Intake of Selected Foods and Nutrients and Breast Cancer Risk: An Age-and Menopause-specific Analysis." *Nutrition and Cancer* 28 (1997): 258–263.

Brekelmans, C. T., et al. "Rotterdam Committee for Medical and Genetic Counseling: Effectiveness of Breast Cancer Surveillance in *BRCA1/2* Gene Mutation Carriers and Women with High Familial Risk." *Journal of Clinical Oncology* 19, no. 4 (2001): 924–924.

Brinton, L. A., et al. "Breastfeeding and Breast Cancer Risk." *Cancer Causes and Control* 6 (1995): 199–208.

Brinton, L., et al. "Modification of Oral Contraceptive Relationships on Breast Cancer Risk by Selected Factors among Younger Women." *Contraception* 55 (1997): 197–203.

Burke, W., et al. "Recommendations for Follow-up Care of Individuals with an Inherited Predisposition to Cancer. II. BRCA1 and BRCA2." Cancer Genetics Studies Consortium. *Journal of the American Medical Association* 277, no. 12 (1997): 997–1003.

Burke, G. L., M. Z. Vitolins, and D. Bland. "Soybean Isoflavones as an Alternative to Traditional Hormone Replacement Therapy: Are We There Yet?" *Journal of Nutrition* 130 (2000): 664S–665S.

Byers, T., and N. Guerrero. "Epidemiologic Evidence for Vitamin C and Vitamin E in Cancer Prevention." *American Journal of Clinical Nutrition* 62 (1995): 1385S–1392S.

Byrne, C., et al. "Predictors of Dietary Heterocyclic Amine Intake in Three Prospective Cohorts." *Cancer Epidemiology Biomarkers and Prevention* 7 (1998): 523–529.

Byrne, C., G. Ursin, and R. Ziegler. "A Comparison of Food Habit and Food Frequency Data as Predictors of Breast Cancer in the NHANES I / NHEFS Cohort." *Journal of Nutrition* 126 (1996): 2757–2764.

Calle, E. E., et al. "Occupation and Breast Cancer Mortality in a Prospective Cohort of U.S. Women." *American Journal of Epidemiology* 148 (1998): 191–197.

Campbell, C., L. O. Luedecke, and T. D. Shultz. "Yogurt Consumption and Estrogen Metabolism in Healthy Premenopausal Women." *Nutrition Research* 19 (1999): 531–543.

Cantor, K. "Drinking Water and Cancer." *Cancer Causes and Control* 8 (1997): 292–308.

Caygill, C., A. Charlett, and M. Hill. "Fat, Fish, Fish Oil, and Cancer." *British Journal of Cancer* 74 (1996): 159–164.

Chehab, F. F., et al. "Early Onset of Reproductive Function in Normal Female Mice Treated with Leptin." *Science* 275 (1997): 88–90.

Chen, C.-L., et al. "Leisure-time Physical Activity in Relation to Breast Cancer among Young Women (Washington, United States)." *Cancer Causes and Control* 8 (1997): 77–84.

Chiechi, L. M. "Dietary Phytoestrogens in the Prevention of Long-term Postmenopausal Diseases." *International Journal of Gynecology & Obstetrics* 67 (1999): 39–40.

Chu, S. Y., et al. "Cigarette Smoking and the Risk of Breast Cancer." *American Journal of Epidemiology* 131 (1990): 244–253.

Cigolini, M., et al. "Moderate Alcohol Consumption and Its Relation to Visceral Fat and Plasma Androgens in Healthy women." *International Journal of Obesity* 20 (1996): 206–212.

Clavel-Chapelon, F., M. Niravong, and R. R. Joseph. "Diet and Breast Cancer: Review of the Epidemiologic Literature." *Cancer Detection and Prevention* 21 (1997): 426–440.

Cleary, M. P., and N. J. Maihle. "The Role of Body Mass Index in the Relative Risk of Developing Premenopausal versus Postmenopausal Breast Cancer." Proceedings of the Society for Experimental Biology and Medicine 216 (1997): 28–43.

Colditz, G. A., B. A. Rosner, and F. E. Speizer. "Risk Factors for Breast Cancer According to Family History of Breast Cancer." *Journal of the National Cancer Institute* 88, no. 6 (1996): 365–371.

Colditz, G. A., and A. L. Frazier. "Models of Breast Cancer Show That Risk Is Set by Events of Early Life: Prevention Efforts Must Shift Focus." *Cancer Epidemiology Biomarkers & Prevention* 4 (1995): 567–571.

Colditz, G. A., et al. "Alcohol Intake in Relation to Diet and Obesity in Women and Men." *American Journal of Clinical Nutrition* 54 (1991): 49–55.

Collaborative Group on Hormonal Factors in Breast Cancer. "Breast Cancer and Hormonal Contraceptives: Collaborative Reanalysis of Individual Data on 53,297 Women with Breast Cancer and 100,239 Women without Breast Cancer from 54 Epidemiological Studies." *The Lancet* 347 (1996): 1713–1727.

Collichio, F. A., R. Agnello, and J. Staltzer. "Pregnancy after Breast Cancer: From Psychosocial Issues through Conception." *Oncology* 12 (1998): 759–765.

Coogan, P. F., et al. "Physical Activity in Usual Occupation and Risk of Breast Cancer (United States)." *Cancer Causes and Control* 8 (1997): 626–631.

D'Avanzo, B., et al. "Nutrient Intake According to Education, Smoking, and Alcohol in Italian Women." *Nutrition and Cancer* 28 (1997): 46–51.

D'Avanzo, B., et al. "Physical Activity and Breast Cancer Risk." *Cancer Epidemiology, Biomarkers and Prevention* 5 (1998): 155–160.

Decarli, A., et al. "Macronutrients, Energy Intake, and Breast Cancer Risk: Implications from Different Models." *Epidemiology* 8 (1997): 425–428.

Decker, E. A. "The Role of Phenolics, Conjugated Linoleic Acid, Carnosine, and Pyrroloquinoline Quinone as

Nonessential Dietary Antioxidants." *Nutrition Review* 53 (1995): 49–58.

den Tonkelaar, I., et al. "Urinary Phytoestrogens and Postmenopausal Breast Cancer Risk." *Cancer Epidemiology, Biomarkers and Prevention* 10 (2001): 223–228.

DeStefani, E., et al. "Dietary Fiber and Risk of Breast Cancer: A Case-Control Study in Uruguay." *Nutrition and Cancer* 28 (1997): 14–19.

Dietz, W. H. "Periods of Risk in Childhood for the Development of Adult Obesity—What Do We Need to Learn?" *Journal of Nutrition* 127 (1997): 1884s–1886s.

Djuric, Z., et al. "Oxidative DNA Damage Levels in Blood from Women at High Risk for Breast Cancer Are Associated with Dietary Intake of Meats, Vegetables, and Fruits." *Journal of the American Dietetic Association* 98 (1998): 524–528.

Domchek, S. M. "The Utility of Ductal Lavage in Breast Cancer Detection and Risk Assessment." *Breast Cancer Research* 4, no. 2 (2002): 51–53.

Dooley, W. C., et al. "Ductal Lavage for Detection of Cellular Atypia in Women at High Risk for Breast Cancer." *Journal of the National Cancer Institute* 93, no. 21 (2001): 1624–1632.

Dorant, E., P. A. V. D. Brandt, and R. A. Goldbohm. "Allium Vegetable Consumption, Garlic Supplement Intake, and Female Breast Carcinoma Incidence." *Breast Cancer Research and Treatment* 33 (1995): 163–170.

Dorgan, J. F. "Physical Activity and Breast Cancer: Is There a Link?" *Journal of the National Cancer Institute* 90 (1998): 1116–1117.

Dorgan, J. F., et al. "Physical Activity and Risk of Breast Cancer in the Framingham Heart Study." *American Journal of Epidemiology* 139 662–669.

Dorgan, J. F., et al. "The Relation of Reported Alcohol Ingestion to Plasma Levels of Estrogens and Androgens in Premenopausal Women." *Cancer Causes and Control* 5 (1994): 53–60.

Egan, K., and E. Giovannucci. "Dietary Mutagens and the Risk of Breast Cancer." *Journal of the National Cancer Institute* 90 (1998): 1687–1689.

Eichholzer, M., and F. Gutzwiller. "Dietary Nitrates, Nitrites, and N-Nitroso Compounds and Cancer Risk: A Review of the Epidemiologic Evidence." *Nutrition Reviews* 56 (1998): 95–105.

Ekbom, A., et al. "Breast Feeding and Breast Cancer in the Offspring." *British Journal of Cancer* 67 (1993): 842–845.

El-Bayoumy, K. "Evaluation of Chemopreventive Agents against Breast Cancer and Proposed Strategies for Future Clinical Intervention Trials." *Carcinogenesis* 15 (1994): 2395–2420.

El-Bayoumy, K., et al. "Dietary Control of Cancer." *Proceedings of the Society for Experimental Biology and Medicine* 216 (1997): 211–223.

Ellison, P. T. "Developmental Influences on Adult Ovarian Hormonal Function." *American Journal of Human Biology* 8 (1996): 725–734.

Enger, S. M., et al. "Breastfeeding History, Pregnancy Experience, and Risk of Breast Cancer." *British Journal of Cancer* 76 (1997): 118–123.

Esther, M. J., et al. "Vitamin D and Breast Cancer Risk: The NHANES I Epidemiologic Follow-up Study, 1971–1975 to 1992." *Cancer Epidemiology, Biomarkers and Prevention* 8 (1999): 399–406.

Ferraroni, M., et al. "Alcohol and Breast Cancer Risk: A Case-Control Study from Northern Italy." *Journal of Epidemiology* 20 (1991): 859–864.

Fisher, B., et al. "Tamoxifen for Prevention of Breast Cancer: Report of the National Surgical Adjuvant Breast and Bowel Project P-1 Study." *Journal of the National Cancer Institute* 90, no. 18 (1998): 1371–1388.

Fleischer, A. C., et al. "Early Detection of Ovarian Carcinoma with Transvaginal Color Doppler Ultrasonography." *American Journal of Obstetrics and Gynecology* 174, no. 1 pt. 1 (1996): 101–106.

Foster, R. D., et al. "Skin-Sparing Mastectomy and Immediate Breast Reconstruction: A Prospective Cohort Study for the Treatment of Advanced Stages of Breast Carcinoma." *Annals of Surgical Oncology* 9, no. 8 (October 2002): 820–821.

Franceschi, S. "Micronutrients and Breast Cancer." *European Journal of Cancer Prevention* 6 (1997): 535–539.

Franceschi, S., et al. "Low-Risk Diet for Breast Cancer in Italy." *Cancer Epidemiology, Biomarkers and Prevention* 6 (1997): 875–879.

Francis, K. "Physical Activity: Breast and Reproductive Cancer." *Comprehensive Therapy* 22 (1996): 94–99.

Frankel, S., et al. "Childhood Energy Intake and Adult Mortality from Cancer: The Boyd Orr Cohort Study." *British Medical Journal* 316 (1998): 499–503.

Freudenheim, J. L., et al. "Lifetime Alcohol Consumption and Risk of Breast Cancer." *Nutrition and Cancer* 23 (1995): 1–11.

Freudenheim, J. L., et al. "Lactation History and Breast Cancer Risk." *American Journal of Epidemiology* 146 (1997): 932–938.

Freudenheim, J. L., et al. "Premenopausal Breast Cancer Risk and Intake of Vegetables, Fruits, and Related Nutrients." *Journal of National Cancer Institute* 88 (1996): 340–348.

Freudenheim, J. L., et al. "Exposure to Breast Milk in Infancy and the Risk of Breast Cancer." *Epidemiology* 5 (1994): 324–331.

Friedenreich, C. M., and K. S. Courneya. "Exercise as Rehabilitation for Cancer Patients." *Clinical Journal of Sport Medicine* 6 (1996): 237–244.

Friedenreich, C. M., and T. E. Rohan. "A Review of Physical Activity and Breast Cancer." *Epidemiology* 6 (1995): 311–317.

Friedenreich, C. M., et al. "A Cohort Study of Alcohol Consumption and Risk of Breast Cancer." *American Journal of Epidemiology* 137 (1993): 512–520.

Gammon, M. D., E. M. John, and J. A. Britton. "Recreation and Occupational Physical Activities and Risk of Breast Cancer." *Journal of the National Cancer Institute* 90 (1998): 100–117.

Gammon, M. D., et al. "Recreational Physical Activity and Breast Cancer Risk among Women under Age 45 Years." *American Journal of Epidemiology* 147 (1998): 273–280.

Gapstur, S. M., et al. "Increased Risk of Breast Cancer with Alcohol Consumption in Postmenopausal Women." *American Journal of Epidemiology* 136 (1992): 1221–1231.

Garro, A. J., and C. S. Lieber. "Alcohol and Cancer." *Annual Review of Pharmacology and Toxicology* 30 (1990): 219–249.

Gertig, D. M., et al. "N-Acetyl Transferase 2 Genotypes, Meat Intake and Breast Cancer Risk." *International Journal of Cancer* 80 (1999): 13–17.

Ginsberg, J., and G. M. Prelevic. "Lack of Significant Hormonal Effects and Controlled Trials of Phyto-oestrogens." *Lancet* 355 (2000): 163–164.

Ginsburg, E. S., et al. "Effects of Alcohol Ingestion on Estrogens in Postmenopausal Women." *Journal of the American Medical Association* 276 (1996): 1747–1751.

Giovannucci, E., et al. "A Comparison of Prospective and Retrospective Assessments of Diet in the Study of Breast Cancer." *American Journal of Epidemiology* 137 (1993): 502–511.

Godard, B., et al. "Risk Factors for Familial and Sporadic Ovarian Cancer among French Canadians: A Case-Control Study." *American Journal of Obstetrics and Gynecology* 179, no. 2 (1998): 403–410.

Goldacre, M. J. "Abortion and Breast Cancer: A Case-control Record Linkage Study." *Journal of Epidemiology and Community Health* 55 (2001): 336–337.

Goodman, M. T., et al. "The Association of Diet, Obesity, and Breast Cancer in Hawaii." *Cancer Epidemiology, Biomarkers, and Prevention* 1 (1992): 269–275.

Gowen, L. C., et al. "BRCA1 Required for Transcription-Coupled Repair of Oxidative DNA Damage." *Science* 281, no. 5379 (1998): 1009–1012.

Grady, D., et al. "Cardiovascular Disease Outcomes during 6.8 Years of Hormone Therapy: Heart and Estrogen/Progestin Replacement Study Follow-up (HERS II)." *Journal of the American Medical Association* 288 (2002): 49–57.

Grant, W. B. "An Estimate of Premature Cancer Mortality in the United States Due to Inadequate Doses of Solar Ultraviolet-B Radiation, a Source of Vitamin D." *Cancer* 94, no. 6 (March 15, 2002): 1867–1875.

Greenwald, P. "The Potential of Dietary Modification to Prevent Cancer." *Preventive Medicine* 25 (1996): 41–43.

Gutman, H., et al. "Sarcoma of the Breast: Implications for Extent of Therapy." *Surgery* 116, no. 3 (September 1994): 505–509.

Haenszel, W., and M. Kurihara. "Studies of Japanese Migrants: Mortality from Cancer and Other Diseases among Japanese in the United States." *Journal of National Cancer Institute* 40 (1968): 43–68.

Hahn, N. I. "Are Phytoestrogens Nature's Cure for What Ails Us? A Look at the Research." *Journal of the American Dietetic Association* 98 (1998): 974–976.

Haile, R. W., et al. "A Case-Control Study of Reproductive Variables, Alcohol, and Smoking in Premenopausal Bilateral Breast Cancer." *Breast Cancer Research and Treatment* 37 (1996): 49–56.

Hankinson, S. E., et al. "A Prospective Study of Reproductive Factors and Risk of Epithelial Ovarian Cancer." *Cancer* 76, no. 2 (1995): 284–290.

Hankinson, S. E., et al. "Alcohol, Height, and Adiposity in Relation to Estrogen and Prolactin Levels in Premenopausal Women." *Journal of the National Cancer Institute* 87 (1995): 1297–1302.

Hartmann, L. C., et al. "Efficacy of Bilateral Prophylactic mastectomy in Women with a Family History of Breast Cancer." *New England Journal of Medicine* 340, no. 2 (1999): 77–84.

Hartmann, L. C., et al. "Efficacy of Bilateral Prophylactic Mastectomy in *BRCA1* and *BRCA2* Gene Mutation Carriers." *Journal of the National Cancer Institute* 93, no. 21 (2001): 1633–1637.

Herbert, J. R., and A. Rosen. "Nutritional, Socioeconomic, and Reproductive Factors in Relation to Female Breast Cancer Mortality: Findings from a Cross-National Study." *Cancer Detection and Prevention* 20 (1996): 234–244.

Herman, C., et al. "Soybean Phytoestrogen Intake and Cancer Risk." *Journal of Nutrition* 125 (1995): 757S–770S.

Hill, M. "Nitrate Toxicity: Myth or Reality." *British Journal of Nutrition* 81 (1999): 343–344.

Hoffman-Goetz, L., et al. "Possible Mechanisms Mediating an Association between Physical Activity and Breast Cancer." *Cancer* 83 (1998): 621–628.

Holmberg, L., et al. "Alcohol Intake and Breast Cancer Risk: Effect of Exposure from 15 Years of Age." *Cancer Epidemiology, Biomarkers, and Prevention* 4 (1995): 843–847.

Holmberg, L., et al. "Diet and Breast Cancer Risk." *Archives of Internal Medicine* 154 (1994): 1805–1811.

Holmes, M. D., and W. C. Willett. "Can Breast Cancer Be Prevented by Dietary and Lifestyle Changes?" *Annals of Medicine* 27 (1995): 429–430.

Holmes, M. D., et al. "Dietary Factors and the Survival of Women with Breast Carcinoma." *Cancer* 86 (1999): 826–835.

Hulley, S., et al. "Noncardiovascular Disease Outcomes during 6.8 Years of Hormone Therapy. Heart and Estrogen/Progestin Replacement Study Follow-up (HERS II)." *Journal of the American Medical Association* 288 (2002): 58–66.

Hunter, D. J., and W. C. Willett. "Diet, Body Size, and Breast Cancer." *Epidemiologic Reviews* 15 (1993): 110–129.

Hunter, D. J., and W. C. Willett. "Nutrition and Breast Cancer." *Cancer Causes and Control* 7 (1996): 56–68.

Hunter, D. J., et al. "A Prospective Study of the Intake of Vitamins C, E, and A and the Risk of Breast Cancer." *The New England Journal of Medicine* 329 (1993): 234–240.

Hunter, D. J., et al. "Cohort Studies of Fat Intake and the Risk of Breast Cancer—A Pooled Analysis." *The New England Journal of Medicine* 334 (1996): 356–361.

Hunter, D. J., et al. "Non-dietary Factors as Risk Factors for Breast Cancer, and as Effect Modifiers of the Association of Fat Intake and Risk of Breast Cancer." *Cancer Causes and Control* 8 (1997): 49–56.

Ingram, D. "Diet and Subsequent Survival in Women with Breast Cancer." *British Journal of Cancer* 69 (1994): 592–595.

Institute of Medicine (US) Committee on the Early Detection of Breast Cancer. *Mammography and Beyond: Developing Technologies for the Early Detection of Breast Cancer.* Washington, D.C.: National Academy Press, 2001.

Ip, C. "Review of the Effects of Trans Fatty Acids, Oleic Acid, n-3 Polyunsaturated Fatty Acids, and Conjugated Linoleic Acid on Mammary Carcinogenesis in Animals." *American Journal of Clinical Nutrition* 66 (1997): 1523S–1529S.

Ip, C., and J. A. Scimeca. "Conjugated Linoleic Acid and Linoleic Acid Are Distinctive Modulators of Mammary Carcinogenesis." *Nutrition and Cancer* 27 (1997): 131–135.

Iwase, H., et al. "Clinical Significance of *AIB1* Expression in Human Breast Cancer." *Breast Cancer Research and Treatment* 80, no. 3 (August 2003): 339–345.

Jain, M. "Dairy Foods, Dairy Fats and Cancer: A Review of Epidemiological Evidence." *Nutrition Research* 18 (1998): 905–937.

Jain, M., and A. B. Miller. "Tumor Characteristics and Survival of Breast Cancer Patients in Relation to Premorbid Diet and Body Size." *Breast Cancer Research and Treatment* 42 (1997): 43–55.

Jain, M., A. B. Miller, and T. To. "Premorbid Diet and the Prognosis of Women with Breast Cancer." *Journal of the National Cancer Institute* 86 (1994): 1390–1397.

Jarvinen, R., et al. "Diet and Breast Cancer Risk in a Cohort of Finnish Women." *Cancer Letters* 114 (1997): 251–253.

Kaaks, R. "Nutrition, Hormones, and Breast Cancer: Is Insulin the Missing Link?" *Cancer Causes and Control* 7 (1996): 605–625.

Karlan, B. Y., and L. D. Platt. "Ovarian Cancer Screening: The Role of Ultrasound in Early Detection." *Cancer* 76, (1995): 2011–2015.

Katsouyanni, K., et al. "A Case-Control Study of Lactation and Cancer and the Breast." *British Journal of Cancer* 73 (1996): 814–818.

Katsouyanni, K., et al. "Ethanol and Breast Cancer: An Association that May Be Both Confounded and Casual." *International Journal of Cancer* 58 (1994): 356–361.

Kauff, N. D., et al. "Risk-Reducing Salpingo-oophorectomy in Women with a *BRCA1* or *BRCA2* Mutation." *New England Journal of Medicine* 346, no. 21 (2002): 1609–1615.

Kazer, R. R. "Insulin Resistance, Insulin-like Growth Factor I and Breast Cancer: A Hypothesis." *International Journal of Cancer* 62 (1995): 403–406.

Kennedy, E., S. Bowman, and R. Powell. "Dietary-Fat Intake in the U.S. Population." *Journal of the American College of Nutrition* 18 (1999): 207–212.

Kerber, R. A., and M. L. Slattery. "The Impact of Family History on Ovarian Cancer Risk: The Utah Population Database." *Archives of Internal Medicine* 155, no. 9 (1995): 905–912.

Kerlikowske, K., et al. "Effect of Age, Breast Density , and Family History on the Sensitivity of First Screening Mammography." *Journal of the American Medical Association* 276, no. 1 (1996): 33–38.

Khan, A. D., et al. "Age at Menarche and Nutritional Supplementation." *American Institute of Nutrition* 125 (1995): 1090s–1096s.

King, M. C., et al. "National Surgical Adjuvant Breast and Bowel Project: Tamoxifen and Breast Cancer Incidence among Women with Inherited Mutations in BRCA1 and BRCA2: National Surgical Adjuvant Breast and Bowel Project (NSABP-P1) Breast Cancer Prevention Trial." *Journal of the American Medical Association* 286, no. 18 (2001): 2251–2256.

King, S. E., and D. Schottenfeld. "The 'Epidemic' of Breast Cancer in the U.S.—Determining the Factors." *Oncology* 10 (1996): 453–464.

Knekt, P., et al. "Intake of Dairy Products and the Risk of Breast Cancer." *British Journal of Cancer* 73 (1996): 687–691.

Knekt, P., et al. "Intake of Fried Meat and Risk of Cancer: A Follow-up Study in Finland." *International Journal of Cancer* 59 (1994): 756–760.

Knize, M., et al. "Food Heating and the Formation of Heterocyclic, Aromatic Amine and Polycyclic Aromatic Hydrocarbon Mutagens/Carcinogens." *Advances in Experimental Medicine and Biology* 459 (1999): 179–193.

Kohlmeier, L., and M. Mendez. "Controversies Surrounding Diet and Breast Cancer." *Proceedings of the Nutrition Society* 56 (1997): 369–382.

Kopp, P. "Resveratrol, a Phytoestrogen Found in Red Wine: A Possible Explanation for the Conundrum of the 'French Paradox'?" *European Journal Endocrinology* 138 (1998): 619–620.

Kramer, B. S., et al. "A National Cancer Institute Sponsored Screening Trial for Prostatic, Lung, Colorectal, and Ovarian Cancers." *Cancer* 71 (1993): 589–593.

Kramer, M. M., and C. L. Wells. "Does Physical Activity Reduce Risk of Estrogen-Dependant Cancer in Women?" *Medicine and Science in Sports and Exercise* 28 (1998): 322–334.

Kuhl, C. K., et al. "Breast MR Imaging Screening in 192 Women Proved or Suspected to be Carriers of Breast Cancer Susceptibility Gene: Preliminary Results." *Radiology* 215, no. 1 (2000): 267–279.

Kurzer, M. S. "Hormonal Effect of Soy Isoflavones: Studies in Premenopausal and Postmenopausal Women." *Journal of Nutrition* 130 (2000): 660S–661S.

Kurzer, M. S., and X. Xu. "Dietary Phytoestrogens." *Annual Review of Nutrition* 17 (1997): 353–381.

Lacey, J. V., et al. "Menopausal Hormone Replacement Therapy and Risk of Ovarian Cancer." *Journal of the American Medical Association* 288 (2002): 334–341.

Laing, A. E., et al. "Breast Cancer Risk Factors in African-American Women: The Howard University Tumor Registry Experience." *Journal of the National Medical Association* 85 (1993): 931–939.

Lamartiniere, C. A. "Protection against Breast Cancer with Genistein: A Component of Soy." *American Journal of Clinical Nutrition* 71 (2000): 1705s–1707s.

Lazovich, D. "Induced Abortion and Breast Cancer Risk." *Epidemiology* 11 (2000): 76–80.

Leddy, S. K. "Incentives and Barriers to Exercise in Women with a History of Breast Cancer." *Oncology Nursing Forum* 24 (1997): 885–890.

Lee, I.-M. "Exercise and Physical Health: Cancer and Immune Function." *Research Quarterly for Exercise and Sport* 66 (1995): 286–291.

Lee, I.-M., R. S. Paffenbarger, Jr., and C. H. Hennekens. "Physical Activity, Physical Fitness and Longevity." *Aging Clinical Experimental Research* 9 (1997): 2–11.

Leiss, J. K., and D. A. Savitz. "Home Pesticide Use and Childhood Cancer: A Case-Control Study." *American Journal of Public Health* 85 (1995): 249–252.

Lerman, C., et al. "Prophylactic Surgery Decisions and Surveillance Practices One Year following *BRCA1/2* Testing." *Preventive Medicine* 31, no. 1 (2000): 75–80.

Levi, F., et al. "Alcohol and Breast Cancer in the Swiss Canton of Vaud." *European Journal of Cancer* 32A (1996): 2108–2113.

Lewin, J. M., et al. "Clinical Comparison of Full-Field Digital Mammography and Screen-Film Mammography for Detection of Breast Cancer." *American Journal of Roentgenology* 179, no. 3 (2002): 671–677.

Lewin, J. M., et al. "Comparison of Full-Field Digital Mammography with Screen-Film Mammography for Cancer Detection: Results of 4,945 Paired Examinations." *Radiology* 218, no. 3 (2001): 873–880.

Lewis, R. G., R. C. Fortmann, and D. E. Camann. "Evaluation of Methods for Monitoring the Potential Exposure of Small Children to Pesticides in the Residential Environment." *Archives of Environmental Contamination and Toxicology* 26 (1994): 37–46.

Lipkin, M., and H. L. Newmark. "Vitamin D, Calcium, and Prevention of Breast Cancer: A Review." *Journal of the American College of Nutrition* 18 (1999): 392S–397S.

Longnecker, M. P., et al. "Intake of Carrots, Spinach, and Supplements Containing Vitamin A in Relation to Risk of Breast Cancer." *Cancer Epidemiology, Biomarkers and Prevention* 6 (1997): 887–892.

Longnecker, M. P., et al. "Risk of Breast Cancer in Relation to Lifetime Alcohol Consumption." *Journal of the National Cancer Institute* 87 (1995): 923–929.

Lynch, H. T., et al. "Hereditary Ovarian Cancer: Heterogeneity in Age at Diagnosis." *Cancer* 67, no. 5 (1991): 1460–1466.

Mackay, H. J., and C. J. Twelves. "Protein Kinase C: A Target for Anticancer Drugs?" *Endocrine Related Cancer* 10, no. 3 (September 2003): 347–357.

Maskarinec, G., and L. Meng. "An Investigation of Soy Intake and Mammographic Characteristics in Hawaii." *Breast Cancer Research* 3 (2001): 134–141.

McDonnell, S. K., et al. "Efficacy of Contralateral Prophylactic Mastectomy in Women with a Personal and Family History of Breast Cancer." *Journal of Clinical Oncology* 19, no. 19 (2001): 3938–3943.

McTiernan, A. "Exercise and Breast Cancer—Time to Get Moving?" *The New England Journal of Medicine* 336 (1997): 1311–1312.

McTiernan, A., et al. "Occurrence of Breast Cancer in Relation to Recreational Exercise in Women Age 50–64 Years." *Epidemiology* 7 (1996): 598–604.

Meijers-Heijboer, E. J., et al. "Presymptomatic DNA Testing and Prophylactic Surgery in Families with a *BRCA1* or *BRCA2* Mutation." *Lancet* 355, no. 9220 (2000): 2015–2020.

Meijers-Heijboer, H., et al. "Breast Cancer after Prophylactic Bilateral Mastectomy in Women with a *BRCA1* or *BRCA2* Mutation." *New England Journal of Medicine* 345, no. 3 (2001): 159–164.

Melbye, M., et al. "Induced Abortion and the Risk of Breast Cancer." *The New England Journal of Medicine* 336 (1997): 81–85.

Messina, M. "Soy, Soy Phytoestrogens (Isoflavones), and Breast Cancer." *American Journal of Clinical Nutrition* 70 (1999): 574–575.

Mezzetti, M., et al. "Population Attributable Risk for Breast Cancer: Diet, Nutrition, and Physical Exercise." *Journal of the National Cancer Institute* 90 (1998): 389–394.

Miller, A. B., et al. "Canadian National Breast Screening Study-2: 13-Year Results of a Randomized Trial in Women Aged 50–59 Years." *Journal of the National Cancer Institute* 92, no. 18 (2000): 1490–1499.

Miller, R. W. "Special Susceptibility of the Child to Certain Radiation-induced Cancers." *Environmental Health Perspectives* 103 (1995): 41–44.

Mittendorf, R., et al. "Strenuous Physical Activity in Young Adulthood and Risk of Breast Cancer." *Cancer Causes and Control* 6 (1995): 347–353.

Mock, V., et al. "Effects of Exercise on Fatigue, Physical Functioning, and Emotional Distress during Radiation Therapy for Breast Cancer." *Oncology Nursing Forum* 24 (1997): 991–1000.

Modan, B., et al. "National Israel Ovarian Cancer Study Group: Parity, Oral Contraceptives, and the Risk of Ovarian Cancer among Carriers and Noncarriers of a *BRCA1* or *BRCA2* Mutation." *New England Journal of Medicine* 345, no. 4 (2001): 235–240.

Murkies, A., et al. "Phytoestrogens and Breast Cancer in Postmenopausal Women: A Case-Control Study." *Menopause* 7 (2000): 289–296.

Muto, M. G., et al. "Screening for Ovarian Cancer: The Preliminary Experience of a Familial Ovarian Cancer Center." *Gynecologic Oncology* 51, no. 1 (1993): 12–20.

Narod, S. A., et al. "Risk modifiers in Carriers of *BRCA1* Mutations." *International Journal of Cancer* 64, no. 6 (1995): 394–398.

Narod, S. A., et al. "Oral Contraceptives and the Risk of Hereditary Ovarian Cancer. Hereditary Ovarian Cancer Clinical Study Group." *New England Journal of Medicine* 339, no. 7 (1998): 424–428.

Narod, S. A., et al. "Tubal Ligation and Risk of Ovarian Cancer in Carriers of *BRCA1* or *BRCA2* Mutations: A Case-Control Study." *Lancet* 357, no. 9267 (2001): 1467–1470.

Newcomb, P. A., and M. T. Mandelson. "A Record-Based Evaluation of Induced Abortion and Breast Cancer Risk (United States)." *Cancer Causes and Control* 11 (2000): 777–781.

Newcomb, P. A., et al. "Lactation and a Reduced Risk of Premenopausal Breast Cancer." *The New England Journal of Medicine* 330, no. 2 (1994): 81–87.

Newman, V., et al. "Dietary Supplement Use by Women at Risk for Breast Cancer Recurrence." *Journal of the American Dietetic Association* 98 (1998): 285–292.

Nieman, D. C., et al. "Moderate Exercise Training and Natural Killer Cell Cytotoxic Activity in Breast Cancer Patients." *International Journal of Sports Medicine* 16 (1995): 334–337.

NIH consensus conference. Ovarian Cancer: Screening, Treatment, and Follow-up. NIH Consensus Development Panel on Ovarian Cancer. *Journal of the American Medical Association* 273, no. 6 (1995): 491–497.

NIH editors (press release). "NHLBI Stops Trial of Estrogen plus Progestin Due to Increased Breast Cancer Risk, Lack of Overall Benefit." Bethesda, Md.: National Institutes of Health, July 9, 2002.

Noguchi, M. "Minimally Invasive Surgery for Small Breast Cancer." *Journal of Surgical Oncology* 84, no. 2 (October 2003): 94–101.

Nonet, G. H., et al. "Dairy Products and Breast Cancer: The IGF-I, Estrogen, and bGH Hypothesis." *Medical Hypotheses* 48 (1997): 453–461.

O'Driscoll, D., et al. "Screening with Breast Ultrasound in a Population at Moderate Risk Due to Family History." *Journal of Medical Screening* 8, no. 2 (2001): 106–109.

Olsson, H., et al. "Proliferation of the Breast Epithelium in Relation to Menstrual Cycle Phase, Hormonal Use, and Reproductive Factors." *Breast Cancer Research and Treatment* 40, no. 2 (1996): 187–196.

O'Shaughnessy, J. A., et al. "Ductal Lavage and the Clinical Management of Women at High Risk for Breast Carcinoma: A Commentary." *Cancer* 94, no. 2 (2002): 292–298.

Paley, P. J., et al. "Occult Cancer of the Fallopian Tube in *BRCA-1* Germline Mutation Carriers at Prophylactic Oophorectomy: A Case for Recommending Hysterectomy at Surgical Prophylaxis." *Gynecologic Oncology* 80, no. 2 (2001): 176–180.

Parodi, P. W. "Conjugated Linoleic Acid and Other Anticarcinogenic Agents of Bovine Milk Fat." *Journal of Dairy Science* 82 (1999): 1339–1349.

Pedersen, A. B., et al. "Menstrual Differences Due to Vegetarian and Nonvegetarian Diets." *American Journal of Clinical Nutrition* 53 (1991): 879–885.

Perera, F. P. "Molecular Epidemiology: Insights into Cancer Susceptibility, Risk Assessment, and Prevention." *Journal of the National Cancer Institute* 88 (1996): 496–509.

Piantadosi, S. "Vitamin A Analogue for Breast Cancer Prevention: A Grade of F or Incomplete?" *Journal of the National Cancer Institute* 91 (1999): 1794.

Piver, M. S., et al. "Familial Ovarian Cancer: A Report of 658 Families from the Gilda Radner Familial Ovarian Cancer Registry 1981–1991." *Cancer* 71, suppl. 2 (1993): 582–588.

Piver, M. S., et al. "Primary Peritoneal Carcinoma after Prophylactic Oophorectomy in Women with a Family History of Ovarian Cancer: A Report of the Gilda Radner Familial Ovarian Cancer Registry." *Cancer* 71, no. 9 (1993): 2751–2755.

Pollak, M. "IGF-I Physiology and Breast Cancer." *Recent Results in Cancer Research* 152 (1998): 63–70.

Potischman, N., et al. "Diet during Adolescence and Risk of Breast Cancer among Young Women." *Journal of the National Cancer Institute* 90 (1998): 226–233.

Puskin, J. S., and C. B. Nelson. "Estimates of Radiogenic Cancer Risks." *Health Physics* 69 (1995): 93–101.

Rebbeck, T. R., et al. "Breast Cancer Risk after Bilateral Prophylactic Oophorectomy in *BRCA1* Mutation Carriers." *Journal of the National Cancer Institute* 91, no. 17 (1999): 1475–1479.

Rebbeck, T. R., et al. "The Prevention and Observation of Surgical End Points Study Group: Prophylactic Oophorectomy in Carriers of BRCA1 or BRCA2 Mutations." *New England Journal of Medicine* 346, no. 21 (2002): 1616–1622.

Reitsamer, R., et al. "Sentinel Lymph Node Biopsy in Breast Cancer Patients after Neoadjuvant Chemotherapy." *Journal of Surgical Oncology* 84, no. 2 (October 2003): 63–67.

Risch, H. A. "Hormonal Etiology of Epithelial Ovarian Cancer, with a Hypothesis concerning the Role of Androgens and Progesterone." *Journal of the National Cancer Institute* 90, no. 23 (1998): 1774–1786.

Rock, C. L., et al. "Nutrient Intakes from Foods and Dietary Supplements in Women at Risk for Breast Cancer Recurrence." *Nutrition and Cancer* 29 (1997): 133–139.

Rockhill, B., et al. "Physical Activity and Breast Cancer Risk in a Cohort of Young Women." *Journal of the National Cancer Institute* 90 (1998): 1155–1160.

Rohan, T. E., W. Fu, and J. E. Hiller. "Physical Activity and Survival from Breast Cancer." *European Journal of Cancer Prevention* 4 (1995): 419–424.

Rose, D., J. M. Connolly, and X. Liu. "Diet and Breast Cancer: Opportunities for Prevention and Intervention." *Etiology of Breast and Gynecological Cancers* 396 (1997): 147–158.

Rose, D. P., et al. "Effects of Dietary Fish Oil on Fatty Acids and Eicosanoids in Metastasizing Human Breast Cancer Cells." *Nutrition and Cancer* 22, no. 2 (1994): 131–141.

Scheuer, L., et al. "Outcome of Preventive Surgery and Screening for Breast and Ovarian Cancer in BRCA Mutation Carriers." *Journal of Clinical Oncology* 20, no. 5 (2002): 1260–1268.

Segar, M. L., et al. "The Effect of Aerobic Exercise on Self-Esteem and Depressive and Anxiety Symptoms among Breast Cancer Survivors." *Oncology Nursing Forum* 25 (1998): 107–113.

Sellers, T. A., et al. "The Role of Hormone Replacement Therapy in the Risk for Breast Cancer and Total Mortality in Women with a Family History of Breast Cancer." *Annals of Internal Medicine* 127, no. 11 (1997): 973–980.

Serra-Majem, L., et al. "Changes in Diet and Mortality from Selected Cancers in Southern Mediterranean Countries." *European Journal of Clinical Nutrition* 47 (1993): S25–S34.

Setchell, K. D. R., and A. Cassidy. "Dietary Isoflavones: Biological Effects and Relevance to Human Health." *Journal of Nutrition* 129, suppl. (1999): 758S–767S.

Simcox, N. J., et al. "Pesticides in Household Dust and Soil: Exposure Pathways for Children of Agricultural Families." *Environmental Health Perspectives* 103 (1995): 1126–1134.

Smith, R. E., and B. C. Good. "Chemoprevention of Breast Cancer and the Trials of the National Surgical Adjuvant Breast and Bowel Project and Others." *Endocrine Related Cancer* 10, no. 3 (September 2003): 389–396.

Synderwine, E. G. "Some Perspectives on the Nutritional Aspects of Breast Cancer Research." *Cancer* 74S (1994): 1070–1077.

Steenland, K., S. Nowlin, and S. Palu. "Cancer Incidence in the National Health and Nutrition Survey I Follow-up Data: Diabetes, Cholesterol, Pulse, and Physical Activity." *Cancer Epidemiology, Biomarkers and Prevention* 4 (1995): 807–811

Steinmetz, K. A., and J. D. Potter. "Vegetables, Fruit, and Cancer Prevention: A Review." *Journal of the American Dietetic Association* 96 (1996): 1027–1039.

Stoll, B. A. "Can Supplementary Dietary Fibre Suppress Breast Cancer Growth?" *British Journal of Cancer* 73 (1996): 557–559.

Stoutjesdijk, M. J., et al. "Magnetic Resonance Imaging and Mammography in Women with a Hereditary Risk of Breast Cancer." *Journal of the National Cancer Institute* 93, no. 14 (2001): 1095–1102.

Struewing, J. P., et al. "Prophylactic Oophorectomy in Inherited Breast/Ovarian Cancer Families." *Journal of the National Cancer Institute* Monographs 17 (1995): 33–35.

Thomsen, S., and D. Tatman. "Physiological and Pathological Factors of Human Breast Disease That Can Influence Optical Diagnosis." *Annals of the New York Academy of Sciences* 838 (1998): 171–193.

Tilanus-Linthorst, M. M., et al. "First Experiences in Screening Women at High Risk for Breast Cancer with MR Imaging." *Breast Cancer Research and Treatment* 63, no. 1 (2000): 53–60.

Tretli, S., and M. Gaard. "Lifestyle Changes during Adolescence and Risk of Breast Cancer: An Ecologic Study of the Effect of World War II in Norway." *Cancer Causes and Control* 7 (1996): 507–512.

Trichopoulou, A., et al. "Consumption of Olive Oil and Specific Food Groups in Relation to Breast Cancer Risk in Greece." *Journal of the National Cancer Institute* 87 (1995): 110–116.

Troisi, R. L., et al. "Relation of Body Fat Distribution to Reproductive Factors in Pre- and Postmenopausal Women." *Obesity Research* 3 (1995): 143–151.

Upadhyay, G., et al. "Functional Expression of Sodium Iodide Symporter (NIS) in Human Breast Cancer Tissue." *Breast Cancer Research and Treatment* 77, no. 2 (January 2003): 157–165.

Ursin, G., et al. "Does Oral Contraceptive Use Increase the Risk of Breast Cancer in Women with *BRCA1/BRCA2* Mutations More Than in Other Women?" *Cancer Research* 57, no. 17 (1997): 3678–3681.

Vachon, C. M., et al. "Association of Parity and Ovarian Cancer Risk by Family History of Breast or Ovarian Cancer in a Population-Based Study of Postmenopausal Women." *Epidemiology* 13, no. 1 (2002): 66–71.

Verhoeven, D. T. H., et al. "Vitamins C and E, Retinol, Beta-Carotene and Dietary Fiber in Relation to Breast Cancer Risk: A Prospective Cohort Study." *British Journal of Cancer* 75 (1997): 149–155.

Veronesi, U., et al. "Prevention of Breast Cancer with Tamoxifen: Preliminary Findings from the Italian Randomized Trial among Hysterectomised Women: Italian Tamoxifen Prevention Study." *Lancet* 352, no. 9122 (1998): 93–97.

Viel, J.-F., et al. "Alcoholic Calories, Red Wine Consumption and Breast Cancer among Premenopausal Women." *European Journal of Epidemiology* 13 (1997): 639–643.

Warner, E., et al. "Comparison of Breast Magnetic Resonance Imaging, Mammography, and Ultrasound for Surveillance of Women at High Risk for Hereditary Breast Cancer." *Journal of Clinical Oncology* 19, no. 15 (2001): 3524–3531.

Weiner, Z., et al. "Screening for Ovarian Cancer in Women with Breast Cancer with Transvaginal Sonography and Color Flow Imaging." *Journal of Ultrasound Medicine* 12, no. 7 (1993): 387–393.

Willett, W. "Diet, Nutrition, and Avoidable Cancer." *Environmental Health Perspectives* 103 (1995): 165–170.

Writing Group for the Women's Health Initiative Investigators. "Risks and Benefits of Estrogen Plus Progestin in Healthy Postmenopausal Women: Principal Results from the Women's Health Initiative Randomized Controlled Trial." *Journal of the American Medical Association* 28 (2002): 321–333.

Wu, A. H., et al. "Tofu and Risk of Breast Cancer in Asian-Americans." *Cancer Epidemiology, Biomarkers and Prevention* 5 (1996): 901–906.

Wu, A. H., et al. "Soy Intake and Risk of Breast Cancer in Asians and Asian-Americans." *American Journal of Clinical Nutrition* 68, suppl. (1998): 1437S–1443S.

Wu, A. H., et al. "Menstrual and Reproductive Factors and Risk of Breast Cancer in Asian-Americans." *British Journal of Cancer* 73 (1996): 680–686.

Yasui, T., et al. "Hormone Replacement Therapy in Postmenopausal Women." *Journal of Medical Investigation* 50, no. 3–4 (August 2003): 136–145.

Zahm, S. H., and S. S. Devesa. "Childhood Cancer: Overview of Incidence Trends and Environmental Carcinogens." *Environmental Health Perspective* 103 (1995): 177–184.

Zand, R. S. R., D. J. A. Jenkins, and E. P. Diamandis. "Steroid Hormone Activity of Flavonoids and Related Compounds." *Breast Cancer Research and Treatment* 62 (2000): 34–49.

Zhang, S., et al. "Dietary Carotenoids and Vitamins A, C, and E and Risk of Breast Cancer." *Journal of the National Cancer Institute* 91 (1999): 547–556.

INDEX

Boldface page numbers indicate extensive treatment of a topic.

A

abdomen, fluid in 15–16
ablation
    cryoablation **78**
    radiofrequency ablation **187**
    ultrasound ablation 248
ABNOBAviscum (mistletoe extract) 157
ABS. *See* American Brachytherapy Society
ACCC. *See* Association of Community Cancer Centers
accessory breast tissue **1**
AC chemotherapy
    in clinical trials 260
    effectiveness of 94
acetaminophen, for pain control 176, 177
acini **1**
acitretin **1**
ACS. *See* American Cancer Society
acupressure **1**
    in clinical trials 259
acupuncture **1–2**
acustimulation **2**
Ad5CMV-*p53* gene therapy, in clinical trials 253
adenocarcinoma **2**
adenoma **2**
adenovirus **2**
adhesive capsulitis 108
adjuvant, definition of 279
adjuvant treatment **2,** 214
    chemotherapy 62, 63, 71
    in clinical trials 242, 245, 255, 258–262
    hormonal 121–122
    in older women 3–4
    for pain control 177
adolescents
    lifestyle of, and breast cancer risk 72

Look Good . . . Feel Better Program for 139
    and smoking **199,** 200
adrenal glands 279
Adriamycin (doxorubicin) **2,** 272
    in clinical trials 240–255, 257–261, 263, 264–265, 267–268
    for lung metastasis 140
Adrucil. *See* fluorouracil
advance directives **2–3**
advocacy
    patient 164
    Patient Advocate Foundation 178
African-American women
    breast cancer in **3,** 185
    Sisters Network, Inc., and 199
age **3**
    and alcohol consumption 4–5
    and breast cancer 31, 41
age bias **3–4**
agonists, definition of 279
agranulocyte, definition of 279
AICR. *See* American Institute for Cancer Research
air transportation 105, 164
Alabama, cancer centers in 232
Alaska Natives, breast cancer in **164–165**
Albert Einstein Comprehensive Cancer Center, contact information for 235
alcohol **4–5**
    age and 4–5
    benefits of 5
    and breast cancer 32, 41, 72, 137
    wine 222
aldesleukin (IL-2)
    in biological therapy 22
    in clinical trials 243, 244, 254, 265–266
    side effects of 23
alkaline phosphatase (ALP) 5, 27
alkaline phosphatase test **5**

Alkeran. *See* ʟ-phenylalanine mustard
alkylating agents **5–6.** *See also specific agents*
    side effects of 6
allicin **6**
allinase, in garlic 111
allium compounds 180
allogeneic, definition of 279
allogeneic bone marrow transplant 29. *See also* bone marrow transplant
allyl sulfides 180
alopecia (hair loss) 68–69, **117**
ALP. *See* alkaline phosphatase
alpha-carotene 180
alpha-tocopherol 62
alternative medicine. *See* complementary and alternative medicine
American Academy of Medical Acupuncture 2
American Board of Plastic and Reconstructive Surgeons, contact information for 227
American Brachytherapy Society (ABS) 6
    contact information for 227
American Brain Tumor Association, contact information for 227
American Cancer Society (ACS) 6
    on breast self-exams 54
    Cancer Survivors Network of 60
    contact information for 228
    exercise recommendations of 101
    on ginseng 113–114
    local transportation programs of 105
    Look Good . . . Feel Better Program of 139
    on macrobiotic diet 145
    on mammograms 147, 150
    Reach to Recovery program of **187**

screening guidelines of 42
    as support group resource 206
    temporary housing programs of 105
    Web site of **6–7**
American College of Radiology
    contact information for 230
    mammogram reporting system of 150–151
American ginseng 113
American Institute for Cancer Research (AICR) 7
    contact information for 230
American Society of Clinical Oncology (ASCO) 7
    contact information for 230
American Society of Plastic and Reconstructive Surgeons. *See* American Society of Plastic Surgeons
American Society of Plastic Surgeons (ASPS) **7,** 181
amethopterin. *See* methotrexate
aminoglutethimide (Cytadren, Elipten) **7,** 270
amitriptyline, for pain control 177
A33 monoclonal antibody **7**
amputation, for metastatic bone cancer 28
AMSA. *See* amsacrine
amsacrine (*m*-acridinylamine methans-sulfon anisidide, AMSA) 270
amygdalin, purified form of 135–136
analgesics. *See also* pain control
    nonopioid 177
    opioid 176–177
anaplastic, definition of 279
anastrozole. *See* Arimidex
androgens **7–8**
    side effects of 8
anemia **8,** 188
    chemotherapy and 67
    Fanconi, genes for 48
    hemolytic 8